Resent Results in Cancer Research **169**

Managing Editors
P. M. Schlag, Berlin · H.-J. Senn, St. Gallen

Associate Editors
P. Kleihues, Zürich · F. Stiefel, Lausanne
B. Groner Frankfurt · A. Wallgren, Göteborg

Founding Editor
P. Rentchnik, Geneva

S. González-Moreno (Ed.)

Advances in Peritoneal Surface Oncology

With 45 Figures in 57 Separate Illustrations, 12 in Color and 19 Tables

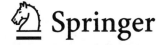

Santiago González-Moreno, MD, PhD
Department of Surgical Oncology
Centro Oncológico MD Anderson International España
Calle Gómez Hemans 2
28033 Madrid
Spain
sgonzalez@mdanderson.es

Library of Congress Control Number: 2006937141

ISSN 0080-0015
ISBN 978-3-540-30759-4 Springer Berlin Heidelberg New York

This work is subject to copyright. All rights are reserved, whether the whole or part of the material is concerned, specifically the rights of translation, reprinting, reuse of illustrations, recitations, broadcasting, reproduction on microfilm or in any other way, and storage in data banks. Duplication of this publication or parts thereof is permitted only under the provisions of the German Copyright Law of September 9, 1965, in its current version, and permission for use must always be obtained from Springer-Verlag. Violations are liable for prosecution under the German Copyright Law.

Springer is part of Springer Science+Business Media

http//www.springer.com
© Springer-Verlag Berlin Heidelberg 2007

The use of general descriptive names, trademarks, etc. in this publication does not imply, even in the absence of a specific statement, that such names are exempt from the relevant protective laws and regulations and therefore free for general use.

Product liability: The publishers cannot guarantee the accuracy of any information about dosage and application contained in this book. In every case the user must check such information by consulting the relevant literature.

Editor: Dr. Ute Heilmann, Heidelberg
Desk Editor: Dörthe Mennecke-Bühler, Heidelberg
Cover-design: Frido Steinen Broo, eStudio Calamar, Spain
Production & Typesetting: Verlagsservice Teichmann, Mauer
Printed on acid-free paper – 21/3151xq – 5 4 3 2 1 0

Preface

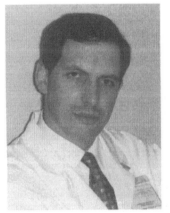

As a result of decades of basic and clinical research, scientific interest in peritoneal surface malignancy has been translated into actual clinical practice, allowing selected patients with peritoneal carcinomatosis or primary peritoneal neoplasms to be treated with curative intent. The use of cytoreductive surgery in combination with perioperative intraperitoneal chemotherapy for this purpose is now a reality around the world in dedicated, specialized centers. Peritoneal surface oncology has progressively emerged as a distinct area of interest, with a specific and steadily increasing body of knowledge, spanning from basic science or diagnostic pathology to surgical technique and regional chemotherapy administration. In recent years, the interest of clinicians and researchers in this field has only grown. The present volume in the series Recent Results in Cancer Research offers an authoritative compilation of the current state of the art.

This volume opens with a concise but comprehensive review of the historical developments and research landmarks that have led to the present status of the field, written by Dr. Paul H. Sugarbaker, a privileged witness and one of the main actors in this history. Looking back to the past undoubtedly helps point out future research directions and strategies.

Nobody has studied in depth the pathogenesis of peritoneal carcinomatosis at cellular, ultrastructural, and molecular levels like Dr. Yutaka Yonemura. He and his colleagues (Chap. 2) offer us a magnificent description of the process leading to overt peritoneal dissemination, starting from single cancer cells gaining access to the free peritoneal cavity. In gastrointestinal cancer, these cells detach from the primary malignancy after reaching the serosal surface. A positive peritoneal fluid cytology and/or serosal involvement are well-known high-risk factors for cancer recurrence in the peritoneal surfaces, having a profound impact on prognosis. Drs. Ludeman and Shepherd (Chap. 3) stress the paramount importance of an adequate pathologic assessment and the reporting of such crucial prognostic factors in evaluation of a primary tumor resection specimen by the diagnostic pathologist. It is in this setting of free microscopic peritoneal disease where adjuvant intraperitoneal chemotherapy should theoretically show its maximum efficacy, having a profound impact on patient survival. As described by Dr. Sugarbaker in Chap. 7, a number of sound, randomized, controlled trials have actually demonstrated this advantage in colorectal, gastric, and ovarian cancer. However, the clinical oncology community has largely overlooked these results, showing that the transition from clinical research to common practice does not require well-designed phase III studies alone. This area should be identified as one of the challenges and priorities in peritoneal surface oncology for the years to come.

The conduct of randomized trials in surgical oncology is a formidable endeavor. Drs. Verwaal and Zoetmulder from Amsterdam, authors of a landmark phase III trial establishing the superiority of cytoreduction combined with hyperthermic intraperitoneal chemotherapy and subsequent systemic chemotherapy over the common practice of palliative surgery and systemic chemotherapy in peritoneal carcinomatosis of colorectal origin, share with us the lessons learned from the design and conduct of this trial in Chap. 9. Ethical issues and patient refusal to be randomized to an arm without the combined radical treatment, clearly perceived as the treatment of choice, have hampered the conduct of similar phase III studies by other institutions and collaborative groups. A new phase III trial to revalidate the conclusions of the Dutch trial will not be possible because of these reasons. The aforementioned randomized trial and numerous rigorous phase II studies that are available provide enough scientific evidence to support the use of cytoreductive surgery and perioperative intraperitoneal chemotherapy as the standard of care for selected patients with peritoneal carcinomatosis of colorectal origin. These trials are reviewed in detail by Drs. Elias and Goere in Chap. 11. Dr. Elias and his group have undoubtedly made a tremendous contribution to the advance of clinical research in this setting, bringing the treatment of carcinomatosis of colorectal origin to a new level of excellence with the use of hyperthermic intraperitoneal oxaliplatin (alone or combined with irinotecan), which has resulted in unprecedented survival results. These results will need to be further ratified in larger trials, but he already points out future directions for further advancement in the treatment of this disease process.

The pharmacological and clinical principles of perioperative intraperitoneal chemotherapy administration, with and without hyperthermia, along with the basic studies that support this practice for the different cytotoxic drugs employed, are comprehensively reviewed by Drs. de Bree and Tsiftsis in Chaps. 4 and 5. Aside from illustrating the bases of current intraperitoneal chemotherapy practices for peritoneal carcinomatosis, these chapters should constitute a unique methodological reference for researchers interested in exploring the perioperative intraperitoneal delivery of new chemotherapeutic agents. The various technological solutions developed for the administration of hyperthermic intraoperative intraperitoneal chemotherapy are described and discussed in detail in Chap. 6 by Dr. Lowy's group, led by Dr. Sarnaik.

As outlined by Dr. Sugarbaker in Chap. 1, progress in peritoneal surface oncology has not occurred without difficulties. Perhaps the most important challenge that we face today has to do with the wide heterogeneity in clinical research methodology and actual clinical practices employed by the different groups around the world, resulting in scientific reports and efforts that are difficult to compare and unify. Drs. Gilly, Glehen and colleagues offer a concise overview of this problem in Chap. 8, and their proposal to overcome what they consider a difficult challenge. The progressive building of a consensus is a complex task that will bring this problem to an end, which we see coming closer after the fruitful works of the latest biannual International Workshop on Peritoneal Surface Malignancy held in Madrid in 2004 and most recently in Milan in December 2006. As a palpable first achievement in this direction, I especially appreciate the willingness of all authors in this book to use the unified nomenclature that was made consensual in these meetings (i.e., the acronym "HIPEC" for hyperthermic intraperitoneal chemotherapy).

Pseudomyxoma peritonei (PMP) and peritoneal mesothelioma (PM) are uncommon diseases whose standard of care nowadays, when feasible, is cytoreductive surgery combined with perioperative intraperitoneal chemotherapy. In Chap. 10, Drs. Lambert, Lambert, and Mansfield provide a perspective rarely found in the scientific literature on PMP. They outline the difficulties associated with the development of experimental models and possible opportunities for basic research in this disease. These initiatives should help us to understand the peculiar biological behavior observed in this condition that has largely served as a paradigm of peritoneal spread of a gastrointestinal neoplasm. Hopefully, this knowledge can be translated into new therapeutic options for PMP and other instances of peritoneal carcinomatosis of gastrointestinal origin. PM is a challenging disease, starting from its very histopathological characterization and diagnosis. Dr. Ordóñez, one of the leading world experts in this field, offers us in Chap. 12 an excellent review of the histopathological, immunohistochemical, and electron microscopical diagnostic features of this disease in its different varieties. Dr. Deraco and his colleagues have developed significant expertise in the management of this disease, which they describe in detail in Chap. 13, along with future directions for clinical research.

The difficult and often discouraging management of peritoneal carcinomatosis of gastric origin has not prevented Dr. Yonemura and coworkers (Chap. 14) from pursuing new therapeutic options and continuing an intense clinical research activity in this disease. Neoadjuvant intraperitoneal and systemic chemotherapy (NIPS) followed by complete cytoreduction and perioperative intraperitoneal chemotherapy constitutes a valid treatment option for these patients, as described in Chap. 14.

Ovarian cancer has traditionally been an example of treatable peritoneal dissemination. The paradigm of optimal debulking surgery followed by systemic chemotherapy is now shifting, at least in the United States, towards a bidirectional (intraperitoneal plus intravenous) postoperative chemotherapy approach. Dr. Markman has been in the forefront of clinical research regarding intraperitoneal chemotherapy for ovarian cancer for over two decades. Finally, his efforts have resulted in a recognized clinical application. We are honored to include his expert review of this topic in Chap. 15.

I cannot finalize this preface without expressing my deep gratitude to all the expert colleagues and friends from around the world who enthusiastically accepted the invitation I conveyed to them one day to write one or more chapters for this book. The result of their effort is in your hands now, and I hope you will enjoy and learn from its thoughtfully selected, masterly written contents. Springer is to be congratulated for the vision to dedicate a whole volume to an emerging field like peritoneal surface oncology, and I appreciate the opportunity granted to me to serve as its editor. Special thanks go to Ms. Dörthe Mennecke-Bühler, Springer medicine desk editor, for her diligent work and her constant support and guidance, which have made my editing job very bearable. I would not have arrived at this moment without the help of Dr. Paul H. Sugarbaker, who trained me in peritoneal surface oncology for 2 years and has been an invaluable mentor ever since, for which I am indebted and deeply grateful. Finally, I would like to dedicate this effort to all our patients who, in the midst of the suffering that goes along with a terrible condition like peritoneal carcinomatosis, blindly put their confidence and hope in us to help them through this difficult event in their lives.

Santiago González-Moreno
Department of Surgical Oncology
Centro Oncológico MD Anderson International España
Madrid, Spain

Contents

1 **Management of Peritoneal Surface Malignancy: A Short History**
Paul H. Sugarbaker.. 1

2 **The Natural History of Free Cancer Cells in the Peritoneal Cavity**
Yutaka Yonemura, Taiichi Kawamura, Etsurou Bandou, Gorou Tsukiyama, Yoshio Endou, and Masahiro Miura...... 11

3 **Pathological Evaluation and Implications of Serosal Involvement in Gastrointestinal Cancer**
Linmarie Ludeman and Neil A. Shepherd................... 25

4 **Principles of Perioperative Intraperitoneal Chemotherapy for Peritoneal Carcinomatosis**
Eelco de Bree and Dimitris D. Tsiftsis..................... 39

5 **Experimental and Pharmacokinetic Studies in Intraperitoneal Chemotherapy: From Laboratory Bench to Bedside**
Eelco de Bree and Dimitris D. Tsiftsis..................... 53

6 **Technology for the Delivery of Hyperthermic Intraoperative Intraperitoneal Chemotherapy: A Survey of Techniques**
Amod A. Sarnaik, Jeffrey J. Sussman, Syed A. Ahmad, Benjamin C. McIntyre, and Andrew M. Lowy.............. 75

7 **Adjuvant Intraperitoneal Chemotherapy: A Review**
Paul H. Sugarbaker.. 83

8 **Clinical Research Methodology in Peritoneal Surface Oncology: A Difficult Challenge**
François-Noël Gilly, Olivier Glehen, Annie C. Beaujard, Eddy Cotte 91

9 **Lessons Learnt from Clinical Trials in Peritoneal Surface Oncology: Colorectal Carcinomatosis**
Frans A. N. Zoetmulder, Vic J. Verwaal 99

10 **Experimental Models and Questions in Basic Science Research for Pseudomyxoma Peritonei**
Laura A. Lambert, Donald H. Lambert, Paul Mansfield 105

11 **Peritoneal Carcinomatosis of Colorectal Origin: Recent Advances and Future Evolution Toward a Curative Treatment**
Dominique Elias and Diane Goere 115

12 **Pathological Characterization and Differential Diagnosis of Malignant Peritoneal Mesothelioma**
Nelson G. Ordóñez 123

13 **Advances in Clinical Research and Management of Diffuse Peritoneal Mesothelioma**
Marcello Deraco, Dario Baratti, Nadia Zaffaroni, Antonello Domenico Cabras, and Shigeki Kusamura 137

14 **Advances in the Management of Gastric Cancer with Peritoneal Dissemination**
Yutaka Yonemura, Taiichi Kawamura, Etsurou Bandou, Gorou Tsukiyama, Masayuki Nemoto, Yoshio Endou, Masahiro Miura 157

15 **Intraperitoneal Chemotherapy in the Management of Ovarian Cancer**
Maurie Markman 165

List of Contributors

Syed A. Ahmad, MD
Division of Surgical Oncology
Department of Surgery
University of Cincinnati
College of Medicine
Barrett Cancer Center
234 Goodman Street
Cincinnati, OH 45219-0772
USA

Etsurou Bandou, MD, PhD
Gastric Surgery Division
Shizuoka Cancer Center
Shizuoka 411-8777
Japan

Dario Baratti, MD
Department of Surgery
National Cancer Institute
Via Venezian 1
20133 Milan
Italy

Annie C. Beaujard, MD
HCL, Department of Oncologic Surgery
Centre Hospitalier et
Universitaire Lyon Sud
Pierre Bénite
69495 Pierre Bénite Cedex
France

Antonello Domenico Cabras, MD
Department of Pathology
National Cancer Institute
Via Venezian 1
20133 Milan
Italy

Eddy Cotte, MD
HCL, Department of Oncologic Surgery
Centre Hospitalier et Universitaire Lyon Sud
69495 Pierre Bénite Cedex
France

Eelco de Bree, MD
Assistant Professor of Surgery
Department of Surgical Oncology
Medical School of Crete University Hospital
Herakleion
Greece

Marcello Deraco, MD
Department of Surgery
National Cancer Institute
Via Venezian 1
20133 Milan
Italy

Dominique Elias, MD, PhD
Professor, Department of Surgical Oncology
Gustave Roussy Institute
39 Rue Camille Desmoulins
94805 Villejuif Cédex
France

Yoshio Endou, PhD
Department of Experimental Therapeutics
Cancer Research Institute
Kanazawa University
Kanazawa
Japan

François-Noël Gilly, MD, PhD
HCL, Department of Oncologic Surgery
Centre Hospitalier et Universitaire Lyon Sud
69495 Pierre Bénite Cedex
France
and
Université Lyon 1, EA 3738
Faculté de Médecine Lyon Sud, BP 12
69921 Oullins Cedex
France

Olivier Glehen, MD, PhD
HCL, Department of Oncologic Surgery
Centre Hospitalier et Universitaire Lyon Sud
69495 Pierre Bénite Cedex
France

Diane Goere, MD
Department of Surgical Oncology
Gustave Roussy Institute
39 Rue Camille Desmoulins
94805 Villejuif Cedex
France

Taiichi Kawamura, MD, PhD
Gastric Surgery Division
Shizuoka Cancer Center
Shizuoka 411-8777
Japan

Shigeki Kusamura, MD, PhD
Department of Surgery
National Cancer Institute
Via Venezian 1
20133 Milan
Italy

Donald H. Lambert, MD, PhD
Professor
Department of Anesthesia
Boston University Medical School
Boston Medical Center
88 East Newton Street, H2817
Boston, MA 02110
USA

Laura A. Lambert, MD
Assistant Professor
Department of Surgical Oncology
University of Texas
M.D. Anderson Cancer Center
1400 Holcombe Boulevard
Houston, TX 77030
USA

Andrew M. Lowy, MD
Division of Surgical Oncology
Department of Surgery
University of Cincinnati College of Medicine
Barrett Cancer Center
234 Goodman Street
Cincinnati, OH 45219-0772
USA

Linmarie Ludeman, MB, ChB, MRCPath
Consultant Histopathologist
Gloucestershire Royal Hospital
Great Western Road
Gloucester GL1 3NN
UK

Paul Mansfield, MD
Professor, Department of Surgical Oncology
University of Texas
M.D. Anderson Cancer Center
1400 Holcombe Boulevard
Houston, TX 77030
USA

Maurie Markman, MD
University of Texas
M.D. Anderson Cancer Center
Mail Box 121
1515 Holcombe Boulevard
Houston, TX 77030
USA

Benjamin C. McIntyre, MD
Division of Surgical Oncology
Department of Surgery
University of Cincinnati College of Medicine
Barrett Cancer Center
234 Goodman Street
Cincinnati, OH 45219-0772
USA

List of Contributors

Masahiro Miura, PhD
Department of Anatomy
School of Medicine
Ooita University
Ooita
Japan

Masayuki Nemoto, MD
Gastric Surgery Division
Shizuoka Cancer Center
Shizuoka
Japan

Nelson G. Ordóñez, MD
The University of Texas
M.D. Anderson Cancer Center
1515 Holcombe Boulevard
Houston, TX 77030
USA

Amod A. Sarnaik, MD
Division of Surgical Oncology
Department of Surgery
University of Cincinnati College of Medicine
Barrett Cancer Center
234 Goodman Street
Cincinnati, OH 45219-0772
USA

Neil A Shepherd, DM, FRCPath
Professor, Consultant Histopathologist
Gloucestershire Royal Hospital
Great Western Road
Gloucester, GL1 3NN
UK
and
Visiting Professor of Pathology
Cranfield University
Bedfordshire MK45 4DT
UK

Paul H. Sugarbaker, MD, FACS, FRCS
Washington Cancer Institute
106 Irving Street NW
Suite 3900
Washington, DC 20010
USA

Jeffrey J. Sussman, MD
Division of Surgical Oncology
Department of Surgery
University of Cincinnati College of Medicine
Barrett Cancer Center
234 Goodman Street
Cincinnati, OH 45219-0772
USA

Dimitris Tsiftsis, MD, PhD
Professor of Surgery and Head of Department
Department of Surgical Oncology
Medical School of Crete University Hospital
Herakleion
Greece

Gorou Tsukiyama, MD, PhD
Gastric Surgery Division
Shizuoka Cancer Center
Shizuoka 411-8777
Japan

Vic J. Verwaal, MD, PhD
Netherlands Cancer Institute
Plesmanlaan 166
1066 CX Amsterdam
The Netherlands

Yutaka Yonemura, MD, PhD
Gastric Surgery Division
Shizuoka Cancer Center
1007 Shimo-Nagakubo
Suntou-gun
Nagaizumi-Machi
Shizuoka 411-8777
Japan

Nadia Zaffaroni, PhD
Department of Experimental Oncology
National Cancer Institute
Via Venezian 1
20133 Milan
Italy

Frans A.N. Zoetmulder
The Netherlands Cancer Institute
Antoni van Leeuwenhoek Ziekenhuis
Plesmanlaan 121
1066 CX Amsterdam
The Netherlands

1 Management of Peritoneal Surface Malignancy: A Short History

Paul H. Sugarbaker

1.1 Introduction

The development of management plans for peritoneal carcinomatosis and peritoneal mesothelioma originates in pharmacological, surgical, and technical advances. The major new pharmacological information was the description of the peritoneal space to plasma barrier [1]. These studies described the behavior of large molecules such as cancer chemotherapy agents that were instilled directly into the peritoneal cavity in a large volume of fluid. The surgical technical innovation was the description of peritonectomy procedures [2]. A new concept of the peritoneal lining as an organ that can be resected to prepare the peritoneal space for subsequent intraperitoneal chemotherapy was a crucial addition to the intraperitoneal chemotherapy treatments. Finally, as increasing numbers of patients were treated with this combined approach the nuances required in the management of these patients evolved [3]. This more knowledgeable management was dependent on the organization of peritoneal surface oncology treatment centers. This institutional commitment to the further development of treatments for peritoneal surface malignancy allowed the accumulation of data that could be shared by all of the groups. In addition, regular interactions of the peritoneal surface oncology groups in the United States, Europe, Korea, and Japan led to an exchange of ideas and treatment results that greatly accelerated the evolution of effective management plans [4]. An essential part of this exchange was the development of quantitative prognostic indicators that permit knowledgeable patient selection within a single institution and the sharing of data on similar populations of patients between institutions [5]. The combined treatment of peritonectomy procedures and intraperitoneal chemotherapy put together with more knowledgeable patient management and data accumulation using prognostic indicators has resulted in a worldwide interest in this potentially curative approach to a disease process that in the past was always fatal. Newer and more beneficial treatments and a reduction in the morbidity and mortality associated with these treatments are reported in the peer-reviewed literature on a regular basis.

1.2 Peritoneal Space to Plasma Barrier

The original pharmacological principles regarding the physiological behavior of large molecules placed directly into the peritoneal space in a large volume of physiological fluid were developed for the most part at the National Institutes of Health, Bethesda, Maryland, USA. The early publications by Flessner, Dedrick, and Schultz in the experimental laboratory and Meyers and Collins and Speyer et al. in the clinic aroused great interest in this new route of administration for cancer chemotherapy [6–8]. The importance of drug selection and proper dosimetry of intraperitoneal chemotherapy for vesicant drugs such as doxorubicin and for liver-metabolized drugs such as 5-fluorouracil was described by Sugarbaker et al. [9, 10]. The importance of molecular size in maintaining this peritoneal space to plasma barrier was clarified early on by Meyers and Collins [7].

Little has changed over the course of the last three decades in the pharmacological principles established by these early investigators. Some clarifications of the use of chemotherapy within the peritoneal space have occurred [11]. First, it was made clear that the extent of peritonectomy had little to do with the continued presence of the peritoneal space to plasma barrier. Vazquez et al. established that the percentage of the parietal peritoneum removed had little or no impact on the pharmacology of intraperitoneal chemotherapy with 5-fluorouracil [12]. Second, it was made clear that the volume of intraperitoneal fluid used to dilute the chemotherapy solution and thereby fill the peritoneal space had a profound impact on the pharmacology of intraperitoneal drug instillation [13, 14]. Both Elias and Sidaris and Sugarbaker et al. showed that a volume of fluid determined by body surface area must be prescribed along with a chemotherapy dose determined by body size. Only if both volume and dose of chemotherapy were controlled could the systemic exposure be predicted and the intraperitoneal and systemic effects remain constant from patient to patient. Third, it was demonstrated that the use of hyperthermic intraperitoneal chemotherapy had little or no effect on subsequent 5-fluorouracil chemotherapy used in the early postoperative period [15].

1.3 A Requirement for Complete Cytoreduction Using Peritonectomy Procedures

Perhaps the most clearly demonstrated clinical finding with the combined treatment for colon and appendiceal carcinomatosis is the absolute requirement for clearing the peritoneal space of malignant disease in order for intraperitoneal chemotherapy to affect long-term survival [3]. A similar observation has been made for gastric cancer with carcinomatosis [16]. With ovarian cancer and peritoneal mesothelioma significant reduction in the tumor volume is necessary and peritonectomy procedures are indicated; however, complete visible clearing of the peritoneal space is not necessary for the intraperitoneal chemotherapy to result in long-term benefit.

The peritonectomy procedures were described initially by Sugarbaker in 1995 [2]. Yonemura and colleagues published similar procedures especially adapted for the management of carcinomatosis from gastric cancer [17]. Additional procedures included the total anterior parietal peritonectomy [18]. Extensive visceral resections including total gastrectomy have allowed an extension of the surgical technology of peritonectomy and the resulting optimal cytoreduction to a larger number of cancer patients [19].

Surgical technical advances associated with complete cytoreduction with peritonectomy have involved the use of self-retaining retractors and ball-tip high-voltage electrosurgery. A recent advance whose results have not yet been completely realized is the resurfacing of these extensive raw tissue surfaces with antisclerotic agents. Also needed is instruction at treatment centers in the advanced surgical technology required for peritonectomy.

1.4 Long-Term Intraperitoneal Chemotherapy

The earliest efforts at intraperitoneal chemotherapy consisted of instillations initiated several weeks after a surgical procedure in patients determined to have peritoneal dissemination. Also, long-term neoadjuvant combined intraperitoneal 5-fluorouracil and systemic mitomycin C for colorectal or appendiceal carcinomatosis was reported on by Esquivel and colleagues [20]. Long-term intraperitoneal chemotherapy for 1 year after the resection of colon or rectal cancer at high risk for local-regional recurrence was reported by Sugarbaker et al. This was perhaps the first randomized and controlled trial showing that long-term intraperitoneal chemotherapy could reduce the incidence of peritoneal surface progression when used in an adjuvant setting [21]. Long-term intraperitoneal chemotherapy showed benefit in ovarian cancer as reported by Alberts and coworkers as a phase III investigation [22]. In a well-designed study these clinical researchers used equivalent doses of intraperitoneal cisplatin versus intravenous cisplatin in patients receiving systemic cyclophosphamide for ovarian cancer. Statistically significant improved survival was shown in the 654 randomized patients. Markman and colleagues showed the same improvement in survival when intraperitoneal paclitaxel was used [23]. More recently, Armstrong and colleagues in a third Gynecologic Oncology Group multi-institutional trial showed that bidirectional chemotherapy with cisplatin and paclitaxel was superior to a systemic treatment regimen [24]. This resulted in an NCI clinical alert urging those involved in the management of ovarian cancer to consider intraperitoneal chemotherapy when managing these patients.

As a result of these three efforts of the Gynecologic Oncology Group a revised plan of management for optimal treatment of patients with peritoneal dissemination of gastrointestinal, peritoneal mesothelioma, and gynecologic malignancy has occurred. A new exploration of long-term bidirectional chemotherapy with selected drugs being given intravenously and high-molecular-weight drugs being given intraperitoneally is currently targeted as a highest-priority clinical research effort.

1.5 Early Postoperative Intraperitoneal Chemotherapy

The initial reports of large numbers of patients with colorectal and appendiceal malignancy realizing long-term benefit from cytoreductive surgery combined with intraperitoneal chemotherapy were for treatment regimens using early postoperative intraperitoneal chemotherapy [3]. The most profound changes in the natural history of a peritoneal surface malignancy as a result of combined treatment seem to be in the minimally aggressive peritoneal surface malignancies such as appendiceal cancer [25]. Also, Elias and Pocard showed benefits from cytoreductive surgery with early postoperative intraperitoneal chemotherapy in colorectal cancer patients [26].

Early postoperative intraperitoneal chemotherapy remains the favored treatment plan for several chemotherapy agents when the intraperitoneal route of administration is favored. Drugs that have a high rate of hepatic metabolism of the chemotherapy agent so that a large proportion of the drug is detoxified with a single pass through the liver are appropriate. These agents include 5-fluorouracil and doxorubicin [8–11]. Also, taxanes, especially paclitaxel, are appropriate for early postoperative intraperitoneal chemotherapy. This drug is not significantly augmented by heat, works as a cell cycle-specific drug that should be used over the long term, and is much better tolerated from the perspective of nausea and vomiting after administration if it is given in divided doses over the first 5 days postoperatively. Recent clinical investigators are testing combinations of heated intraoperative intraperitoneal chemotherapy and early postoperative intraperitoneal chemotherapy as a perioperative multidrug treatment plan to determine an optimal combination of these treatment strategies [27].

1.6 Heated Intraoperative Intraperitoneal Chemotherapy

The earliest clinical efforts with heated intraoperative intraperitoneal chemotherapy were those of Spratt et al. in 1980 [28]. Shortly thereafter, in 1988, Koja and colleagues at Tottori University, Japan applied the treatments to patients with gastric cancer and peritoneal seeding [29]. The landmark reports by Fujimoto from Chiba University, Japan and Yonemura from Kanazawa University, Japan should also be mentioned [30–33]. The studies from Japan involved gastric cancer patients with demonstrated peritoneal seeding or gastric cancer with adjuvant intraperitoneal chemotherapy. The combination of cytoreductive surgery with heated intraoperative intraperitoneal chemotherapy has now been demonstrated in a phase III trial to improve the survival of colon cancer patients with peritoneal seeding [34]. Also, a large retrospective multi-institutional study suggests that approximately 25% of colon cancer patients with this combined therapy will be alive and disease-free at 5 years [35]. All of the natural history studies suggest that these patients have a median survival limited to 6 months or less [36–38].

Some of the most significant but perhaps underappreciated studies come from the use of early postoperative intraperitoneal chemotherapy in an adjuvant setting. In a phase III study Yu and colleagues from Taegu used early postoperative intraperitoneal mitomycin C and 5-fluorouracil to improve survival of stage III and resectable stage IV gastric cancer patients [39].

An adjuvant study in colorectal cancer that has not received sufficient recognition is the study by Scheithauer and colleagues [40]. These investigators compared intravenous to intraperitoneal 5-fluorouracil after a potentially curative resection of colon cancer. They showed statistically significant benefit with this local-regional approach. Vaillant and coworkers in France showed improvement, although not statistically significant, in stage II but not stage III colon cancer patients [41].

1.7 More Knowledgeable Use of Quantitative Prognostic Indicators for Combined Treatment

In the early efforts to manage carcinomatosis, patients were scored as carcinomatosis present versus carcinomatosis absent. In a group of patients with peritoneal seeding no survival at 3 years was expected in patients with gastrointestinal cancer. In the absence of peritoneal seeding surgical resection of gastrointestinal cancer combined with systemic chemotherapy became the standard of care. It soon became obvious that not all patients with carcinomatosis were the same. Four different scoring systems by which to quantitate carcinomatosis have been described. Perhaps the original one was the „P factor" utilized in the Japanese classification of gastric cancer. P1 (cancer seedlings limited to the stomach itself), P2 (cancer seedlings limited to the space above the transverse colon), and P3 (cancer seedlings located throughout the peritoneal space) have stood the test of time as a useful quantitation of gastric carcinomatosis [42]. For more precise quantitation of the distribution and volume of carcinomatosis the Peritoneal Cancer Index has been utilized. This scoring system combines the distribution of carcinomatosis and the lesion size of the nodules present throughout the abdomen and especially emphasizes cancerous involvement of the small bowel and its mesentery. The Peritoneal Cancer Index can be scored with a CT, using the findings at the time of abdominal exploration of the abdomen and pelvis and after the maximal efforts at cytoreduction have occurred. Other methodologies for quantitating peritoneal cancer dissemination are the Gilly Staging System from Lyon, France and the simplified peritoneal cancer index utilized at the Netherlands Cancer Institute [43].

It was clear as the multiple publications on colorectal and gastric cancer appeared that an assessment of the completeness of cytoreduction was necessary. It has been suggested that the completeness of cytoreduction will vary as the invasive character of the malignancy and its response to perioperative intraperitoneal chemotherapy will vary. A completeness of cytoreduction scoring system has been reported [43].

It is obvious to those working long-term in this field that early interventions in patients who have not had extensive prior surgery provide the best results in terms of survival and lowest morbidity and mortality. Some means of assessing the extent of prior surgery was found to be necessary. The prior surgical score was presented by Sugarbaker and colleagues and shown to have a major impact in determining survival of appendiceal malignancy patients and ovarian cancer patients [5, 25, 44].

Finally, an important adjunct to the assessment of prognosis in these patients is renewed interest in the histomorphology of peritoneal surface malignancy. The work of Ronnett and colleagues clearly shows that the invasive character of a malignant process has a profound effect on the success of combined treatment [45]. Similar emphasis on histomorphology in the outcome of combined treatment in peritoneal mesothelioma patients has been demonstrated by Cerruto et al. and Deraco et al. [46, 47].

1.8 Development of Peritoneal Surface Oncology Treatment Centers

To the credit of Heald and colleagues, promoters of the refined techniques for rectal cancer excision, the importance of a treatment center in the United Kingdom for pseudomyxoma peritonei patients was made clear. In 1998 this became a reality. Moran and colleagues have added greatly to the quality of care of appendiceal malignancy patients in the UK. In 2002 a second center was established under the direction of Sarah O'Dwyer and colleagues in Manchester, UK. Other designated treatment centers have appeared throughout Europe.

1.9 Future Directions

A summary of the evolution of treatments for peritoneal carcinomatosis is shown in Table 1.1. New efforts to further develop and improve the outcome of patients with peritoneal surface malignancy are under way. It has become clear that early treatments, usually before any systemic chemotherapy is administered, may be optimal for these patients. Certainly, a watch and wait policy with referral of symptomatic patients to a peritoneal surface oncology center is no longer acceptable. Second, the perioperative treatments are now many and varied. Because of the efforts of Elias and colleagues a bidirectional approach is becoming the standard of care [13]. As reviewed by Sugarbaker and colleagues, some chemotherapy agents are most appropriate for intravenous use with heat targeting to the peritoneal cavity [11]. Others are more valuable because of their large molecular size and the heat augmentation to be used as part of a hyperthermic intraoperative intraperitoneal chemotherapy regimen (HIPEC).

Neoadjuvant treatments are now being explored, especially in Japan, for gastric cancer. The high response rate of combined systemic and intravenous chemotherapy reported by Yonemura et al. presents an exciting new direction in which to go with a very poor prognosis group of patients [48]. Also, continued use of adjuvant therapies for patients with peritoneal seeding using a combination of intraperitoneal and systemic agents remains to be fully explored.

Finally, to allow treatments to be extended beyond the operating theater a new interest in the use of antisclerosis agents to diminish adhesions postoperatively has occurred. Numerous agents are now available including methylcellulose, polylactide sheets, polyethylene glycol spray, and 5-fluorouracil early postoperative irrigations. Continued studies to maintain the integrity of the peritoneal cavity are needed.

1.10 Respect for the Peritoneum as a First Line of Defense of Carcinomatosis

Finally, there is a realization that a comprehensive approach to the management of gastrointestinal cancer, gynecologic malignancy, and peritoneal mesothelioma is possible. Not only systemic treatments but also cytoreductive surgery and intraperitoneal chemotherapy need to be considered for every patient. The peritoneum is now being accepted as an organ from which cancer can be resected for cure. Also, the amazing properties of the peritoneum to present a first line of defense to the organism in the dissemination of intraperito-

Table 1.1 Evolution of treatments for peritoneal carcinomatosis from gastrointestinal cancer

Authors	Year	Event	Reference
Spratt et al.	1980	Suggested a hyperthermic peritoneal perfusion system with the administration of intraperitoneal chemotherapy. University of Louisville, Kentucky.	28
Speyer et al.	1981	Pharmacology of intraperitoneal 5-fluorouracil in humans. National Institutes of Health, Bethesda, Maryland.	8
Koga et al.	1984	Experimental study with prophylactic continuous hyperthermic peritoneal perfusion with mitomycin C. A significant prolongation of survival was obtained when 41.5°C hyperthermia was combined with mitomycin C. Tottori University, Japan.	50
Flessner et al.	1984	Pharmacokinetic studies established the peritoneal plasma barrier. National Institutes of Health, Bethesda, Maryland.	6
Sugarbaker et al.	1985	Randomized controlled study of intravenous versus intraperitoneal 5-fluorouracil documented a diminished incidence of peritoneal carcinomatosis in colon cancer patients. National Institutes of Health, Bethesda, Maryland.	21
Koga et al.	1988	First study of adjuvant intraoperative hyperthermic peritoneal perfusion with mitomycin C in gastric cancer. Tottori University, Japan.	29
Fujimoto et al.	1988	Used intraoperative hyperthermic peritoneal perfusion with mitomycin C combined with extended surgery in patients with gastric cancer and established peritoneal carcinomatosis. After the treatment, 12.8% survived 1 year as compared with 0% after surgery alone. Chiba University, Japan.	30
Sugarbaker and Jablonski	1989	Trial of early postoperative intraperitoneal mitomycin C and 5-fluorouracil in the management of carcinomatosis. Washington Hospital Center, Washington, DC.	3
Sugarbaker	1995	Peritonectomy procedures. Washington Hospital Center, Washington, DC.	2
Yonemura et al.	1996	Suggested peritoneal cavity expander for optimization of intraoperative intraperitoneal hyperthermic chemotherapy delivery in patients with gastric cancer. Kanazawa University, Japan.	16
Yu et al.	1998	Positive results of randomized study on adjuvant early postoperative intraperitoneal chemotherapy for gastric cancer. Kyungpook National University, Taegu, Korea.	39
Moran and Cecil	1998	Pseudomyxoma peritonei treatment center designated for the United Kingdom. North Hampshire Hospital, Basingstoke, England.	51
Urano et al.	1999	In vivo chemohyperthermia parameters defined. Memorial Sloan-Kettering, New York.	52
Zoetmulder et al.	2002	Randomized trial showing superiority of comprehensive treatment for carcinomatosis from colon cancer. Netherlands Cancer Institute, Amsterdam.	34

neal cancer have been appreciated. The great harm that can be done when surgeons fail to appreciate this first line of defense has been described for appendiceal and ovarian cancer patients. Also, increase in the morbidity and mortality of these combined treatments after extensive prior surgery has been well described for colon cancer patients [49].

Acknowledgements. Supported by Foundation for Applied Research in Gastrointestinal Oncology.

References

1. Jacquet P, Sugarbaker PH (1996) Peritoneal-plasma barrier. In: Sugarbaker PH (ed) Peritoneal carcinomatosis: principles of management. Kluwer, Boston, pp 53–63
2. Sugarbaker PH (1995) Peritonectomy procedures. Ann Surg 221:29–42
3. Sugarbaker PH, Jablonski KA (1995) Prognostic features of 51 colorectal and 130 appendiceal cancer patients with peritoneal carcinomatosis treated by cytoreductive surgery and intraperitoneal chemotherapy. Ann Surg 221:124–132
4. Sugarbaker PH, Garofalo A, Gonzalez-Moreno S (2006) Progress in peritoneal surface malignancy. Eur J Surg Oncol (in press)
5. Jacquet P, Sugarbaker PH (1996) Current methodologies for clinical assessment of patients with peritoneal carcinomatosis. J Exp Clin Cancer Res 15:49–58
6. Flessner MF, Dedrick RL, Schultz JS (1985) Exchange of macromolecules between peritoneal cavity and plasma. Am J Physiol 248:H15–H25
7. Myers CE, Collins JM (1983) Pharmacology of intraperitoneal chemotherapy. Cancer Invest 1:395–407
8. Speyer JL, Sugarbaker PH, Collins JM, Dedrick RL, Klecker RW Jr, Meyers CE (1981) Portal levels and hepatic clearance of 5-fluorouracil after intraperitoneal administration in humans. Cancer Res 41:1916–1922
9. Sugarbaker PH, Graves T, DeBruijn EA, Cunliffe WJ, Mullins RE, Hull WE, Oliff L, Schlag P (1990) Rationale for early postoperative intraperitoneal chemotherapy (EPIC) in patients with advanced gastrointestinal cancer. Cancer Res 50:5790–5794
10. Sugarbaker PH (1991) Early postoperative intraperitoneal adriamycin as an adjuvant treatment for advanced gastric cancer with lymph node or serosal invasion. In: Sugarbaker PH (ed) Management of gastric cancer. Kluwer, Boston, pp 277–284
11. Sugarbaker PH, Mora JT, Carmignani P, Stuart OA, Yoo D (2005) Update on chemotherapeutic agents utilized for perioperative intraperitoneal chemotherapy. Oncologist 10:112–122
12. De Lima Vazquez V, Stuart OA, Sugarbaker PH (2003) Extent of a parietal peritonectomy does not change intraperitoneal chemotherapy pharmacokinetics. Cancer Chem Pharmacol 52:108–112
13. Elias DM, Sideris L (2003) Pharmacokinetics of heated intraoperative intraperitoneal oxaliplatin after complete resection of peritoneal carcinomatosis. Surg Oncol Clin N Am 12:755–769
14. Sugarbaker PH, Stuart OA, Carmignani CP (2005) Pharmacokinetic changes induced by the volume of chemotherapy solution in patients treated with hyperthermic intraperitoneal mitomycin C. Cancer Chemother Pharmacol (Epub August 11)
15. Jacquet P, Averbach A, Stephens AD, Stuart OA, Chang D, Sugarbaker PH (1998) Heated intraoperative intraperitoneal mitomycin C and early postoperative intraperitoneal 5-fluorouracil: pharmacokinetic studies. Oncology 55:130–138
16. Yonemura Y, Fujimura T, Nishimura G, Falla R, Sawa T, Katayama K, Tsugawa K, Fushida S, Miyazaki I, Tanaka M, Endou Y, Sasaki T (1996) Effects of intraoperative chemohyperthermia in patients with gastric cancer with peritoneal dissemination. Surgery 119:437–444
17. Yonemura Y, Fujimura T, Fushida S, Fujita H, Bando E, Taniguchi K, Nishimura G, Miwa K, Ohyama S, Sugiyama K, Sasaki T, Endo Y (1999) Peritonectomy as a treatment modality for patients with peritoneal dissemination from gastric cancer. In: Nakajima T, Yamaguchi T (eds) Multimodality therapy for gastric cancer. Springer-Verlag, Tokyo
18. De Lima Vazquez V, Sugarbaker PH (2003) Total anterior parietal peritonectomy. J Surg Oncol 83:261–263
19. Sugarbaker PH (2002) Cytoreduction including total gastrectomy for pseudomyxoma peritonei. Br J Surg 89:208–212
20. Esquivel J, Vidal-Jove J, Steves MA, Sugarbaker PH (1993) Morbidity and mortality of cytoreductive surgery and intraperitoneal chemotherapy. Surgery 113:631–636
21. Sugarbaker PH, Gianola FJ, Speyer JL, Wesley R, Barofsky I, Meyers CE (1985) Prospective randomized trial of intravenous versus intraperitoneal 5-fluorouracil in patients with advanced primary colon or rectal cancer. Surgery 98:414–421
22. Alberts DS, Liu PY, Hannigan EV, O'Toole R, Williams SD, Young JA, Franklin EW, Clarke-Pearson DL, Malviya VK, DuBeshter B, Adelson MD, Hoskins WJ (1996) Intraperitoneal cisplatin plus intravenous cyclophosphamide versus intravenous cisplatin plus intravenous cyclophosphamide for stage III ovarian cancer. N Engl J Med 335:1950–1955
23. Markman M, Bundy BN, Alberts DS, Fowler JM, Clark-Pearson DL, Carson LF, Wadler S, Sickel J (2001) Phase III trial of standard-dose intravenous cisplatin plus paclitaxel versus moderately high-dose carboplatin followed by intravenous paclitaxel and intraperitoneal cisplatin in small-volume stage III ovarian carcinoma: an intergroup study of the Gynecologic Oncology Group, Southwestern Oncology Group, and Eastern Cooperative Oncology Group. J Clin Oncol 19:1001–1007
24. Armstrong DK, Bundy B, Wenzel L, Huang HQ, Baergen R, Lele S, Copeland LJ, Walker JL, Burger RA; Gynecologic Oncology Group (2006) Intraperitoneal cisplatin and paclitaxel in ovarian cancer. N Engl J Med 354:34–43
25. Sugarbaker PH (1999) Results of treatment of 385 patients with peritoneal surface spread of appendiceal malignancy. Ann Surg Oncol 6:727–731
26. Elias DM, Pocard M (2003) Treatment and prevention of peritoneal carcinomatosis from colorectal cancer. Surg Oncol Clin N Am 12:543–559
27. Yonemura Y, Bandou E, Sawa T, Yoshimitsu Y, Endou

Y, Sasaki T, Sugarbaker PH (2006) Neoadjuvant treatment of gastric cancer with peritoneal dissemination. Eur J Surg Oncol 32:661–665
28. Spratt JS, Adcock RA, Muskovin M, Sherrill W, McKeown J (1980) Clinical delivery system for intraperitoneal hyperthermic chemotherapy. Cancer Res 40:256–260
29. Koga S, Hamazoe R, Maeta M, Shimizu N, Murakami A, Wakatsuki T (1988) Prophylactic therapy for peritoneal recurrence of gastric cancer by continuous hyperthermic peritoneal perfusion with mitomycin C. Cancer 61:232–237
30. Fujimoto S, Shrestha RD, Kokubun M, Ohta M, Takahashi M, Kobayashi K, Kiuchi S, Okui K, Miyoshi T, Arimizu N, Takamizawa H (1988) Intraperitoneal hyperthermic perfusion combined with surgery effective for gastric cancer patients with peritoneal seeding. Ann Surg 208:36–41
31. Fujimoto S, Takahashi M, Mutou T, Kobayashi K, Toyosawa T (1999) Successful intraperitoneal hyperthermic chemoperfusion for the prevention of postoperative peritoneal recurrence in patients with advanced gastric carcinoma. Cancer 85:529–534
32. Yonemura Y, Fujimura T, Fushida S, Takegawa S, Kamata T, Katayama K, Kosaka T, Yamaguchi A, Miwa K, Miyazaki I (1991) Hyperthermo-chemotherapy combined with cytoreductive surgery for the treatment of gastric cancer with peritoneal dissemination. World J Surg 15:530–535
33. Fujimura T, Yonemura Y, Muraoka K, Takamura H, Hirono Y, Sahara H, Ninomiya I, Matsumoto H, Tsugawa K, Nishimura G, Sugiyama K, Miwa K, Miyazaki I (1994) Continuous hyperthermic peritoneal perfusion for the prevention of peritoneal recurrence of gastric cancer: randomized controlled study. World J Surg 18:150–155
34. Verwaal VJ, van Ruth S, de Bree E, van Slooten GW, van Tinteren H, Boot H, Zoetmulder FAN (2003) Randomized trial of cytoreduction and hyperthermic intraperitoneal chemotherapy versus systemic chemotherapy and palliative surgery in patients with peritoneal carcinomatosis of colorectal cancer. J Clin Oncol 21:3737–3743
35. Glehen O, Kwiatkowski F, Sugarbaker PH, Elias D, Levine EA, De Simone M, Barone R, Yonemura Y, Cavaliere F, Quenet F, Gutman M, Tentes AA, Lorimier G, Bernard JL, Bereder JM, Porcheron J, Gomez-Portilla A, Shen P, Deraco M, Rat P (2004) Cytoreductive surgery combined with perioperative intraperitoneal chemotherapy for the management of peritoneal carcinomatosis from colorectal cancer: a multi-institutional study. J Clin Oncol 22:3284–3292
36. Chu DZ, Lang NP, Thompson C, Osteen PK, Westbrook KC (1989) Peritoneal carcinomatosis in nongynecologic malignancy. A prospective study of prognostic factors. Cancer 63:364–367
37. Sadeghi B, Arvieux C, Glehen O, Beaujard AC, Rivoire M, Baulieux J, Fontaumard E, Brachet A, Caillot JL, Faure JL, Porcheron J, Peix JL, Francois Y, Vignal J, Gilly FN (2000) Peritoneal carcinomatosis from non-gynecologic malignancies: results of the EVOCAPE 1 multicentric prospective study. Cancer 88:358–363
38. Jayne DG, Fook S, Loi C, Seow-Choen F (2002) Peritoneal carcinomatosis from colorectal cancer. Br J Surg 89:1545–1550
39. Yu W, Whang I, Chung HY, Averbach A, Sugarbaker PH (2001) Indications for early postoperative intraperitoneal chemotherapy of advanced gastric cancer: results of a prospective randomized trial. World J Surg 25:985–990
40. Scheithauer W, Kornek GV, Marczell A, Karner J, Salem G, Greiner R, Burger D, Stoger F, Ritschel J, Kovats E, Vischer HM, Schneeweiss B, Depisch D (1998) Combined intravenous and intraperitoneal chemotherapy with fluorouracil + leucovorin vs. fluorouracil + levamisole for adjuvant therapy of resected colon carcinoma. Br J Cancer 77:1349–1354
41. Vaillant JC, Nordlinger B, Deuffic S, Arnaud JP, Pelissier E, Favre JP, Jaeck D, Fourtanier G, Grandjean JP, Marre P, Letoublon C (2000). Adjuvant intraperitoneal 5-fluorouracil in high-risk colon cancer: A multicenter phase III trial. Ann Surg 231:449–456
42. Japanese Research Society for Gastric Cancer (1995) Japanese classification of gastric carcinoma, 1st edn. Kanehara & Co., Tokyo
43. Glehen O, Gilly FN (2003) Quantitative prognostic indicators of peritoneal surface malignancy: carcinomatosis, sarcomatosis, and peritoneal mesothelioma. Surg Oncol Clin N Am 12: 649–671
44. Look M, Chang D, Sugarbaker PH (2004). Long-term results of cytoreductive surgery for advanced and recurrent epithelial ovarian cancers and papillary serous carcinoma of the peritoneum. Int J Gynecol Cancer 14:35–41
45. Ronnett BM, Shmookler BM, Sugarbaker PH, Kurman RJ (1997). Pseudomyxoma peritonei: new concepts in diagnosis, origin, nomenclature, relationship to mucinous borderline (low malignant potential) tumors of the ovary. In: Fechner RE, Rosen PP (eds) Anatomic pathology. ASCP Press, Chicago, pp 197–226
46. Cerruto CA, Brun EA, Sugarbaker PH (2006) Prognostic significance of histo-morphologic parameters in diffuse malignant peritoneal mesothelioma. Arch Pathol Lab Med 130: 1654–1661
47. Deraco M, Nonaka D, Baratti D, Casali P, Rosai J, Younan R, Salvatore A, Cabras AD, Kusamura S (2006). Prognostic analysis of clinicopathologic factors in 49 patients with diffuse malignant peritoneal mesothelioma treated with cytoreductive surgery and intraperitoneal hyperthermic perfusion. Ann Surg Oncol 13:229–237
48. Yonemura Y, Bandou E, Sawa T, Yoshimitsu Y, Endou Y, Sasaki T, Sugarbaker PH (2006). Neoadjuvant treat-

ment of gastric cancer with peritoneal dissemination. Eur J Surg Oncol 32:661–665
49. Verwaal VJ, van Tinteren H, Ruth SV, Zoetmulder FAN (2004) Toxicity of cytoreductive surgery and hyperthermic intra-peritoneal chemotherapy. J Surg Oncol 85:61–67
50. Koga S, Hamazoe R, Maeta M, Shimizu N, Kanayama H, Osaki Y (1984) Treatment of implanted peritoneal cancer in rats by continuous hyperthermic peritoneal perfusion in combination with an anticancer drug. Cancer Res 44:1840–1842
51. Moran BJ, Cecil TD (2003) The etiology, clinical presentation, and management of pseudomyxoma peritonei. Surg Oncol Clin N Am 12:585–603
52. Urano M, Kuroda M, Nishimura Y (1999). For the clinical application of thermochemotherapy given at mild temperatures. Int J Hyperthermia 15:79–107

2 The Natural History of Free Cancer Cells in the Peritoneal Cavity

Yutaka Yonemura, Taiichi Kawamura, Etsurou Bandou, Gorou Tsukiyama, Yoshio Endou, Masahiro Miura

Recent Results in Cancer Research, Vol. 169
© Springer-Verlag Berlin Heidelberg 2007

2.1 Molecular Mechanisms Involved in Peritoneal Dissemination

Peritoneal dissemination is established through a multistep process [1]. The first step is the detachment of cancer cells from the serosal surface of the primary tumor; the detached cancer cells are referred to as «peritoneal free cancer cells» (Fig. 2.1b, process 1). E-cadherin is the key molecule for the homophilic cell–cell adhesion [2], and the deleted expression of E-cadherin or abnormalities on the E-cadherin gene have a role in the detachment of cancer cells [3]. Namely, cancer cells with reduced expression of E-cadherin easily detach from the serosal surface and become peritoneal free cancer cells. In gastric cancer, abnormal expression of E-cadherin is more frequently found in poorly differentiated adenocarcinoma than in differentiated adenocarcinoma, and peritoneal dissemination is the main form of metastasis in poorly differentiated adenocarcinoma of the stomach [4].

S100-A4 is known to be involved in cancer cell motility by virtue of its ability to activate nonmuscle myosin [5]. Gastric cancer with reduced E-cadherin and high expression of S100-A4 often shows serosal invasion, peritoneal dissemination, and an infiltrating type in growth pattern [6]. Furthermore, these tumors show a strong correlation with poorly differentiated adenocarcinoma histology [6]. Accordingly, the expression pattern of S100A4 and E-cadherin may be a powerful predictor of peritoneal dissemination.

Peritoneal free cancer cells attach to the mesothelial cells (Fig. 2.1, process 2), invade into the submesothelial tissue (processes 4 and 5), proliferate (process 6), and grow to become established metastases with vascular neogenesis.

Two different processes are proposed in the formation of peritoneal dissemination, designated as «transmesothelial» (Fig. 2.1a) and «translymphatic» metastasis (Fig. 2.1b).

Transmesothelial metastasis originates from the direct attachment of peritoneal free cancer cells on the distant mesothelium (Fig. 2.1a). The normal peritoneal mesothelial cells strongly attach to each other without separation space and act as a barrier against the invasion of peritoneal free cancer cells into the submesothelial tissue. The tissue between the mesothelial cell layer and the submesothelial capillary is designated as the «peritoneal-blood barrier» (Fig. 2.1), which prohibits the movement of oxygen and nutrients from the submesothelial capillary to the peritoneal cavity [7]. Accordingly, most free cancer cells attached to the mesothelial cells die off because of the poor nutrient environment [8]. However, once free cancer cells loosely attach to the mesothelial cells with adhesion molecules like CD-44, cytokines produced by cancer cells contract mesothelial cells by the phosphorylation of their cell skeleton [9, 10]. As a result, cancer cells migrate into the submesothelial space through the cleaved space between mesothelial cells and strongly attach to the exposed base-

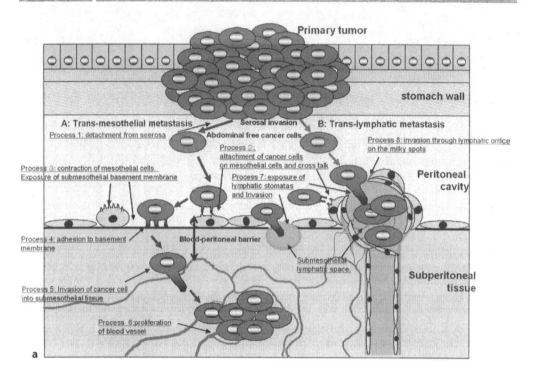

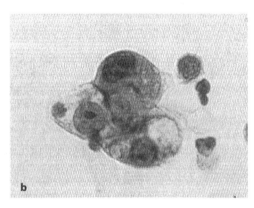

Fig. 2.1 a Multistep processes in the peritoneal dissemination. Process 1: detachment from serosa: E-cadherin. S100A4, motility factors (AMF/AMFR, HGF/c-Met, Rho); process 2: adhesion to mesothelial cells (CD-44); process 3: contraction of mesothelial cells (CD44, CEA.), cytokines (interleukins, EGF, HGF, VEGF-C); process 4: adhesion molecules (integrins, CD44); process 5: invasion: motility factors, matrix metalloproteinases, urokinase, UKPR; process 6: vascular neogenesis: VEGF, VEGF-C, bFGF, lymphangiogenesis, lymphatic dilatation: VEGF-C, VEGF-D; process 7: exposure of lymphatic stomatas or lymphatic orifices. **b** Peritoneal free cancer stained with Papanicolaou staining

ment membrane by the expression of integrin molecules. Integrins are the receptors of the components of the basement membrane and are expressed on the membrane of cancer cells. There is a close relation between overexpression of integrins and the metastatic ability of cancer cells [11, 12]. In an experimental peritoneal dissemination model, cancer cells with a highly metastatic ability overexpress integrin $\alpha 2/\alpha 3/\beta 1$ [13].

When cancer cells express motility factors and matrix proteinases, they can invade the subperitoneal tissue by degrading the peritoneal blood barrier. MET is a tyrosine kinase type receptor against hepatocyte growth factor (HGF) that increases the motility and proliferative activity of cancer cells [14]. In human gastric cancer, MET expression is associated with poorly differentiated adenocarcinoma and peritoneal dissemination [15, 16].

When cancer cells invade near the subperitoneal capillary, they can proliferate via autocrine or paracrine loop by the production of growth factors from cancer cells or stromal cells. Furthermore, angiogenic factors like VEGF-A and VEGF-C secreted from peritoneal free cancer cells induce vascular neogenesis in the subperitoneal tissue [17]. As a result, the width of the peritoneal-blood barrier shortens and a soil ready for metastasis is established.

The second metastatic process to the peritoneum is translymphatic metastasis (Fig. 2.1b). Peritoneal free cancer cells migrate into the lymphatic orifices (stomatas), opening on the peritoneal surface, and proliferate in the submesothelial lymphatic space just beneath the lymphatic stomatas. Peritoneal dissemination via translymphatic metastasis is established earlier than that via transmesothelial metastasis, because transmesothelial metastasis requires more metastatic steps than translymphatic metastasis.

There are many lymphatic orifices on the greater omentum, appendices epiploicae of the colon (Fig. 2.2a and b, Parts 1, 4, 6), inferior surface of the diaphragm (Fig. 2.2a, Parts 2, 3), falciform ligament (Fig. 2.2c, Part 9), Douglas' pouch (Fig. 2.2a and d, Part 5), and small bowel mesentery (Fig. 2.2b, Parts 7,8). The greater omentum (Fig. 2.2a, Part 1), falciform ligament (Fig. 2.3), and Douglas' pouch have many milky spots, which are a lymphatic apparatus consisting of peritoneal macrophages and lymphocytes in a lymph sinus (Fig. 2.3a–c). Lymphatic orifices are found on the milky spots (Fig. 2.3b), and the peritoneal macrophages mobilize into the peritoneal cavity through the lymphatic orifice. Accordingly, milky spots

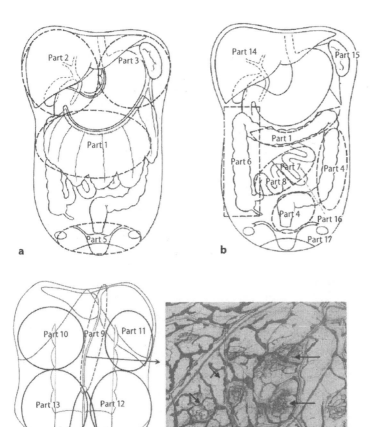

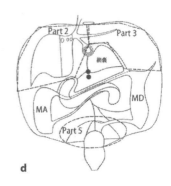

Fig. 2.2 a, b Classification of peritoneal surface, according to the distribution of lymphatic stomatas and milky spots. **c** Classification of peritoneal surface of anterior abdominal wall. On the surface of falciform ligament (*Part 9*), many milky spots stained by 5'Nase staining are found (←). **d** Classification of the peritoneal surface in the undersurface of diaphragm and Douglas' pouch

have an important role in the immunological function of the peritoneal cavity. Peritoneal free cancer cells migrate into the lymphatic sinus of the milky spot and proliferate along with neovascularization (Fig. 2.3d).

On the peritoneum covering Douglas' pouch, rich subperitoneal lymphatic plexuses and milky spots are found (Fig. 2.4a and b). The pelvic subperitoneal lymphatics stream toward the rectum and finally flow into the lymph nodes around the iliac artery (Fig. 2.4b). Peritoneal free cancer cells accumulate on the Douglas' pouch by gravity, and cytokines produced by cancer cells induce contraction of mesothelial cells. As a result, stomatas on the milky spots are exposed, resulting in the migration of cancer cells into the submesothelial lymphatic vessels.

On the diaphragm, numerous lymphatic orifices designated "stomatas" are found, which connect with the submesothelial lymphatic vessels beneath the macula cribriformis, which is a structure like a sieve (Fig. 2.5). Mesothelial cells cover the macula cribriformis, and the holes in the macula cribriformis connect with the underlying lymphatic vessels (Fig. 2.5). Usually stomatas are covered with flat mesothelial cells, but stomatas increase in size because of mesothelial cell contraction induced by the cytokines produced from cancer cells and peritoneal inflammatory cells. Peritoneal free cancer cells migrate into the submesothelial lymphatic space in the diaphragm and proliferate (Fig. 2.5). In addition, negative pressure caused by inspiration enhances the migration of peritoneal free cancer cells through diaphragmatic stomatas.

In contrast, there are no lymphatic stomatas or milky spots on the liver capsule (Fig. 2.2b,

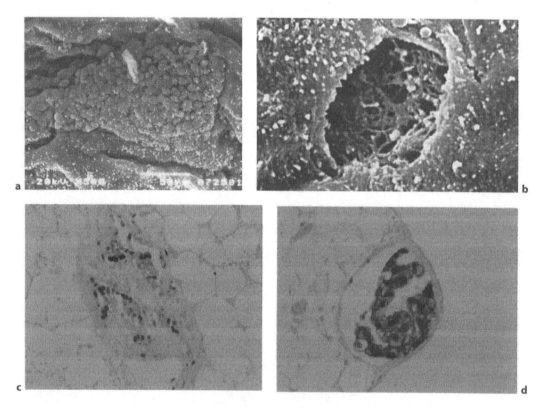

Fig. 2.3 a Electron microscopic finding of human milky spots on the greater omentum. **b** Lymphatic orifice on the milky spots in the greater omentum, which connects with the submesothelial lymphatic vessel. **c** Histological findings of milky spots on human greater omentum, which consist of macrophage, lymphatic vessels, and lymphatic sinus. **d** Histological findings of gastric cancer cell emboli in the lymphatic space on human greater omentum

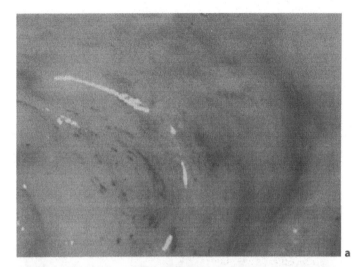
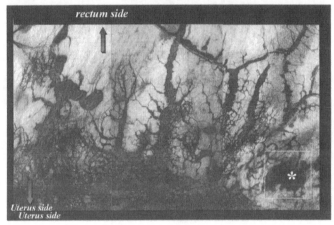

Fig. 2.4 a Milky spots and submesothelial lymphatic vessels stained after intraperitoneal injection of activated carbon particle on the Douglas' pouch. **b** Submesothelial lymphatic plexus of Douglas' pouch, stained with 5'Nase method. * Milky spots stained with activated carbon particles

Part 14), the peritoneum covering the abdominal wall (Fig. 2.2c, Parts 10, 11, 12, 13), or the serosal surface of small bowel and splenic capsule (Fig, 2.2b, Part 15). These peritoneal parts are not affected until late stages of peritoneal dissemination.

Translymphatic metastasis is established in lymphatic stomatas and milky spots. The area of the peritoneum with rich lymphatic orifices occupies about 65% of its total surface [19].

The mechanism of peritoneal dissemination in pseudomyxoma peritonei is different from that of gastric and colon cancer. The mechanism of peritoneal dissemination in pseudomyxoma peritonei is established mainly through a translymphatic process. In pseudomyxoma peritonei, free cancer cells are produced by the perforation or rupture of the primary tumor due to an increased luminal pressure of the appendix (Fig. 2.7). Intraperitoneal free cancer cells of pseudomyxoma are covered with mucin (Fig. 2.6) and hardly adhere to the peritoneal surface via the adhesion molecules expressed on the cell surface. Accordingly, they metastasize through milky spots and lymphatic stomatas on the diaphragm by the negative pressure of inspiration. Invasive ability of pseudomyxoma is also low, and the tumor cells proliferate mainly in the lymphatic space of the milky spots and lymphatic stomatas (Fig. 2.7). Furthermore, the liver and spleen capsules are involved by contact from the metastases in the diaphragm.

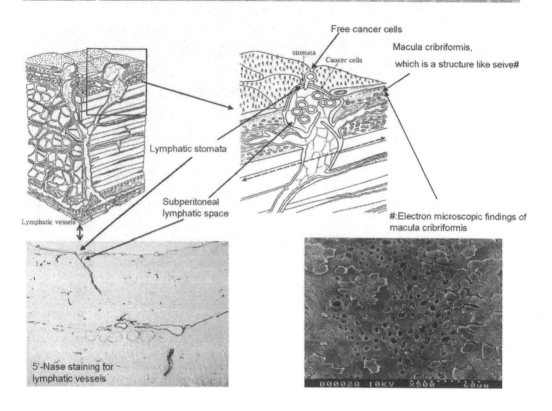

Fig. 2.5 Mechanisms of metastasis through stomatas on the diaphragm. Cancer cells migrate through stomatas and into the submesothelial lymphatic vessels

On the Douglas' pouch, pseudomyxoma cells accumulate by gravity and proliferate, producing mucin. Cancer cells proliferate slowly on the surface of peritoneum without invasion into the submesothelial tissue.

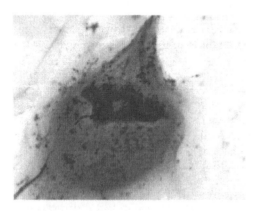

Fig. 2.6 Peritoneal free cancer cells of pseudomyxoma peritonei. Cells are covered with mucin

In contrast, peritoneal metastases from gastric and colon cancer are usually established by both translymphatic and transmesothelial metastasis. Transmesothelial metastasis is established through several steps as shown in Fig. 2.1. Accordingly, concerted expression of metastasis-related genes is essential to overcome each step.

Recently available DNA microarray-based gene expression profiling technology provides a strategy for searching systematically in a combinatory manner for molecular markers of cancer metastasis. In gastric cancer, simultaneous analysis of a large number of genes may offer a powerful and complementary approach to clarify the genes that are closely related to peritoneal dissemination. Matrix metalloproteinase (MMP)-7 [20], Reg IV [21, 22], dopa decarboxylase (DDC), and several adhesion molecules have been reported as candidates for target genes involved in peritoneal dissemination.

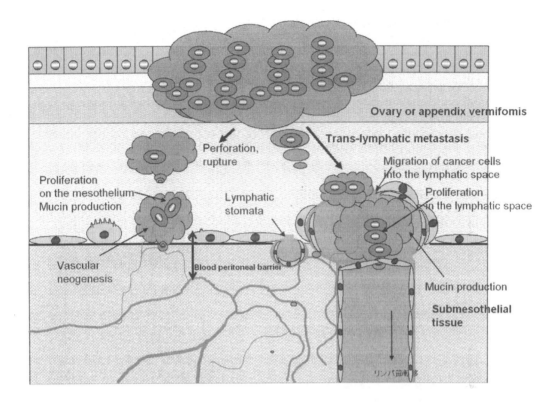

Fig. 2.7 Mechanisms of the formation of peritoneal dissemination of pseudomyxoma peritonei

Among MMPs, MMP-7 and MT1-MMP are expressed mainly by cancer cells, whereas the other MMPs are expressed by both stromal cells and cancer cells [24]. MMP-7 can degrade a wide range of extracellular matrices and can activate other proMMPs, resulting in the cleavage of all kinds of stromal substrates [24]. Yonemura et al. reported that MMP-7 is exclusively expressed in peritoneal dissemination from gastric cancer and that antisense-oligonucleotides specific for MMP-7 mRNA suppressed the invasion of a highly metastatic gastric cancer cell line in vitro [24]. Furthermore, intraperitoneal administration of the antisense oligonucleotides improved the survival of mice bearing peritoneal dissemination. These results strongly suggest an important role of MMP-7 in the genesis of peritoneal dissemination in gastric cancer.

The Reg gene was found as a growth factor of islet B-cells [25, 26a]. Reg protein is normally expressed in the gastrointestinal tract and is induced in inflammatory bowel disease and gastrointestinal cancers. Pleiotropic functions in cancer cells include promoting proliferation and resistance to apoptosis [26b]. Oue et al. reported a close association between the high expression of Reg IV and the invasive ability of gastric cancer [21]. Miyagawa et al. reported that Reg IV is a potential novel marker for peritoneal dissemination [22]. Reg IV and its receptor might be useful therapeutic targets for the management of peritoneal dissemination.

Expression of DDC, which is responsible for the synthesis of the key neurotransmitters dopamine and serotonin, is upregulated in the peritoneal dissemination of gastric cancer. Sakakura et al. reported significant high signals of DDC mRNA expression in pellets of peritoneal lavage fluid by real-time reverse transcriptase-polymerase chain reaction (RT-PCR) methodology; therefore, DDC may potentially be a novel marker of peritoneal dissemination of gastric cancer [28].

In the adhesion molecules, integrins are reported as the markers for peritoneal dissemination [11, 13]. Kawamura et al. reported that a highly metastatic cell line on the peritoneum overexpresses integrin α1, α2, and β1 [11]. Furthermore, neutralizing antibody for integrin α1, α2, and β1 subunits can inhibit the adhesion of cancer cells to the peritoneum. These results suggest integrins as target molecules to consider in research for the prevention of peritoneal dissemination.

Furthermore, complementary DNA microarray and histochemical analyses revealed differences in the concerted expressions of several genes coding for matrix proteinases, cell adhesion, motility, angiogenesis, and proliferation between the highly metastatic and parental cell lines [27]. Accordingly, multiple genes should be controlled simultaneously for the treatment of peritoneal dissemination.

2.2 Detection of Free Cancer Cells in the Peritoneal Cavity

The Japanese General Rules of Gastric Cancer Treatment recommend that peritoneal lavage cytological examination is done right after laparotomy to confirm the existence or absence of peritoneal free cancer cells. A positive cytology is recorded as "Cy1." Patients with Cy1 status are classified as stage IV, because peritoneal recurrence develops even after curative resection.

The conventional staining method to detect peritoneal free cancer cells is Papanicolaou staining (Fig. 2.1b) Bando et al. reported that 5% (51/1001) of 1001 patients with potentially curable gastric cancer showed peritoneal free cancer cells, and the 5-year survival rate of the patients with P0 (no established macroscopic peritoneal seeding) Cy1 status was only 2% [29]. Wu et al. reported that peritoneal free cancer cells were found in 19% of 134 patients with potentially curable serosa-involved gastric cancer [30].

A positive cytology is significantly associated with wall invasion, histological type, infiltrating growth, and size of serosal invasion [29]. Bando et al. reported that tumor size larger than 6 cm, diameter of serosal invasion greater than 2.5 cm [31], T3/T4 tumors, and an infiltrating growth pattern are independent predictors of peritoneal recurrence [29]. However, the sensitivity of these clinicopathological parameters is low to predict peritoneal recurrence. In contrast, the specificity of peritoneal lavage cytology for peritoneal recurrence is satisfactory but the sensitivity is only 56%.

A significant number of patients with a negative cytology may still develop recurrence in the form of peritoneal dissemination. Bando et al. reported that the results of peritoneal lavage cytology were negative in 49% of all patients who developed peritoneal recurrence [29]. These results point out that the conventional staining methods lack sensitivity.

Recently, more sensitive methods and combination assays using several markers to detect peritoneal dissemination have been proposed. Immunocytological detection of peritoneal free cancer cells has been reported. Cytological samples were stained with monoclonal antibodies against tumor-associated antigens (CEA, CA19-9, Ber EP4), and no unwarranted reactions were found in the control samples. With immunocytochemical detection of peritoneal micrometastasis in gastric cancer it was possible to identify free cancer cells in 35% of the patients, with a 14% improvement over routine cytopathology results [32]. Furthermore, combining the conventional method with immunocytological studies provided more sensitive results than the conventional staining alone [33].

It has been shown that quantification of CEA protein levels in peritoneal wash fluid can be a sensitive and useful predictor of peritoneal recurrence. Nishiyama et al. reported that CEA levels in peritoneal washings were statistically independent of those in sera and could more reliably predict the presence of peritoneal dissemination than a cytological study [35]. Furthermore, the sensitivity rate of their results ranged from 50% to 70% for the prediction of peritoneal dissemination [34, 35].

(RT-PCR using specific primers for cancer-specific antigens was developed for the sensitive detection of micrometastases in the peritoneal cavity. The target genes are CEA [37], MMP-7 [38], and DDC [28]. More recently, real-time fluorescence PCR examination using the LightCycler allowed rapid and sensitive detection of CEA mRNA in peritoneal washing samples. Total assay time to obtain the results is significantly shorter than that with the conventional RT-PCR. This assay system can detect reliably a minimum of 10 cancer cells [39]. However, some false-positive results, which may be attributable to CEA-expressing noncancerous cells, have been encountered. In addition, this system is expensive and time-consuming. Yonemura et al. reported that the CEA RT-PCR assay yielded 40/230 (17%) positives, which included none of 26 patients with benign disease. The incidence of a positive cytology and a positive CEA level in peritoneal wash fluid was 19% and 15%, respectively. Logistic stepwise regression analysis revealed that lymph node status, depth of invasion, venous invasion, the results of peritoneal cytological examination, and CEA RT-PCR assay were independently related to peritoneal recurrence. Peritoneal cytological examination was the most significant predictive factor for peritoneal recurrence, with a sensitivity of 46%, a specificity of 94%, and accuracy of 73%, while the corresponding values of the CEA RT-PCR assay were 31%, 95%, and 73%. However, Yonemura et al. demonstrated that CEA levels in wash fluid are not an independent predictor for peritoneal dissemination, and that their accuracy is inferior to that of cytological examination [36].

When the results were studied according to the combination analyses of peritoneal wash cytology and CEA-RT-PCR, the prognosis of patients with positive CEA-RT-PCR or positive cytology was significantly poorer than that of those with negative CEA-RT-PCR and peritoneal wash cytology (Fig. 2.8). Combining cytological examination with CEA RT-PCR assay resulted in a sensitivity rate for peritoneal recurrence of 57%, an 11% improvement over that of cytology alone. The data indicate that the use of a combination of CEA-RT-PCR and cytological assay is more likely to identify patients who will develop peritoneal recurrence. This may be useful for the classification of patients for suitable therapeutic trials.

2.3 Clinical Implications and Significance of a Positive Cytology

The prognosis of patients with potentially curable gastric cancer and intraperitoneal free cancer cells (P0Cy1) is very poor, because almost all patients with P0Cy1 status die 3 years after gastrectomy because of peritoneal recurrence. Simple gastrectomy without additional lymphadenectomy is the optimal strategy for the treatment [30]. Chemotherapy regimens like intravenous 5-fluorouracil (5-FU) infusion [40] alone or in combination with other anticancer drugs (FAM [41], FAMTX [42]) have been used for these patients. However, there has been no reported study specifically addressing the efficacy of systemic chemotherapy in patients with P0Cy1 status.

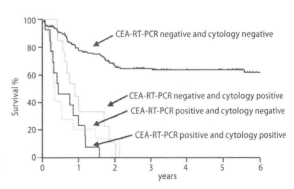

Fig. 2.8 Survival of patients according to the peritoneal wash cytology and CEA-RT-PCR using peritoneal washing fluid in 230 patients who had undergone curative surgery

TS-1 is a new oral fluorinated pyrimidine agent, which contains tegafur, 5-chloro-2,4-dihydroxypyridine (CDHP) and potassium oxonate (Oxo) in a molar ratio of 1:0.4:1 [43]. Dihydropyrimidine dehydrogenase (DPD), which is found in a high concentration in the liver, rapidly degrades 5-FU. CDHP is a specific inhibitor of DPD, and the inhibition of 5-FU by CDHP is very important for the efficacy of 5-FU. In an experimental model, high and constant 5-FU concentrations were maintained by continuous infusion of 5-FU in combination with CDHP [44]. However, in the model, diarrhea due to 5-FU is a severe dose-limiting factor. Oxo is an inhibitor of orotate phosphoribosyltransferase (ORPT) and acts as a protector against 5-FU-induced gastrointestinal toxicity without loss of antitumor activity [44]. Accordingly, TS-1 might be more effective in the treatment of cancer patients than continuous infusion of 5-FU from the point of antitumor potency and toxicity.

Because prolonged exposure is desirable from the standpoint of antitumor mechanisms of 5-FU, oral administration of TS-1 is certainly the most appealing route of administration, as compared with intravenous infusion of 5-FU [45]. Hirata et al. reported that high enough plasma concentrations of 5-FU to kill cancer cells were maintained for a 4-week period of consecutive administration of TS-1 [46].

Yonemura et al. reported the effects of TS-1 for potentially curable patients with peritoneal free cancer cells (P0/Cy1 status) as a postoperative chemotherapy [47]. After radical gastrectomy, 35 patients were treated with oral TS-1 (80 mg/m2) for 28 consecutive days and 14-day rest, and the schedule was repeated every 6 weeks (TS-1 group). The patients treated with TS-1 survived significantly longer than those in the control group. Two-year survival rates of the control group and the TS-1 group were 9% and 53%, respectively (Fig. 2.9). Recurrence was not found in 15 patients (43%) of the TS-1 group and in 3 patients (5%) of the control group. A Cox proportional hazard model showed that TS-1 treatment was an independent prognostic factor, and the relative risk for TS-1 treatment was 0.17-fold lower than that of the control group. Major adverse reactions included myelosuppression and gastrointestinal toxicities, but they were generally mild, and no treatment-related deaths occurred. From these results it can be concluded that TS-1 treatment is safe and effective as adjuvant postoperative chemotherapy for patients with P0/Cy1 status.

Hyperthermic intraperitoneal perfusion chemotherapy (HIPEC) is also reported to be effective for the prevention of recurrence in patients with P0Cy1 status. After radical gastrectomy for patients with potentially curable serosa-involved gastric cancer, the peritoneal cavity was perfused with 6–8 l of heated saline at 42 degrees centigrade with 30 mg of MMC and 150 mg of CDDP for 60 min [48]. Patients treated with HIPEC survived significantly longer than the control group (Fig. 2.10) [48, 49]. In addition, peritoneal recurrence after HIPEC was significantly lower than in the control group.

Peritoneal lavage by preoperative laparoscopy has a role in assessment of the peritoneal cytological status in patients with advanced gastric cancer and may alter their therapeutic approach [50].

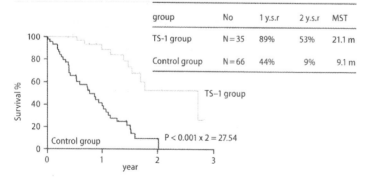

Fig. 2.9 Survival of patients with potentially curable gastric cancer and peritoneal free cancer cells, who were treated with postoperative oral administration of 80 mg/m^2 of TS-1 at the respective dose for 28 days, followed by a 2-week rest. This schedule was repeated every 6 weeks until the occurrence of recurrence, unacceptable toxicities, or patients' refusal

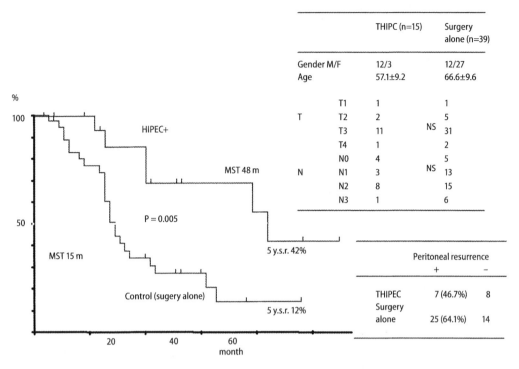

Fig. 2.10 Survival of patients with potentially curable gastric cancer and peritoneal free cancer cells, who were treated with HIPEC and without HIPEC. (Kiyosaki et al. [48])

References

1. Yonemura Y (1998) Gene families associated with formation of peritoneal dissemination. In: Yonemura Y, Shoten M (eds) Peritoneal dissemination. Kanazawa, pp 47–95
2. Vleminckx K, Vakaet I. Jr, Mareel M et al. (1991) Genetic manipulation of E-cadherin expression by epithelial tumor cells reveals an invasion suppressor role. Cell 66:107–119
3. Takeichi M (1990) Cadherins: a molecular family important in selective cell-cell adhesion. Annu Rev Biochem 59:237–252
4. Yonemura Y, Nojima M, Kaji M et al. (1995) E-cadherin and urokinase-type plasminogen activator tissue status in gastric carcinoma. Cancer 76:941–953
5. Davies BR, Davied MP, Gibbs FE et al. (1993) Induction of the metastatic phenotype by transfection of a benign rat mammary epithelial cell line with the gene for p9Ka, a rat calcium-binding protein, but not with the oncogene EJ-ras-1. Oncogene 8:999–1008
6. Yonemura Y, Endou Y, Kimura K et al. (2000) Inverse expression of S100A4 and E-cadherin is associated with metastatic potential in gastric cancer. Clin Cancer Res 6:4234–4242
7. Jacquet P, Sugarbaker PH (1996) Peritoneal-plasma barrier. In Sugarbaker PH (ed) Peritoneal carcinomatosis: principles of management. Kluwer Academic Publisher, Boston, pp 53–63
8. Weiss L (1990) Metastatic inefficiency. Adv Cancer Res 54:159–211
9. Yonemura YC et al. (1997) A possible role of cytokines in the formation of peritoneal dissemination. Int J Oncol 111:349–358D
10. Yonemura Y (1998) Mechanisms of the formation of peritoneal dissemination. In: Yonemura Y, Shoten M (eds) Peritoneal dissemination. Kanazawa, pp 1–46
11. Kawamura T, Endo Y, Yonemura Y et al. (2001) Significance of integrin alpha2/beta1 in peritoneal dissemination of a human gastric cancer xenograft model. Int J Oncol 18:809–815
12. Nishimura S, Chung YS, Yashiro M et al. (1996) Role of alpha 2 beta 1- and alpha 3 beta 1-integrin in the peritoneal implantation of scirrhous gastric carcinoma. Br J Cancer 74:1406–1412
13. Yonemura Y et al. (1996) Roles of VLA-2 and VLA-3 on the formation of peritoneal dissemination in gastric cancer. Int J Oncol 8:925–931
14. Takaishi K, Sasaki T, Kato M et al. (1994) Involvement of Rho p21 small GTP-binding protein and its regulator in the HGF-induced cell motility. Oncogene 9:273–279
15. Kaji M, Yonemura Y, Harada S et al. (1996) Participa-

tion of c-met in the progression of human gastric cancers: anti-c-met oligonucleotides inhibit proliferation or invasiveness of gastric cancer cells. Cancer Gene Ther 3:393–404
16. Taniguchi K, Yonemura Y, Nojima N et al. (1998) The relation between the growth patterns of gastric carcinoma and the expression of hepatocyte growth factor receptor (c-met), autocrine motility factor receptor, and urokinase-type plasminogen activator receptor. Cancer 82:2112–2122
17. Yonemura Y, Eno Y, Tabata K et al. (2005) Role of VEGF-C and VEGF-D on lymphangiogenesis in gastric cancer. Int J Clin Oncol 10:318–327
18. Shimotsuma M, Simpson-Morgan MW, Takahashi T et al. (1992) Activation of omental milky spots and milky spot macrophages by intraperitoneal administration of a streptococcal preparation, OK-432. Cancer Res 52:5400–5402
19. Esperanca MJ, Collins D (1966) Peritoneal dialysis efficiency in relation to body weight. J Ped Surg 1:162–169
20. Inoue H, Matsuyama A, Mimori K et al. (2002) Prognostic score of gastric cancer determined by cDNA microarray. Clin Cancer Res 8:3475–3479
21. Oue N, Hamai Y, Mitani Y et al. (2004) Gene expression profile of gastric carcinoma: identification of genes and tags potentially involved in invasion, metastasis, and carcinogenesis by serial analysis of gene expression. Cancer Res 64:2397–2405
22. Miyagawa K, Sakakura C, Nakashima S et al. (2005) Overexpression of Reg IV in peritoneal dissemination of gastric cancer. Gan to Kagaku Ryoho 32:1707–1708
23. Nishimori H, Yasoshima T, Denno R et al. (2000) A novel experimental model of peritoneal dissemination of human gastric cancer: different mechanisms in peritoneal dissemination and hematogenous metastasis. Jpn J Cancer Res 91:715–722
24. Yonemura Y, Endo Y, Fujita H et al. (2001) Inhibition of peritoneal dissemination in human gastric cancer by MMP-7-specific antisense oligonucleotide. J Exp Clin Cancer Res 20:205–212
25. Unno M, Nata K, Noguchi N et al. (2002) Production and characterization of Reg knockout mice. Reduced proliferation of pancreatic beta-cells in Reg knockout mouse. Diabetes 51:S478–S483
26a. Yonemura Y, Sakurai S, Yamamoto H et al. (2003) REG gene expression is associated with the infiltrating growth of gastric carcinoma. Cancer 98:1394–1400
26b. Macadam RC, Sarela AI, Farmery SM et al. (2000) Death from early colorectal cancer is predicted by the presence of transcripts of the REG gene family. Br J Cancer 83:188–195
27. Yanagihara K, Takigahira M, Tanaka H et al. (2005) Development and biological analysis of peritoneal metastasis mouse models for human scirrhous stomach cancer. Cancer Sci 96:323–332
28. Sakakura, Takemura M, Hagiwara A C et al. (2004) Overexpression of dopa decarboxylase in peritoneal dissemination of gastric cancer and its potential as a novel marker for the detection of peritoneal micrometastases with real-time RT-PCR. Br J Cancer 90:665–671
29. Bando E, Yonemura Y, Takeshita Y et al. (1999) Intraoperative lavage for cytological examination in 1,297 patients with gastric carcinoma. Am J Surg 178:256–262
30. Wu CC, Chen JT, Chang MC et al. (1997) Optimal surgical strategy for potentially curable serosa-involved gastric carcinoma with intraperitoneal free cancer cells. J Am Coll Surg 184:611–617
31. Bando E, Kawamura T, Kinoshita K et al. (2003) Magnitude of serosal changes predicts peritoneal recurrence of gastric cancer. J Am Coll Surg 197:212–222
32. Benevolo M, Mottolese M, Cosimelli M et al. (1998) Diagnostic and prognostic value of peritoneal immunocytology in gastric cancer. J Clin Oncol 16:3406–3411
33. Juhl H, Stritzel M, Wroblewski A et al. (1994) Immunocytological detection of micrometastatic cells: comparative evaluation of findings in the peritoneal cavity and the bone marrow of gastric, colorectal and pancreatic cancer patients. Int J Cancer 57:330–335
34. Asao T, Fukuda T, Yazawa S et al. (1991) Carcinoembryonic antigen levels in peritoneal washings can predict peritoneal recurrence after curative resection of gastric cancer. Cancer 68:44–47
35. Nishiyama M, Takashima I, Tanaka T et al. (1995) Carcinoembryonic antigen levels in the peritoneal cavity: useful guide to peritoneal recurrence and prognosis for gastric cancer. World J Surg 19:133–137
36. Yonemura Y, Endou Y, Fujimura T et al. (2001) Diagnostic value of preoperative RT-PCR-based screening method to detect carcinoembryonic antigen-expressing free cancer cells in the peritoneal cavity from patients with gastric cancer. ANZ J Surg 71:521–528
37. Kodera Y, Nakanishi H, Ito S et al. (2002) Quantitative detection of disseminated free cancer cells in peritoneal washes with real-time reverse transcriptase-polymerase chain reaction: a sensitive predictor of outcome for patients with gastric carcinoma. Ann Surg 235:499–506
38. Yonemura Y, Fujimura T, Ninomiya I et al. (2001) Prediction of peritoneal micrometastasis by peritoneal lavaged cytology and reverse transcriptase-polymerase chain reaction for matrix metalloproteinase-7 mRNA. Clin Cancer Res 7:1647–1653
39. Nakanishi H, Kodera Y, Yamamura Y et al. (2000) Tatematsu M. Rapid quantitative detection of carcinoembryonic antigen-expressing free tumor cells in the peritoneal cavity of gastric-cancer patients with real-time RT-PCR on the lightcycler. Int J Cancer 89:411–417
40. Cullinan SA, Moertel CG, Fleming TR et al. (1985) A comparison of three chemotherapeutic regimens in the treatment of advanced pancreatic and gastric carcinoma. Fluorouracil vs. fluorouracil and doxoru-

bicin vs. fluorouracil, doxorubicin, and mitomycin. JAMA 12.253:2061–2067
41. MacDonald JS, Schein PS, Woolley PV et al. (1980) 5-Fluorouracil, doxorubicin and mitomycin (FAM) combination chemotherapy for advanced gastric cancer. Ann Intern Med 93:533–536
42 Wils JA, Klein HO, Wagener DJ et al. (1991) Sequential high-dose methotrexate and fluorouracil combined with doxorubicin – a step ahead in the treatment of advanced gastric cancer: a trial of the European Organization for Research and Treatment of Cancer Gastrointestinal Tract Cooperative Group. J Clin Oncol 9:827–831
43. Shirasaka T, Nakano K, Takechi T et al. (1996) Antitumor activity of 1 M tegaful,-0.4 M 5-chloro-2,4-dyhydroxypyridine-1 M potassium oxonate (S-1) against human colon carcinoma orthotopically implanted into nude rats. Cancer Res 56:2602–2606
44. Tatsumi K, Fukushima M, Shirasaka T et al. (1987) Inhibitory effect of pyrimidine, barbituric acid and pyrimidine derivatives on 5-fluorouracil degradation in rat liver extracts. Jpn J Cancer Res 78:748–755
45. Van Groeningen CJ, Peters GJ, Schornagel JH et al. (2000) Phase I clinical and pharmacologic study of oral S-1 in patients with advanced gastric solid tumor. J Clin Oncol 18:2772–2779
46. Hirata K, Horikoshi N, Aiba K et al. (1999) Pharmacokinetic study of S-1, a novel oral fluorouracil antitumor drug. Clin Cancer Res 5:2000–2005
47. Yonemura Y et al. (2006) The usefulness of oral TS-1 treatment for potentially curable gastric cancer patients with intraperitoneal free cancer cells. Cancer Treat (in press)
48. Kiyosaki H et al. (2004) Efficacy of prophylactic continuous hyperthermic peritoneal perfusion (CHPP) for the gastric cancer patients with the intraperitoneal cytological positivity for malignancy. 12th International postgraduate course. New frontiers in the diagnosis and management of GI disease. Dec 4, Athens, Abstract, p. 18
49. Yonemura Y, de Aretxabala X, Fujimura T et al. (2001) Intraoperative chemohyperthermic peritoneal perfusion as an adjuvant to gastric cancer: final results of a randomized controlled study. Hepatogastroenterology 48:1776–1782
50. Ribeiro U Jr, Gama-Rodrigues JJ, Bitelman B et al. (1998) Value of peritoneal lavage cytology during laparoscopy staging of patients with gastric carcinoma. Surg Laparoscopy Endoscopy 8:132–135

3 Pathological Evaluation and Implications of Serosal Involvement in Gastrointestinal Cancer

Linmarie Ludeman and Neil A. Shepherd

3.1 Introduction

Involvement of the serosal surface of the gut by gastrointestinal (GI) malignancy correlates with increased risk of locoregional recurrence, transcoelomic spread and a poor prognosis [1–7]. Meticulous pathological assessment of this important parameter has been neglected in the past, because of a surprising failure to recognise the importance of this parameter in the prognosis of GI cancer by pathologists, to a degree engendered by the use of certain traditional staging systems, such as the Dukes classification for colorectal carcinoma, which do not include assessment of the serosa. The latter can be partly explained by the fact that the Dukes classification, at least, was introduced for rectal cancer and there was then little understanding of the importance of serosal involvement in rectal cancer. Only much more recently has this factor even been looked at in rectal cancer. The same comments can be applied to oesophageal cancer: it is only recently that the potential prognostic importance of pleural and peritoneal involvement has been recognised.

There has been a longer, and clearer, understanding of the importance of transcoelomic peritoneal spread in gastric cancer. In the small intestine, adenocarcinoma is a rare tumour and we have very little information on any important prognostic parameters, including serosal involvement. Appendiceal mucinous tumours show a particular propensity to such spread and the understanding and pathological assessment of such tumours have undergone radical changes in recent years. The assessment of serosal involvement by GI cancers now forms an important part of the routine examination of all gastrointestinal tumour resection specimens.

3.2 Anatomy and Microanatomy

The serosa lines the outer aspect of much of the GI tract. In the oesophagus, the parietal pleura makes up a considerable part of the lateral surfaces of a radical oesophagectomy specimen. Furthermore, lower oesophageal cancer shows a particular propensity to spread in the peritoneal cavity and this partially accounts for the importance of staging laparoscopy in the management of this disease. The peritoneum lines much of the circumference of the anterior and posterior stomach. Both small intestine and appendix are lined by serosa for the great majority of their circumference. In the large intestine, the caecum and ascending colon have a retroperitoneal posterior 'surgical margin', as do the descending colon and sigmoid colon, but most of the circumference of the colon is wholly lined by serosa. The rectum has a portion of its anterior surface, superiorly, lined by serosa.

In general it has been considered that the serosal surface provides a local barrier to tumour penetration and this is certainly true in areas where the serosal surface is flat. The serosa itself consists of a layer of mesothelial cells and their associated collagenous basement membrane, underneath which there is loose connective tissue that contains blood vessels, lymphatics and nerves – the subserosa. Whilst involvement of the subserosa by tumour is a common occurrence, this does not have the same potential for transcoelomic spread as true serosal involvement, where there is ulceration of the mesothelial layer by tumour, with tumour cells gaining access to the peritoneal space (vide infra).

3.3 Definition and Pathological Evaluation of Serosal Involvement

The attempt to define 'true' serosal involvement remains problematic, with classification systems each defining local serosal/peritoneal involvement (LPI) in a slightly different way [7–10]. In addition, there are conflicting studies regarding the effect on prognosis of different types of LPI. In the Gloucester, UK, series [6, 7, 11] LPI has been divided into four groups, with group one (LPI 1) indicating tumour well clear of the closest peritoneal surface; group two (LPI 2), where there is a mesothelial reaction with tumour close to but not actually at the surface; group 3 (LPI 3) where there are tumour cells present at the surface with mesothelial reaction and/or ulceration; and group 4 (LPI 4) where there are free tumour cells in the peritoneum with evidence of mesothelial reaction and/or ulceration (Fig. 3.1).

In the Gloucester studies, only groups three and four are regarded as positive for peritoneal involvement, as only these two groups have an adverse effect on prognosis [7]. However, according to others [8–10], serosal involvement by carcinoma includes three types of local peritoneal involvement, all of which are said to be associated with a shorter survival. These three types correspond to LPI types 2–4 in the Gloucester cancer work [6, 7, 11]. Some studies have suggested that only LPI type 4, that is, free tumour cells in the peritoneum, has an adverse effect on prognosis [12, 13]. The situation is complicated by the fact that we have been able to demonstrate that a similar adverse prognosis is applied to cases where tumour is continuous with the serosal surface through an area of suppuration/inflammation, as can be especially seen in cancers of the sigmoid colon also afflicted by diverticular disease and diverticulitis [7].

The pathologist is therefore faced with some conflicting evidence when it comes to defin-

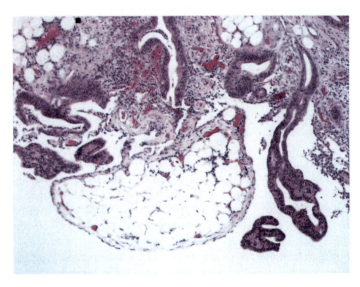

Fig. 3.1 The histological classification of serosal involvement according to the Gloucester, UK, series. There are tumour cells present at the serosal surface with an appropriate mesothelial reaction (LPI 3) but there are also tumour cell groups apparently free with the peritoneal cavity (LPI 4), in this case of colonic carcinoma with extensive local spread

ing what is meant by true serosal involvement. We believe that there is sufficient evidence in the literature now to justify a designation of serosal involvement, with the prognostic and therapeutic implications of that diagnosis, when either LPI 3 or LPI 4 is demonstrated but we do accept that this remains a challenging area for the diagnostic pathologist and a controversial area for those tasked with assessing the therapeutic implications in individual patients.

Although definitions provide some consternation, the microscopic assessment of peritoneal surface involvement is often straightforward, even when there is no obvious ulceration of the serosa, provided the pathologist applies necessary care and attention at the time of macroscopic assessment and dissection. Before any dissection is attempted, the serosal surface overlying the tumour should be carefully inspected to identify areas of possible involvement/LPI. Standard morphological studies have shown that the 'barrier' provided by the serosa and subserosal tissues is more easily penetrated by tumour in the crevices where the mesothelial lining is reflected from the bowel wall onto the mesenteric fat at an acute angle and where there is, therefore, a change in direction of the peritoneum/pleura (Fig. 3.2) [14]. The reason for this phenomenon remains uncertain, although there is likely to be some difference in the microanatomical structure in these areas, making the serosal surface more prone to penetration by tumour [14].

Macroscopically, serosal involvement can be subtle and a telltale sign is loss of the 'shiny' appearance of the serosa, possibly associated with telangiectatic blood vessels. More obvious evidence of peritoneal involvement is provided by a fibrinous exudate and a coarse irregular serosa. At the time of the macroscopic assessment, it has been recommended that at least two blocks are taken from the most suspicious areas for microscopic assessment [6]. If peritoneal involvement is not evident, at least four levels should be cut through those blocks before peritoneal involvement can be ruled out [14].

The presence of free tumour cells in the peritoneal cavity is usually associated with serosal involvement but may be present even without demonstrable involvement of the serosa. Microscopically, isolated clusters of tumour cells can often be seen, apparently floating free within the peritoneal space (Fig. 3.1) [6]. One must resist the notion that these cells represent 'carryover' and an artefact, as it has been demonstrated that peritoneal involvement in such a fashion has a more sinister implication than straightforward 'ulceration' of the peritoneal surface and is regarded as type 4 LPI in the Gloucester, UK work [6, 11].

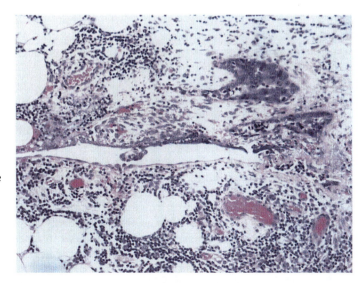

Fig. 3.2 The histology of an advanced adenocarcinoma of the oesophagus. Tumour cell groupings reach the peritoneal surface, typically within a crevice, as seen here, where the mesothelial lining is reflected from the gastro-oesophageal adventitia onto adjacent connective tissue. In oesophageal and colorectal cancer, these crevices are the preferential area of serosal involvement

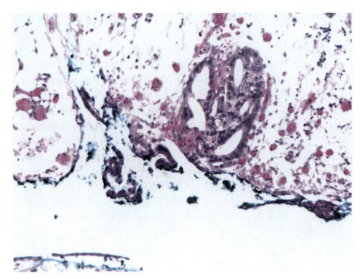

Fig. 3.3 The histology of an intestinal-type gastric adenocarcinoma in which the serosal surface has been painted with green ink. We think such painting has the potential, at least, to falsely identify serosal involvement. Note the separate tumour fragments, within the lumen, coated with paint. These could have been artefactually misplaced into the lumen by the act of painting

At the time of macroscopic and microscopic assessment, it is critical that the pathologist is able to accurately differentiate margin involvement from peritoneal involvement. This is especially the case in oesophageal, colonic and rectal cancer: margin involvement may well be used as a surrogate marker for the quality of surgery. This is one of the prime reasons behind our recommendation that the serosal surface should never be painted at the time of macroscopic assessment (Fig. 3.3) [14]. It does seem that, in the UK at least, pathologists are fast becoming masters of the canvas, with every specimen being liberally covered with paints of many differing colours (often to the detriment of the accurate identification of key pathological features). We think that such a practice should be vociferously discouraged. Only the true surgical margin (whether in the oesophagus, stomach, colon or rectum) should be painted and all serosal surfaces should be left uncoloured. We also have a fear that painting such serosal surface has the potential to introduce artefact and to falsely identify serosal involvement as being present (Fig. 3.3) [14].

Although histochemical and immunohistochemical techniques can provide some dramatic pictures of serosal involvement (Fig. 3.4), we are not convinced that the use of these techniques can be justified on a routine basis.

We feel it is very important to concentrate on meticulous macroscopic assessment, ensuring adequate representation of any potential serosal involvement in tissue blocks, undertaking levels through those blocks, where appropriate, and relying on routine H&E-stained sections for the accurate demonstration of serosal involvement. Having said this, we also firmly believe that much more research is required to enhance our understanding of the cellular and molecular mechanisms that underpin serosal involvement. Furthermore, we require more research studies and clinical trials to further our understanding of the implications of serosal involvement in cancers affecting all parts of the GI tract.

3.4 Cytological Assessment of Serosal Involvement

Although not currently assessed routinely in cases of GI cancers, the value of intraperitoneal tumour cells (IPTC) as a prognostic marker of disseminated disease has been demonstrated repeatedly [14]. The presence of intrapleural and intraperitoneal tumour cells may be assessed cytologically, a technique commonly used in gynaecological oncology [15] but

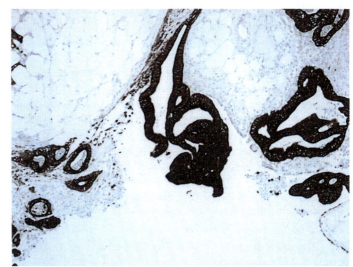

Fig. 3.4 CK20 immunohistochemistry of the colonic adenocarcinoma also seen in Fig. 3.1. Immunohistochemistry provides an impressive demonstration of serosal involvement but cannot be recommended for routine usage

needing wider application in GI oncological assessment. Standard techniques can be used to obtain pleural and peritoneal lavage samples, with routine staining and analysis of the slides [16]. With the use of epithelial marker immunohistochemistry, the positive yield can be increased from 4% to 20%, bearing in mind false positive results in women with epithelial cells from mullerian epithelium [16, 17]. The incidence of positive cytology results range between 4% and 13% pre-resection and 13% and 27% post-resection [18–21]. There is good correlation between histological identification of peritoneal involvement and cytological assessment, suggesting that histology is a valid method of assessing the potential for transcoelomic spread in colorectal carcinoma [11].

3.5 Significance of Serosal Involvement

3.5.1 Oesophagus

Lymph node status and circumferential margin involvement have been consistently shown to be the two independent variables with an important effect on survival after curative surgery for oesophageal carcinoma [14, 22]. However, none of the studies has examined the contribution of serosal (pleural) or peritoneal involvement to prognosis. This is possibly because the local anatomy of the oesophagus, with its relation to other structures in the mediastinum, has been neglected by surgical pathologists. Although most of the oesophagus is covered by adventitia (subserosa), it has to be remembered that the lateral portions of the oesophagus, on either side, are in close approximation to the parietal pleura and therefore there is the potential for pleural involvement in oesophageal carcinoma. A radical oesophageal resection will always include the parietal pleura on either side, immediately beyond the adventitial tissues of the oesophagus. Furthermore, the intra-abdominal portion of the oesophagus is covered by serosa and so can be assessed for serosal/peritoneal involvement (Fig. 3.2).

It is only recently that the potential importance of pleural and peritoneal involvement in oesophageal carcinomas has been recognised. Indeed, the significance of pleural involvement, in terms of locoregional recurrence and prognostic implication, has not, to date, been assessed in any large series [22]. Involvement of the pleura will reflect on local tumour extent (pT4) and will not necessarily imply involvement of the surgical resection margin [14].

The survival benefit gained by radical surgery in the oesophagus is thought to be largely due to a cleared circumferential resection margin [22] and good lymphatic and nodal clearance [23]. However, it has been suggested that positive pleural lavage cytology may be a predictor of local recurrence [24, 25] and, in some centres, pleural involvement is now one of the parameters assessed during pre-operative staging [26, 27]. Also, in oesophageal cancer, especially adenocarcinoma, the high mortality of peritoneal carcinomatosis is likely to be the result of serosal involvement of the intra-abdominal portion of the oesophagus [28]. This underpins the importance of the staging laparoscopy, and thoracoscopy, in the management of oesophageal carcinoma (especially adenocarcinoma) [27]. Of course, laparoscopy will also help to identify spread to other sites, most importantly the liver and perigastric lymph nodes. Whilst we would not deny that involvement of the circumferential surgical margin would seem more important, in terms of prognosis, than serosal involvement in oesophageal carcinoma management, we also believe that much more research is required to assess the implication of pleural and peritoneal involvement in oesophageal carcinoma [14].

3.5.2 Stomach

Unlike other parts of the GI tract, the significance and importance of serosal involvement by gastric carcinoma has been appreciated for years [14]. For instance, in one study, it was shown that serosal involvement and the presence of residual tumour were the only two variables that independently predicted survival [3]. Interestingly enough, nodal involvement was found to lose its significance, once it was corrected for tumour depth and residual tumour [3]. In another study of gastric carcinomas of the middle third of the stomach, serosal involvement and lymphatic invasion were the only two independent prognostic factors to predict survival [5]. Peritoneal seeding was shown to occur in as many as 28% of patients [29] because of the shedding of cancer cells into the peritoneal cavity even in patients with no demonstrable metastatic disease [30].

There is a place, therefore, for intra-operative peritoneal lavage to identify IPTC [31, 32] as positive cytology will result in a poorer prognosis of at least one stage or more. The risk of positive cytology is directly related to the stage of the primary tumour: the percentage of positive cytology is in the order of 10–20% in patients with pT3 and pT4 tumours and increases proportionally to the increase of the area of serosal involvement by the primary tumour [33]. IPTC are commonly present when invasion of the gastric serosa is greater than 3 cm^2 or when adjacent organs or structures are involved [34]. With stage 1 and 2 tumours, in the absence of proven metastatic disease, the risk of finding tumour cells in washings is negligible [30, 35].

A comment is appropriate on the nature and likely site of serosal involvement in gastric cancer. Unsurprisingly, serosal involvement is more likely with diffuse tumours than with intestinal type, not least because the former are more likely to be associated with advanced stage [14]. Unlike with GI cancers at other sites, the stomach is the one organ where involvement of the peritoneum on a flat surface is more likely to be seen (Fig. 3.5). We believe that this is unlikely to reflect any differences in the micro-anatomy of the serosa of the stomach, compared to, say, the oesophagus and the colorectum, and it is more likely to be a manifestation of the biology of the tumour cells, with individual tumour cells, in the diffuse variety of gastric cancer, seemingly having more capability of transgressing the serosal surface and causing transcoelomic disease, and the fact that the stomach is liberally invested with a flat serosal surface. One could also argue that the commonplace advanced nature of gastric cancer at the time of resection, and the proximity of the serosal surface, may also be part of the explanation as to why serosal involvement is more likely to be seen on flat serosal surfaces in gastric cancer. Once again, the mechanisms underpinning this serosal involvement are very poorly understood and require much more basic research.

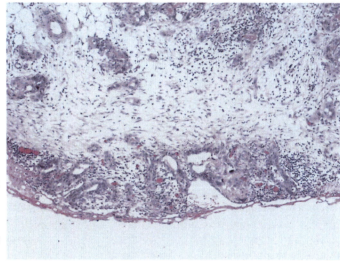

Fig. 3.5 Histological demonstration of involvement of a flat serosal surface in gastric cancer. Unlike GI cancers at other sites, the stomach is the one organ where involvement of the peritoneum on a flat surface is more likely to be seen

3.5.3 Small Intestine

Carcinomas of the small intestine are rare. Therefore, there is little published data evaluating prognostic factors including serosal involvement. As in the large intestine, serosal involvement is staged as pT4, but, unlike the colorectum, the predictive significance of serosal involvement has not been evaluated in any large series. Our own experience, in small intestinal adenocarcinomas and in small intestinal carcinoid tumours, is that serosal involvement is relatively commonly seen, almost certainly itself a manifestation of late presentation and advanced disease. It also stands to reason that serosal involvement by small intestinal adenocarcinomas and carcinoid tumours is an adverse prognostic factor, thereby justifying its accurate identification [14].

3.5.4 Appendix

The commonest tumours of the appendix are the carcinoid tumours and these rarely show serosal involvement, apart from the type known as goblet cell carcinoid or adenocarcinoid. The fact that this tumour does show more propensity to serosal involvement and transcoelomic disease may be an indication of its closer pathogenetic relationship to mucinous glandular tumours, which show a distinct preference for local peritoneal involvement and transperitoneal spread. This having been said, the subject of mucinous appendiceal tumours continues to cause consternation and difficulty for diagnostic pathologists and for those surgeons and oncologists charged with the further management of this disease.

Much of the confusion is due to inconsistent terminology and the lack of large series in which predictive factors are accurately identified [14]. Precise identification and classification of mucinous tumours of the appendix are important, as there is considerable variation in the potential to cause mucinous intraperitoneal disease. Whilst there is, therefore, an increasing burden on the pathologist to identify and classify these tumours appropriately, a significant confounding factor is the fact that there is a spectrum of mucinous tumours rather than rigid categories.

The term pseudomyxoma peritonei (PP) is a description of a clinico-pathological entity [36] in which there is mucinous ascites and mucinous implants in the peritoneum that may, or may not, contain epithelial cells [37]. The spectrum of disease ranges from mucinous ascites (free acellular mucin in the peritoneal cavity), through organising mucinous fluid (mucin containing fibroblasts, capillaries, inflammatory cells and mesothelial cells) and disseminated peritoneal adenomucinosis (mucin with scanty simple to focally proliferative mucinous epithelium with little cytological atypia or mitoses) through to peritoneal mucinous carcinomatosis (pools of mucin within which there are abundant malignant epithelial cells with either cytological or architectural features of malignancy). It is clear from the above that there will be considerable interobserver variation. What constitutes 'little cytological atypia' to one observer may be considered as significant atypia by another. Furthermore, a diagnosis of PP is not meaningful on its own and the term has to be further qualified to be of any useful significance [36].

There are conflicting theories of the pathogenesis of PP and studies have shown contradictory results [37–39]. We believe that PP is caused by rupture of a mucinous appendiceal tumour, with spillage of mucin and/or cells into the peritoneum [36, 37, 40]. There is little support for the theory of neoplastic change in mesothelial cells that have undergone mucinous metaplasia [38, 41, 42]. Even in the presence of a synchronous mucinous ovarian tumour, the most likely origin of the mucin and cells is an appendiceal tumour. Once spillage has occurred, there is accumulation and proliferation of cells within the peritoneal cavity, in areas where implantation is facilitated, such as where there is resorption of fluid or in gravity dependent areas [43]?

There is a spectrum of mucinous appendiceal tumours that have been implicated in the cause of PP. These range from mucosal hyperplasia (with pathology similar to that of hyperplastic/metaplastic polyp of the colon), benign mucinous cystadenoma, where there is modest cytonuclear atypia and proliferation, to frank adenocarcinoma with invasion of the wall of the appendix. As with the term PP, the term 'mucocoele' describes an appendix that has been distended with mucin and does not reveal the cause for the distension. All mucinous lesions of the appendix should therefore be fully described to be prognostically meaningful [44].

Although mucinous tumours of the appendix bear some morphological resemblance to mucinous ovarian tumours of borderline malignant potential, these lesions cannot be considered in a similar manner, as appendiceal lesions will carry a much less favourable prognosis [45]. The following classification of mucinous appendiceal tumours has been suggested to accommodate morphological and prognostic implications [45]:
- Low-grade appendiceal mucinous neoplasm (LAMN) (Fig. 3.6)
- Mucinous adenocarcinoma (MACA) (Fig. 3.7)

The LAMN category includes all lesions with low-grade cytological atypia, minimal architectural complexity and no destructive invasion. Lesions classified as MACA show destructive invasion of the wall of the appendix and/or high-grade cytoarchitectural atypia [45].

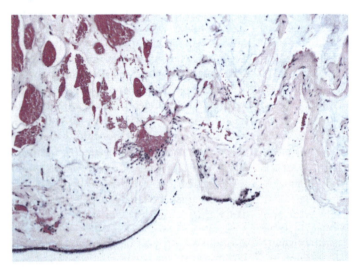

Fig. 3.6 Histology of a typical low-grade appendiceal mucinous neoplasm (LAMN). Above is much mucin within the subserosal tissues of the appendix whilst low-grade glandular neoplasia, with low-grade cytological atypia, minimal architectural complexity and no destructive invasion, has come to line the peritoneal surface below

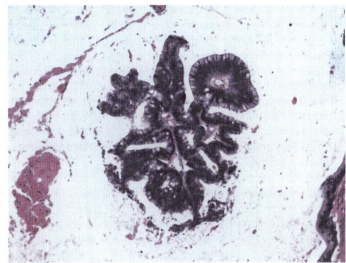

Fig. 3.7 Histology of mucinous adenocarcinoma (MACA) of the appendix. Floating within mucin, in a large mucinous mass in the omentum, metastatic from a primary appendiceal tumour, is this complex glandular lesion with high-grade cytoarchitectural atypia

Not only will the prognosis of PP depend on the nature of the appendiceal lesion, it will also depend on the extent of peritoneal disease: patients with peritoneal mucinous carcinoma (numerous malignant cells in the mucin) will have a worse prognosis and a higher risk of recurrence than patients with peritoneal adenomucinosis [40, 46]. Thorough sampling and examination of the mucin are therefore essential to identify malignant cells within the mucin [14].

Accepting that PP is usually caused by an appendiceal lesion, even in the presence of ovarian pathology, one must ensure exemplary examination of the appendix, even if macroscopically 'normal' [14]. Thus, in any patient with mucinous ascites, the appendix should be removed at the time of surgery, even in the presence of an ovarian tumour [39]. This should then be examined histologically in its entirety, as mucinous lesions may be microscopic or focal and areas of rupture may have sealed off and healed. As discussed above, the nature of the appendiceal lesion will directly influence prognosis.

3.5.5 Colon

We have already indicated that serosal involvement in colonic cancer has been surprisingly neglected until more recently, although we acknowledge that it has been included in a substage of the TNM system for many years and was introduced into one of the modifications of the Dukes system, the Australian Clinicopathological Staging System (ACPS), as early as the 1970s [47–49]. Peritoneal involvement by colonic adenocarcinoma (Figs. 3.1 and 3.4) has been shown to be the parameter of supreme prognostic importance in all-comers with the disease [6] and, especially, in Dukes B colonic cancer [7]. In one of our colonic cancer studies, we showed it to have the strongest independent prognostic significance, even more powerful than the extent of local spread or lymph node involvement [6]. In the ACPS studies of colonic cancer, it has been shown to be the second most important prognostic feature after the number of involved lymph nodes [2, 47–49].

In the staging and predictive assessment of colorectal cancer, there has been a long-term reliance on staging systems based on the Dukes classification, including the ACPS system, which are essentially progressive systems such that the influence of parameters, such as serosal involvement, is lost if there is tumour spread to local lymph nodes (which immediately places the tumour in the C category) [2, 49, 50]. The advantages of systems such as the TNM are apparent here as they include separate assessments for local tumour spread (including local peritoneal involvement as stage pT4a) and for lymph node spread and metastatic disease [2, 11, 49, 50]. Even in the TNM system, only more recently has serosal involvement been separated from involvement of adjacent local organs (now classified as pT4b) and therefore studies using this classification have the potential to obscure the significance of serosal involvement in the presence of involvement of adjacent organs [50].

In a study of nearly 700 patients with colonic cancer, one-third of all patients who died as a result of carcinomatosis first presented with histologically or cytologically confirmed intraperitoneal disease [6]. This serves to confirm the relative importance of intraperitoneal spread in the history of advanced colonic cancer [1, 6]. In primary resections of colonic carcinoma, up to 55% of specimens will show serosal involvement [6, 51] and IPTC have been found in up to 43% of patients with colorectal carcinoma at the time of resection [16]. In a study of the characteristics of colorectal tumours most likely to exfoliate cells into the peritoneal space, macroscopic breach of the peritoneal surface and invasion of the serosal surface were two of the seven factors predicting such exfoliation [52]. A mucinous adenocarcinoma phenotype is also a significant factor leading to serosal involvement [6]. Serosal surface involvement, extent of local spread and lymph node involvement are consistently found to be strong independent prognostic factors [2, 6, 48].

Not only is there controversy as to how to identify and classify serosal involvement in colonic cancer, there is also continuing debate concerning how common the phenomenon is and this will, of course, itself influence the prescient value of the parameter in the different major series. In our Gloucester, UK, series, only a very small proportion of cases (around 5%) represent Dukes stage A with cancer confined within the bowel wall and not fully penetrating the muscularis propia [6, 14]. On the other hand, LPI appears unusually common in the same series, with a rate of up to 57% [6, 7]. We have always maintained that this rate may well be reflective of the true incidence of serosal involvement in colonic cancer in unselected series. We have advanced two main influences here: Firstly, the Gloucester series was a prospective one, set up in 1988 especially to identify this parameter, amongst others, and undertaking meticulous pathological technique so to do. We would argue that some other series may have relied on the fortuitous demonstration of serosal involvement in blocks and sections rather than having specifically and prospectively introduced methodology to identify this parameter.

We have also argued [6, 14] that, on the anti-mesenteric aspect of the colon, that the serosal surface is very close to the outer muscular layer, with often <5 mm between them. Thus, as about 95% of all colonic cancers have fully penetrated the latter, it is not surprising, to us at least, that about half of them, perhaps especially those tumours which are either circumferential or show a large anti-mesenteric component, have spread just that short distance further and have infiltrated and ulcerated the serosa.

The presence of serosal involvement in colonic cancer is a useful indicator of highly significant local disease carrying a significant risk of intraperitoneal dissemination, itself an important factor in the progression of advanced colonic cancer. This having been said, the presence of peritoneal involvement, demonstrated histopathologically, does not necessarily lead to disseminated intraperitoneal dissemination [6, 7]. For instance, in the group of Dukes B colonic cancer patients with LPI as their only adverse prognostic feature, there is still a 75% 5-year survival, equivalent to all-comers with Dukes B colon cancer [7]. Hence, the presence of serosal involvement can only be regarded as a reasonable indicator of potential subsequent intra-peritoneal recurrence, but it cannot be regarded as being implicit of inevitable subsequent (particularly clinically significant) intraperitoneal disease [6].

3.5.6 Rectum

The lower rectum is entirely extraperitoneal but a considerable portion of the upper rectum, especially in women, is invested anteriorly by peritoneum [11]. In previous studies, we have estimated that up to 25% of the total circumference of the rectum, in women, is covered by serosa, whilst this figure falls to about 16% in men [11]. The difference between men and women relates to the position of the peritoneal reflection. In the pouch of Douglas in a woman, the reflection is that much lower.

Especially with the recognition of the importance of local spread to circumferential/mesorectal surgical margins in rectal cancer and, subsequently, especially in the UK and Western Europe, the implementation of initiatives to ensure all surgeons undertake a total mesorectal excision to reduce margin involvement and local recurrence rates [53–55], we believe that involvement of the peritoneum, particularly for upper rectal cancer (Fig. 3.8), may become more important, especially in predicting locoregional recurrence and overall prognosis [11, 14]. In support of this, there are recent data from our own series which identifies LPI as an important factor for locoregional recurrence in upper rectal cancer and as an overall prognostic factor [56]. These data indicate that LPI is the single most predictive factor in locoregional recurrence in about half of all cases, particularly, of course, in cases where total mesorectal excision has been undertaken, thereby reducing the likelihood that direct spread to a surgical margin is an important factor [56]. In this regard, ACPS data are also supportive of this, with a very recent study showing LPI to be predictive of locoregional occurrence and an independent influence on overall survival [57].

3.6 Summary and Conclusions

A large proportion of the luminal GI tract is covered by serosa and we increasingly recognise the importance of involvement of the serosal surface and its influence on locoregional recurrence and survival in most of the main cancers that occur in the GI tract. Thus there is an ever-burgeoning responsibility upon diagnostic histopathologists to introduce appropriate methodology to accurately identify this parameter in GI cancer resection specimens. It is perhaps because of the former reliance

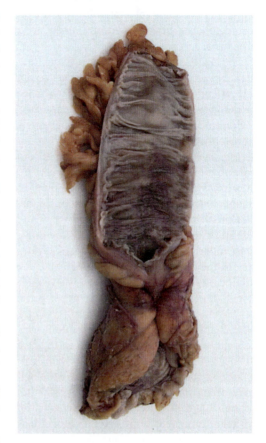

Fig. 3.8 Macroscopic demonstration of upper rectal involvement of the peritoneum. The specimen has been opened to allow fixation above and below the tumour, which has been left unopened to allow correlation of the macroscopic features, at pathological assessment, with the results of pre-operative imaging by MRI. The peritoneal reflection is still clearly defined below. Above this, on the anterior surface of the rectum is an area where there is serosal irregularity and hyperaemia, typical macroscopic features to suggest serosal involvement, which should be confirmed by histological assessment

on rigid sequential staging systems, such as the Dukes classification, that some factors, perhaps most notably involvement of surgical margins, especially in rectal cancer, and serosal involvement, particularly in oesophageal, colonic and rectal cancer, have been relatively neglected. This is surprising because we now know that both of these pathologically derived parameters strongly correlate with subsequent locoregional recurrence and, ultimately, with prognosis.

The significance of serosal involvement has been better recognised in gastric cancer but little attention has been paid to the occurrence in oesophageal cancer. Yet both pleural and peritoneal involvement may be comparatively commonly identified in oesophageal cancer. Serosal involvement and transperitoneal spread are also of considerable prognostic importance in primary appendiceal mucinous tumours. In colonic cancer, serosal involvement is an important predictor of locoregional recurrence and overall survival: in some studies it is the single most important independent prognostic parameter. In the rectum, only more recently has the significance of serosal involvement been appreciated, particularly, of course, for upper rectal cancer. As oncological and surgical concepts have changed in the management of GI cancers and new operations have been introduced to ensure that surgical margin involvement is much less common, we believe that pathologically-determined serosal involvement, whether by meticulous histopathological assessment of resection specimens or by cytological methodology, will become relatively more important as a marker of potential locoregional recurrence and overall survival and as a determinant for alternative novel therapeutic strategies, including intraperitoneal chemotherapy and radical peritoneal surgery.

References

1. Olson RM, Perencevich NP, Malcolm AW, Chaffey JT, Wilson RE (1980) Patterns of recurrence following curative resection of adenocarcinoma of the colon and rectum. Cancer 45:2969–2974
2. Newland RC, Dent OF, Lyttle MN, Chapuis PH, Bokey EL (1994) Pathologic determinants of survival associated with colorectal cancer with lymph node metastases. A multivariate analysis of 579 patients. Cancer 73:2076–2082
3. Jakl RJ, Miholic J, Koller R, Markis E, Wolner E (1995) Prognostic factors in adenocarcinoma of the cardia. Am J Surg 169:316–319
4. Shepherd NA (1995) Pathological prognostic factors in colorectal cancer. In: Kirkham N, Lemoine NR (eds) Progress in Pathology, 2nd edn. Churchill Livingstone, Edinburgh, pp 115–141
5. Sheen-Chen SM, Chou CW, Chen MC, Chen FC, Chen YS, Chen JJ (1997) Adenocarcinoma in the middle third of the stomach-an evaluation for the prognostic significance of clinicopathological features. Hepatogastroenterology 44:1488–1494
6. Shepherd NA, Baxter KJ, Love SB (1997) The prognostic importance of peritoneal involvement in colonic cancer: a prospective evaluation. Gastroenterology 112:1096–1102
7. Petersen VC, Baxter KJ, Love SB, Shepherd NA (2002) Identification of objective pathological prognostic determinants and models of prognosis in Dukes' B colon cancer. Gut 51:65–69
8. Compton C, Fenoglio-Preiser CM, Pettigrew N, Fielding LP (2000) American Joint Committee on Cancer Prognostic Factors Consensus Conference. Cancer 88:1739–1757
9. Compton CC, for members of the Cancer Committee, College of American Pathologists (2000) Updated protocol for the examination of specimens from patients with carcinomas of the colon and rectum, excluding carcinoid tumors, lymphomas, sarcomas, and tumors of the vermiform appendix. A basis for checklists. Arch Pathol Lab Med 124:1016–1025
10. Compton CC (2003) Colorectal carcinoma: diagnostic, prognostic, and molecular features. Mod Pathol 16:376–388
11. Shepherd NA, Baxter KJ, Love SB (1995) Influence of local peritoneal involvement on pelvic recurrence and prognosis in rectal cancer. J Clin Pathol 48:849–855
12. Douard R, Cugnenc P-H, Wind P, Benichou J (2004) Peritoneal involvement and free tumor cells in peritoneal cavity of patients with colon cancer. Am J Clin Pathol 121:154–155
13. Knudsen PJ (1991) The peritoneal elastic lamina. J Anat 177:41–46
14. Ludeman L, Shepherd NA (2005) Serosal involvement in gastrointestinal cancer: its assessment and significance. Histopathology 47:123–131
15. Moore GE, Sako K, Kondo T, Badillo J, Burke E (1961) Assessment of the exfoliation of tumour cells into the body cavities. Surg Gynecol Obstet 112:469–474
16. Leather AJ, Kocjan G, Savage F, Hu W, Yiu CY, Boulos PB, Northover JM, Phillips RK (1994) Detection of free malignant cells in the peritoneal cavity before and after resection of colorectal cancer. Dis Colon Rectum 37:814–819
17. Nekarda H, Schenck U, Ludwig C et al. (1995) Prognostic impact of diagnostic lavage in completely resected gastric cancer [abstract]. Gastric Congress Abstract Proceedings 99
18. Quan SH (1959) Cul-de-sac smears for cancer cells. Surgery 45:258–263
19. Skipper D, Cooper AJ, Marston JE, Taylor I (1987) Exfoliated cells and in vitro growth in colorectal cancer. Br J Surg 74:1049–1052

20. Ambrose NS, MacDonald F, Young J, Thompson H, Keighley MR (1989) Monoclonal antibody and cytological detection of free malignant cells in the peritoneal cavity during resection of colorectal cancer–can monoclonal antibodies do better? Eur J Surg Oncol 15:99–102
21. Yamamoto S, Akasu T, Fujita S, Moriya Y (2003). Long-term prognostic value of conventional peritoneal cytology after curative resection for colorectal carcinoma. Jpn J Clin Oncol 33:33–37
22. Dexter SP, Sue-Ling H, McMahon MJ, Quirke P, Mapstone N, Martin IG (2001) Circumferential resection margin involvement: an independent predictor of survival following surgery for oesophageal cancer. Gut 48:667–670
23. Akiyama H, Tsurumaru M, Udagawa H, Kajiyama Y (1994). Radical lymph node dissection for cancer of the thoracic esophagus. Ann Surg 220:364–372
24. Natsugoe S, Shimada M, Nakashima S, Tokuda K, Matsumoto M, Kijima F, Baba M, Shimizu K, Tanaka S, Aikou T (1999) Intraoperative pleural lavage in esophageal carcinoma. Ann Surg Oncol 6:305–307
25. Jiao X, Zhang M, Wen Z, Krasna MJ (2000) Pleural lavage cytology in esophageal cancer without pleural effusions: clinicopathologic analysis. Eur J Cardiothorac Surg 17:575–579
26. Krasna MJ, Jiao X (2000) Thoracoscopic and laparoscopic staging for esophageal cancer. Semin Thorac Cardiovasc Surg 12:186–194
27. Krasna MJ, Jiao X, Mao YS, Sonett J, Gamliel Z, Kwong K, Burrows W, Flowers JL, Greenwald B, White C (2002) Thoracoscopy/laparoscopy in the staging of esophageal cancer: Maryland experience. Surg Laparosc Endosc Percutan Tech 12:213–218
28. Katayama A, Mafune K, Tanaka Y, Takubo K, Makuuchi M, Kaminishi M (2003) Autopsy findings in patients after curative esophagectomy for esophageal carcinoma. J Am Coll Surg 196:866–873
29. Landry J, Tepper JE, Wood WC, Moulton EO, Koerner F, Sullinger J (1990) Patterns of failure following curative resection of gastric carcinoma. Int J Radiat Oncol Biol Phys 19:1357–1362
30. Burke EC, Karpeh MS Jr, Conlon KC, Brennan MF (1998) Peritoneal lavage cytology in gastric cancer: an independent predictor of outcome. Ann Surg Oncol 5:411–415
31. Suzuki T, Ochiai T, Hayashi H, Nakajima K, Yasumoto A, Hishikawa E, Shimada H, Horiuchi F, Ohki S, Isono K (1999) Importance of positive peritoneal lavage cytology findings in the stage grouping of gastric cancer. Surg Today 29:111–115
32. Japanese Research Society for Gastric Cancer: Miwa Registry-Institute for Stomach Cancer (1996) The report of treatment results of stomach carcinoma in Japan. Miwa Registry-Institute for Stomach Cancer, Tokyo, p 62
33. Kaibara N, Iitsuka Y, Kimura A, Kobayashi Y, Hirooka Y, Nishidoi H, Koga S (1987) Relationship between area of serosal invasion and prognosis in patients with gastric carcinoma. Cancer 60:36–39
34. Ribeiro U Jr, Gama-Rodrigues JJ, Bitelman B, Ibrahim RE, Safatle-Ribeiro AV, Laudanna AA, Pinotti HW (1998) Value of peritoneal lavage cytology during laparoscopic staging of patients with gastric carcinoma. Surg Laparosc Endosc 8:132–135
35. Bonenkamp JJ, Songun I, Hermans J, van de Velde CJ (1996) Prognostic value of positive cytology findings from abdominal washings in patients with gastric cancer. Br J Surg 83:672–674
36. Ronnett BM, Zahn CM, Kurman RJ, Kass ME, Sugarbaker PH, Shmookler BM (1995) Disseminated peritoneal adenomucinosis and peritoneal mucinous carcinomatosis. A clinicopathologic analysis of 109 cases with emphasis on distinguishing pathologic features, site of origin, prognosis, and relationship to "pseudomyxoma peritonei". Am J Surg Pathol 19:1390–1408
37. Young RH, Gilks CB, Scully RE (1991). Mucinous tumors of the appendix associated with mucinous tumors of the ovary and pseudomyxoma peritonei. A clinicopathological analysis of 22 cases supporting an origin in the appendix. Am J Surg Pathol 15:415–429
38. Seidman JD, Elsayed AM, Sobin LH, Tavassoli FA (1993) Association of mucinous tumors of the ovary and appendix. A clinicopathologic study of 25 cases. Am J Surg Pathol 17:22–34
39. Prayson RA, Hart WR, Petras RE (1994) Pseudomyxoma peritonei. A clinicopathologic study of 19 cases with emphasis on site of origin and nature of associated ovarian tumors. Am J Surg Pathol 18:591–603
40. Ronnett BM, Kurman RJ, Zahn CM, Shmookler BM, Jablonski KA, Kass ME, Sugarbaker PH (1995) Pseudomyxoma peritonei in women: a clinicopathologic analysis of 30 cases with emphasis on site of origin, prognosis, and relationship to ovarian mucinous tumors of low malignant potential. Hum Pathol 26:509–524
41. Sandenbergh HA, Woodruff JD (1977) Histogenesis of pseudomyxoma peritonei. Review of 9 cases. Obstet Gynecol 49:339–345
42. Kahn MA, Demopoulos RI (1992) Mucinous ovarian tumors with pseudomyxoma peritonei: a clinicopathological study. Int J Gynecol Pathol 11:15–23
43. Sugarbaker PH, Yan H, Shmookler B (2001) Pedunculated peritoneal surface polyps in pseudomyxoma peritonei syndrome. Histopathology 39:525–528
44. Higa E, Rosai J, Pizzimbono CA, Wise L (1973) Mucosal hyperplasia, mucinous cystadenoma and mucinous cystadenomcarcinoma of the appendix. A re-evaluation of appendiceal "mucocele". Cancer 32:1525–1541
45. Misdraji J, Yantiss RK, Graeme-Cook FM, Balis UL, Young RH (2003) Appendiceal mucinous neoplasms: a clinicopathologic analysis of 107 cases. Am J Surg Pathol 27:1089–1103

46. Ronnett BM, Yan H, Kurman RJ, Shmookler BM, Wu L, Sugarbaker PH (2001) Patients with pseudomyxoma peritonei associated with disseminated peritoneal adenomucinosis have a significantly more favorable prognosis than patients with peritoneal mucinous carcinomatosis. Cancer 92:85–91
47. Newland RC, Dent OF, Chapuis PH, Bokey L (1995). Survival after curative resection of lymph node negative colorectal carcinoma. A prospective study of 910 patients. Cancer 76:564–571
48. Chapuis PH, Dent OF, Fisher R, Newland RC, Pheils MT, Smyth E, Colquhoun K (1985) A multivariate analysis of clinical and pathological variables in prognosis after resection of large bowel cancer. Br J Surg 72:698–702
49. Davis NC, Newland RC (1983) Terminology and classification of colorectal adenocarcinoma: the Australian clinico-pathological staging system. Aust NZ J Surg 53:211–221
50. Hermanek P, Henson DE, Hutter RVP, Sobin LH (1993) TNM supplement: a commentary on uniform use. Springer-Verlag, Berlin
51. Shepherd NA, Baxter KJ, Love SB (1993) Local peritoneal involvement in colonic cancer: a neglected prognostic parameter. J Pathol 169:128A
52. Hase K, Ueno H, Kuranaga N, Utsunomiya K, Kanabe S, Mochizuki H (1998) Intraperitoneal exfoliated cancer cells in patients with colorectal cancer. Dis Colon Rectum 41:1134–1140
53. Quirke P, Durdey P, Dixon MF, Williams NS (1986) Local recurrence of rectal adenocarcinoma due to inadequate surgical resection. Histopathological study of lateral tumour spread and surgical excision. Lancet 2:996–999
54. Birbeck KF, Macklin CP, Tiffin NJ, Parsons W, Dixon MF, Mapstone NP, Abbott CR, Scott N, Finan PJ, Johnston D, Quirke P (2002) Rates of circumferential resection margin involvement vary between surgeons and predict outcomes in rectal cancer surgery. Ann Surg 235:449–457
55. Nagtegaal ID, Marijnen CA, Kranenberg EK, van de Velde CJ, van Krieken JH (2002) Circumferential margin involvement is still an important predictor of local recurrence in rectal carcinoma: not one millimetre but two millimetres is the limit. Am J Surg Pathol 26:350–357
56. Mitchard JR, Love SB, Shepherd NA (in preparation) The significance of peritoneal involvement in predicting local recurrence in rectal cancer
57. Keshava A, Chapuis PH, Chan C, Lin BPC, Bokey EL, Dent OF (2007) The significance of involvement of a free serosal surface for recurrence and survival of clinicopathological stage B and C rectal cancer. Colorectal Dis (in press)

4 Principles of Perioperative Intraperitoneal Chemotherapy for Peritoneal Carcinomatosis

Eelco de Bree and Dimitris D. Tsiftsis

Peritoneal carcinomatosis represents an advanced form of intra-abdominal and pelvic malignant tumours that has been generally associated with a grim prognosis. The peritoneal component of cancer is often the major source of morbidity and mortality. Despite advances in its diagnosis, peritoneal surface malignancy has always been a major problem in cancer management. Surgery alone can never be therapeutic. Even if all visible tumour deposits can be removed, most likely microscopic residual disease will be left behind and progression of peritoneal disease will occur. On the other hand, systemic chemotherapy, alone or in combination with surgery, is generally not so effective such that patients will ultimately die of their disease. In most cases, peritoneal metastases are usually relatively resistant to intravenously administered cytotoxic drugs. A clear dose-effect relation exists, but the intravenously administered dose that is significantly effective generally exceeds the dose that causes lethal systemic toxicity. Moreover, drug penetration from plasma into the superficial peritoneal tumour deposits and into the malignant ascites that contains free tumour cells seems to be impaired (Sugarbaker et al. 1996).

4.1 The Rationale for Intraperitoneal Chemotherapy

Although usually considered as systemic disease, peritoneal carcinomatosis can be better understood as regional dissemination. Intra-abdominal malignancies with tumour implants on peritoneal surfaces may remain confined to the peritoneal cavity for a prolonged period of time. This means that even though it is considered certainly a poor prognostic sign, it is not proof of distant metastases, providing a rationale for regional cancer treatment. Patients with additional haematogenous metastases are usually excluded from regional treatment modalities, since systemic disease is insufficiently treated by a regional approach and should be treated in a systemic way.

Intraperitoneal chemotherapy is a regional treatment modality that was used for peritoneal carcinomatosis as early as 1955 (Weisberger et al. 1955). During the last decades it has been subjected to an increasing number of experimental and clinical investigations. The major advantage of intraperitoneal chemotherapy is the regional dose intensity provided, which may overcome the obstacle of relative drug resistance. Assuming the above mentioned dose-effect relation, this will result in a higher efficacy of the cytotoxic drug.

4.2 The Pharmacokinetic Advantage

After intraperitoneal delivery high regional concentrations can be achieved, while systemic drug levels are low. The concentration differential arises because of the relatively slow rate of movement of the drug from the peritoneal cavity into the plasma (peritoneal clearance). This pharmacokinetic process is based on the characteristics of the peritoneal–plasma barrier, which maintains the continuous high ratio of chemotherapeutic drug concentration between peritoneal cavity and plasma (Jacquet and Sugarbaker 1996; Flessner 2005). The physical nature of the peritoneal–plasma barrier has not been fully elucidated. At present, it is suspected that a complex diffusion barrier exists that consists of peritoneal mesothelium, subserosal tissue and blood vessel walls. The capillary wall appears to offer the dominant resistance to the transfer of large molecules. The mesothelium and peritoneal interstitium impede their movement to a lesser extent. The movement of large drug molecules and hydrophilic agents through this barrier is limited, while the high drug extraction by the liver after absorption from the peritoneal cavity and transport to the portal vein system provides decreased systemic drug exposure. The area under the concentration-time curve (AUC) gradient of the drugs from the peritoneal cavity to peripheral blood expresses most adequately the pharmacological advantage of intraperitoneal drug administration. Depending on their molecular weight, their affinity to lipids, and first-pass effect and clearance by the liver, the intraperitoneal-to-plasma drug AUC ratio may exceed a factor of 1,000. An additional advantage is that the blood drainage of the peritoneal surface through the portal vein to the liver provides, besides the already mentioned first-pass effect, an increased exposure of potential hepatic micrometastases to cytotoxic drugs administered intraperitoneally (Speyer et al. 1981). Certain drugs are also transported through lymphatics to the systemic circulation, and consequently higher drug AUCs are achieved in the lymph compared to plasma. This provides a strong rationale for treatment of concurrent occult or clinical lymph node metastases by intraperitoneal chemotherapy (Lindner et al. 1993).

A valid question is whether the removal of involved peritoneum influences the characteristics of the peritoneal-plasma barrier. This subject was extensively studied by the Sugarbaker group. Initially, they reported that extensive removal of peritoneum during cytoreductive surgery does not seem to affect the pharmacokinetics of intraperitoneal chemotherapy (Jacquet and Sugarbaker 1996). In a more recent study (Jacquet et al. 1998b), the pharmacokinetics of mitomycin C during hyperthermic intraperitoneal chemotherapy (HIPEC) were studied after limited parietal peritonectomy and more than two peritonectomy procedures. After more extensive removal of the peritoneum higher peak plasma drug levels, a higher AUC for the drug in plasma and a decreased ratio of AUC for perfusate to AUC for plasma were noted. The differences were small but statistically significant, which suggests a change in impaired function of this virtual barrier by the removal of peritoneal surfaces. However, in their latest study on this issue (de Lima Vazquez et al. 2003), they did not observe a significant difference between plasma and peritoneal fluid mitomycin C concentrations after total parietal peritonectomy in comparison to that after partial (<60%) parietal peritonectomy. The mean AUC ratio was 20.5 in the total peritonectomy group and 25.7 in the less extensive peritonectomy patients. The mean total amount of drug and the peritoneal fluid volume recovered from the peritoneal cavity at the end of HIPEC were both greater in the total parietal peritonectomy patients (p-values of 0.095 and 0.0317, respectively). Although the results of these studies are somehow inconsistent, even if small differences in the clearance of mitomycin C exist as a result of more extensive parietal peritonectomy procedures, it is unlikely that modification of drug dose is necessary. Moreover, removal of visceral organs seems not to alter the property of the peritoneal-plasma barrier. Others studied the impact of complete evisceration, causing removal of at least half of the peritoneal surface, on clearance of glucose, urea and inulin in dogs (Rubin et al. 1988). No differences were noted in comparison to the same parameters measured in normal dogs. Conclusively, these studies suggest that the peritoneum is of little or no importance to the delayed drug clearance. Hence, the barrier could be referred to as the peritoneal fluid–plasma barrier rather than the peritoneum–plasma barrier.

4.3 Drug Tissue Distribution and Tumour Penetration Depth

High intraperitoneal drug concentration and exposure are the two main factors affecting the treatment of free intraperitoneal tumour cells. However, the AUC for peritoneal fluid may not be correlated with the drug amount in tumour deposits. For invasive peritoneal tumour deposits of adenocarcinoma, which grow towards the subperitoneal space, it is more important to achieve satisfactory local tissue penetration and concentration of the drug than high intraperitoneal fluid drug concentrations only (de Bree et al. 2002b). The agent has to penetrate the peritoneal tumour as well at the site of the peritoneal cavity as into the peritoneal layer and subperitoneal tissue. Since the blood capillaries, in which resorption of the drug towards the systemic blood circulation takes place, are located in this subperitoneal area, systemic concentrations may express penetration capacity of the agent. Therefore, high concentration gradients and increased intraperitoneal-to-plasma drug AUC ratios are not automatically associated with higher efficacy, but may even be undesirable and may demonstrate that the drug is unable to reach this subperitoneal target area. The ideal situation is high local tissue concentration with poor diffusion through the capillary wall, resulting in low systemic drug concentration. Some investigators have advocated the synchronous intraperitoneal administration of vasoconstrictors like epinephrine to decrease drug drainage through the peritoneal and tumoural vascular networks (Chauffert et al. 2003). In experimental models, they demonstrated an increased penetration of cisplatin and oxaliplatin into the metastatic peritoneal tumour nodules.

A disadvantage of intracavitary chemotherapy remains the limited tissue penetration by the therapeutic agent. Unfortunately, for many agents it is difficult to accurately measure tissue penetration depth and concentration after intraperitoneal chemotherapy and, when possible, there is a large inter-individual variation. Nevertheless, the penetration depth of drugs that are intraperitoneally delivered is estimated to be 3–5 mm at maximum (Ozols et al. 1979; McVie et al. 1985; Los et al. 1991; Fujimoto et al. 1992; Panteix et al. 1993; van der Vaart et al.1998). This implies the need for extensive cytoreductive surgery to precede intraperitoneal delivery of drugs.

In in vitro studies penetration depth depends on drug concentration, exposure time, cellular adhesion capacity and packing density of tumour cells. Greater penetration has been observed in tumour tissue with round, loosely packed cells than in epithelioid, tightly packed cells (Grantah et al. 2006). Moreover, penetration differs considerably among drugs. The penetration through tumour tissue of the anthracyclines adriamycin and mitoxantrone was much less and slower than that of methotrexate and 5-fluorouracil in an in vitro tumour model (Tunggual et al. 1999). The particularly poor tissue penetration of anthracyclines may be explained by their sequestration in acidic endosomes of cells and their binding to DNA. Among the anthracycline analogues, the best penetration capacity has been observed for adriamycin and epirubicin and the poorest drug penetration for mitoxantrone (Kyle et al. 2004). In a similar laboratory study (Tannock et al. 2002), penetration was best for etoposide, followed by cisplatin, paclitaxel and gemcitabine, and poorest for vinblastine. Available data on penetration depth of individual drugs in vivo are presented below in the next chapter.

Intraperitoneal chemotherapy may be combined simultaneously with systemic chemotherapy to optimize treatment efficacy in case of residual tumour after cytoreductive surgery. The intraperitoneally delivered cytotoxic agent penetrates the residual tumour nodules from the site of the peritoneal surface, while intravenous drug administration provides drug distribution by capillary blood flow into the tumour deposits (Hofstra et al. 2002; Markman et al. 2002; Rothenberg et al. 2003). For the same reason, substantial drug absorption from the peritoneal cavity to the systemic compartment may be even beneficial when it leads to adequate plasma concentrations without major systemic toxicity. Hence, peritoneal fluid-to-plasma maximal concentration and AUC ratios of certain agents may not accurately represent the pharmacokinetic advantage of intraperitoneal drug administration.

4.4 Timing of Intraperitoneal Chemotherapy

Homogeneous distribution and drug exposure to the entire seroperitoneal surface is required for optimal efficacy. This implies the need for lysis of intra-abdominal adhesions and the use of large volumes of fluid containing the chemotherapeutic agent. Intraperitoneal chemotherapy has been administered in the preoperative, intraoperative, and early and late postoperative periods. From a distributional point of view, the optimal time is either before or during surgery to avoid limitation of homogeneous distribution by postoperative adhesion formation. Preoperative administration has the objective of facilitating subsequent cytoreductive surgery but requires small-volume disease and the absence of extensive adhesions from previous operations. Intraperitoneal chemotherapy is generally used intra- or postoperatively, because the peritoneal surface is usually grossly affected and cytoreductive surgery is required. Intraoperative and early postoperative intraperitoneal therapy are intended to consolidate the effect of surgery by destroying residual small tumour noduli and microscopic intraperitoneal malignant cell nests. In postoperative intraperitoneal chemotherapy, drugs have to be administered during the first postoperative days, before any new surgery-related adhesions are produced. Late postoperative intraperitoneal chemotherapy, longer than 2 weeks after surgery, is associated with diminished therapeutic effect, probably due to uneven peritoneal distribution, caused by postoperative adhesions, and peritoneal cavity access catheter-related problems (Averbach and Sugarbaker 1996). The prerequisites for effective intraperitoneal chemotherapy are summarized in Table 4.1. The different techniques are discussed comprehensively in another chapter of this book.

4.5 Hyperthermia

Besides the realization of optimal conditions for homogeneous drug distribution, another

Table 4.1 Usual preconditions and patient selection for effective intraperitoneal chemotherapy

Absence of haematogenous metastases
Adequate general condition of patient
Lysis of intra-abdominal adhesions
Minimal residual disease after cytoreductive surgery
Large volume carrier solution
Adequate drug choice (see Table 4.2)

advantage of intraoperative application of intraperitoneal chemotherapy is the ability to perform this treatment modality under hyperthermic conditions, which are poorly tolerated by a conscious patient. The selective effect of hyperthermia on malignant cells and its ability to enhance the efficacy of chemotherapeutic agents make it a valuable adjunct to intraperitoneal chemotherapy in the management of peritoneal carcinomatosis (de Bree et al. 2002a).

4.5.1 Direct Cytotoxic Effect of Hyperthermia

The direct cytotoxic effect of heat has been known since ancient times. The father of modern medicine, Hippocrates (470–377 b.c.), stated in his Aphorisms: 'Where drugs do not cure, iron does; where iron does not cure, heat does; where real heat does not cure, cure is impossible' (Fig. 4.1). Since the beginning of recorded history in medicine there have been descriptions of the use of heat to treat malignancies, initially in the form of cauterization for local tumour destruction. During the Dark and Middle Ages it was common for tumours to be treated with direct heat to destroy the tumour or suppress further growth. In the latter half of the nineteenth century and early twentieth century, several cases of spontaneous regression of advanced malignancies after high fever were reported (Sticca and Dach 2003). These reports led several investigators to take a closer look at the association between hyperthermia and malignancy.

In 1893, Coley was the earliest investigator to report on induced hyperthermia. Patients with advanced sarcoma were treated by induced

4 Principles of Perioperative Intraperitoneal Chemotherapy for Peritoneal Carcinomatosis

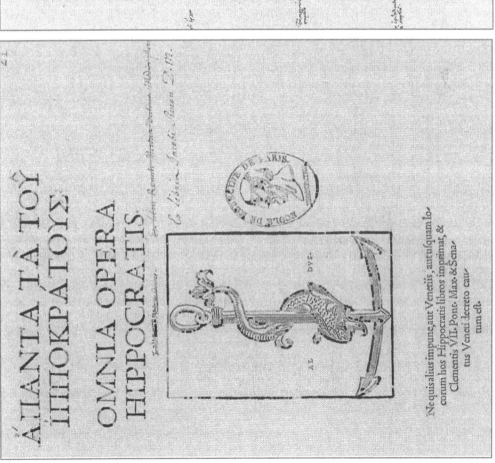

Fig. 4.1 *Left:* Cover of the book containing all work from Hippocrates as published in 1526 by Aldine Press, Venice. *Right:* page 172 from Hippocrates' *Aphorisms* showing lines 14 and 15 in ancient Greek: 'Where drugs do not cure, iron does; where iron does not cure, heat does; where real heat does not cure, cure is impos-

hyperthermia with injections of erysipelas toxin. Several complete responses were noted. This led others to evaluate hyperthermia as a primary treatment for malignancy. During the following decades, clinical responses were observed after hyperthermic therapy for inoperable tumours in several series (Sticca and Dach 2003).

After the initial reports of spontaneous tumour regression due to episodes of hyperthermia, several investigators started to document the selective effects of heat on malignant cells, as well as the basis of this interaction on the cellular and molecular levels. There is an abundance of experimental and clinical evidence to indicate that malignant cells are selectively destroyed by hyperthermia in the range of 41°C to 43°C. The cellular and molecular basis for this selectivity has been well studied (Cavaliere et al. 1967; Overgaard 1977; Sticca and Dach 2003). While inhibited RNA synthesis and mitosis arrest are reversible and non-selective results of hyperthermia, an increase in the number of lysosomes and lysosomal enzyme activity are selective effects in malignant cells. These heat induced lysosomes are more labile in malignant cells, and therefore result in increased destructive capacity. The microcirculation in most malignant tumours exhibits a decrease in blood flow or even complete vascular stasis in response to hyperthermia, which is in contrast to an increased flow capacity found in normal tissues (Dudar and Jain 1984). This, in combination with depression or complete inhibition of oxidative metabolism in tumour cells subjected to hyperthermia and unaltered anaerobic glycolysis, leads to accumulation of lactic acid and lower pH in the microenvironment of the malignant cell. This effect is selective for malignant cells and may be due to the increased sensitivity of mitochondrial membranes in malignant cells. The increased acidity then increases the activity of the lysosymes, which are increased in number. This results in accelerated cell death of the more fragile malignant cells subjected to hyperthermia (Overgaard 1977).

Although many of the clinical studies using hyperthermia as primary treatment modality for advanced malignancy showed occasional enduring complete responses, the majority of patients either did not respond or had transient responses with early recurrences. This, along with the recognition that hyperthermia enhances other kinds of cancer treatment, like chemotherapy and radiation therapy, has largely led to the abandonment of hyperthermia alone as a primary anticancer treatment.

4.5.2 Thermal Enhancement of Chemotherapeutic Drugs

Hyperthermia enhances chemotherapy efficacy in a number of ways (Sticca and Dach 2003). The combination of heat and neoplastic drugs frequently results in increased cytotoxicity over that predicted for an additive effect. The synergism between both kinds of treatment is dependent on several factors including increased drug uptake in malignant cells, which is due to increased membrane permeability and improved membrane transport. There is also evidence that heat may alter cellular metabolism and change drug pharmacokinetics and excretion, both of which can increase the cytotoxicity of certain chemotherapeutic agents. Additional factors include increased drug penetration in tissue, temperature-dependent increases in drug action and inhibition of repair mechanisms. In many cases, this enhancement of activity and penetration depth of drugs is already seen above 39–40°C (Storm 1989; Panteix et al. 1993; Jacquet et al. 1998a; Benoit et al. 1999; Sticca and Dach 2003).

The synergism of heat and drugs has been well documented, especially for selected chemotherapeutic agents used during HIPEC. Several agents have been shown to have an apparently improved therapeutic index and efficacy when used with hyperthermia in in vitro and in vivo experimental studies. Generally, the highest thermal enhancement ratios have been observed for alkylating agents like melphalan, cyclophosphamide and ifosfamide (Takemoto et al. 2003). Thermal enhancement of cytotoxicity for a variety of drugs is discussed in detail below in the next chapter.

It seems that hyperthermia enhances not only the anti-tumour effect of many drugs, but also their acute and late systemic side-effects.

This has been observed for various drugs in experimental animal models for whole body hyperthermia, eroding the potential therapeutic gain of such a combined treatment (Wondergem et al. 1991). However, in HIPEC the heat is applied locoregionally and hence such an adverse effect of hyperthermia on drugs' toxicity is not, or in a much lesser extent, to be expected.

4.5.3 Tissue Penetration Depth of Hyperthermia During HIPEC

Hyperthermia used during HIPEC has a limited penetration depth, emphasizing the need for adequate cytoreductive surgery. In a recent study (van Ruth et al. 2003), a wide inter-individual variability was noted. With an intraperitoneal temperature between 40°C and 41°C, a temperature of 39°C or higher was reached to a mean depth of 3.1 mm at the beginning and 5.1 mm at the end of the procedure. Remarkable is the large decline in the first millimetres, between intraperitoneal and subperitoneal temperature. The rich vascularization of the peritoneum and the relatively cool blood flow lead to loss of heat. This dependence of hyperthermia is known as the 'heat sink effect'. The temperature gradient seems to be larger in the beginning in comparison to the gradient at the end of the procedure, probably because of the increased core temperature resulting in decreased heat loss.

4.6 Drug Choice

The choice of the chemotherapeutic drug is very important and certain aspects have to be considered (Table 4.2). It is important for the agent to lack severe local toxicity after intraperitoneal administration. Moreover, the drug should have a well-established activity against the malignancy treated. Drugs that have to be metabolized systemically into their active form are inappropriate for intraperitoneal use. Whereas in instillation intraperitoneal chemotherapy all categories of active drugs can be used, in HIPEC procedures a direct cytotoxic agent is needed. Anti-metabolites are not suitable for this application, because the exposure duration is too short to be effective. Experimental or clinical evidence should be available suggesting that for the particular drug a concentration- or exposure-dependent cytotoxicity exists. Otherwise, when low target drug levels are equally effective, systemic chemotherapy may be sufficient. Agents with a large molecular weight have more favourable pharmacokinetics, because of limited and delayed absorption from the peritoneal cavity. Drugs highly metabolized in the liver to non-toxic metabolites are preferred because the first-pass effect from the liver decreases further the systemic drug exposure. Additional rapid renal clearance of the drug that has passed the liver may decrease systemic drug exposure. Finally, existence of a synergistic effect of the drug with hyperthermia is preferred for HIPEC. In vivo studies on different agents indicate that the drug of choice at physiological temperatures may not be the drug of choice at elevated temperatures (Urano et al. 1999). A theoretical prerequisite for HIPEC is the heat stability of the drug that is to be administered, but fortunately nearly all drugs are stable under these moderate hyperthermic conditions.

Chapter 5 offers a comprehensive listing of different cytotoxic drugs suitable for intra-

Table 4.2 Specific features of cytotoxic agents favourable for intraperitoneal delivery

Lack of local toxicity of the agent
Documented activity against malignancy to be treated
No need for metabolism into active form
Experimental or clinical evidence for concentration- or exposure-dependent cytotoxicity of the agent
Slow clearance from the peritoneal cavity (i.e. high molecular weight, water rather than lipid solubility)
Significant and rapid hepatic metabolism to non-cytotoxic metabolite (first-pass effect from the liver)
Rapid renal clearance
Direct cytotoxic agent (no antimetabolites, only for HIPEC)
Synergistic effect with hyperthermia (only for HIPEC)

peritoneal administration. For each drug, the reported experimental and clinical studies supporting its use in different malignant peritoneal disease settings are described in detail.

4.7 Carrier Solutions

The volume of chemotherapy solution may have a significant impact on pharmacokinetics. When 10–12.5 mg/m2 mitomycin C was added to 2, 4 or 6 l of 1.5% dextrose peritoneal dialysis solution for 90 min of HIPEC, the intraperitoneal and plasma concentrations were highest for the smaller volumes (Sugarbaker et al. 2006). The mean intraperitoneal-to-plasma AUC ratio was similar for all volumes. When both the volume of chemotherapy solution (1.5 l/m2) and the total dose of mitomycin C were determined from the body surface area, the pharmacokinetics of intraperitoneal mitomycin C were more consistent. The results of this study indicate that the volume of the drug solution should be calculated based on the body surface area in order to achieve less variety in pharmacokinetics and to be able to optimise dosage, while making toxicity predictions easier.

In intraperitoneal chemotherapy the choice of the carrier solution in which the chemotherapeutic drug is dissolved can play an important role in the clearance of the drug from the peritoneal cavity to plasma. The appropriate selection of the carrier solution may enhance the performance of the chemotherapeutic agent, improving tissue penetration and increasing exposure of tumour nodules and residual tumour cells within the peritoneal cavity to the drug. The ideal carrier solution should provide the following: (1) exposure of cancerous surfaces within the peritoneal cavity to high levels of cytotoxic agent for as long as possible, (2) prolonged high intraperitoneal volume, (3) slow clearance from the peritoneal cavity and (4) absence of adverse effects to peritoneal membranes even after prolonged exposure (Mohamed and Sugarbaker 2003). Current techniques for intraperitoneal chemotherapy administration most often use isotonic salt solutions or dextrose-based peritoneal dialysis solutions. The isotonic low-molecular-weight solutions are relatively quickly absorbed from the peritoneal cavity. The decreased amount of carrier solution impairs the exposure of the entire seroperitoneal surface to the drug. The agents with a low molecular weight clear themselves rapidly from the peritoneal cavity, and so the choice of a carrier solution is less critical. For high-molecular-weight drugs with delayed absorption from the peritoneal cavity, the choice of the carrier solution is an important factor in optimizing prolonged intraperitoneal chemotherapy. Because of the short duration of HIPEC, the role of the carrier solution is not as important as in the case of intraperitoneal instillation chemotherapy. The intraperitoneal fluid volume can easily be adjusted during HIPEC by reducing the fluid level in the reservoir of the circulation system. However, large fluid shifts during HIPEC using normal saline as carrier solution may increase the incidence of heart fibrillation perioperatively as observed in some series (Tsiftsis et al. 1999; de Bree et al. 2003a).

The inability of isotonic salt or dextrose solutions to maintain a prolonged high intraperitoneal fluid volume limits their effectiveness as carrier solutions for instillation intracavitary chemotherapy, so a number of other carrier solutions have been studied in both animal models and humans. Studies using hypertonic carrier solutions are limited. In an animal model, prolonged intraperitoneal volume was achieved with the use of 3% sodium chloride solution as carrier for instillation chemotherapy, as compared to 0.9% and 0.3% sodium chloride solutions (Pestieau et al. 2001). By slowing down the clearance of intraperitoneal fluid and thereby maintaining a large distribution, hypertonic solutions may be beneficial. In another animal study (Litterst et al. 1982), it was shown that slightly hypertonic carrier solutions may prolong the peritoneal retention of drugs within the peritoneal cavity, probably by inducing a fluid shift inwards to the peritoneal cavity. A possible disadvantage of this strategy is the dilution of the drug within the peritoneal cavity, which reduces drug concentration and AUC.

In vitro and animal studies have demonstrated that increased drug accumulation in tumour cells and enhanced cytotoxicity can be achieved by using hypotonic solutions (Groos and Masters 1986; Kondo et al. 1996; Tsujitani et al. 1999). Although these experimental studies were promising, clinical success with hypotonic carrier solutions for intraperitoneal chemotherapy has been limited. In a phase I study, intraoperative prophylactic instillation chemotherapy with a hypotonic cisplatin solution was well tolerated in patients with gastric cancer and serosal invasion (Tsujitani et al. 2002). Hypotonic intraperitoneal cisplatin administration seemed not to increase the plasma level of platinum. In the only HIPEC study concerning the comparison of different carrier solutions, 16 patients with peritoneal carcinomatosis were treated by complete cytoreductive surgery and HIPEC with oxaliplatin in successive dextrose solutions of 300, 200, 150 and 100 mOsm/l at an intra-abdominal temperature of 42–44°C for 30 min (Elias et al. 2002). In contradiction to the experimental studies, absorption of oxaliplatin and intratumoural oxaliplatin were not significantly increased by using hypotonic compared with isotonic solutions. The relatively short duration of chemoperfusion may be of importance. Remarkable was the very high incidence of unexplained postoperative peritoneal bleeding (31%) and unusually severe thrombocytopenia in the 150 and 100 mOsm/l groups. Further clarification of safety and efficacy of hypotonic carrier solutions in clinical studies is required before their use can be recommended.

Advances in continuous ambulatory peritoneal dialysis for renal failure provided new solutions for intraperitoneal use. The ability of high-molecular-weight solutions, such as icodextrin and hetastarch, to maintain intraperitoneal volumes over prolonged periods make them attractive carrier solutions for intraperitoneal chemotherapy. To avoid net fluid flow into the peritoneal cavity and consequently the decrease of intraperitoneal drug concentration caused by using hypertonic solutions, isotonic solutions such as 4% icodextrin or 6% hetastarch are preferred. An additional benefit of solutions such as 4% icodextrin is their ability to reduce the incidence of postoperative intra-abdominal adhesions (diZerega et al. 2002). Experimental and clinical studies have demonstrated that the use of such solutions provides prolonged availability of cytotoxic drugs at the seroperitoneal surfaces (Pestieau et al. 2001). In a recent rat model, paclitaxel and docetaxel were administered intraperitoneally by using hetastarch or dextrose peritoneal dialysis solution (Mohamed et al. 2003a, 2003c). Peritoneal fluid amount, peritoneal fluid drug concentrations and AUC ratios were significantly higher with hetastarch, while plasma drug concentrations were similar or even lower. Drug concentrations were significantly higher in local tissues many hours after intraperitoneal drug delivery. In a clinical study (Mohamed et al. 2003b), patients were randomized to receive early postoperative intraperitoneal chemotherapy with paclitaxel in 6% hetastarch or 1.5% dextrose peritoneal dialysis solution after cytoreductive surgery for peritoneal surface malignancy. While no differences in pharmacokinetics of paclitaxel, expressed in concentrations and AUCs in peritoneal fluid and plasma, and in chemotherapy-related complications were observed between the groups, peritoneal fluid volume and total amount of paclitaxel remaining in the peritoneal fluid at the end of the dwell time were significantly greater. Therefore, the investigators concluded that over time a larger number of residual cancer cells on the peritoneal surface could be exposed to the same concentration, supporting the concept that high-molecular-weight carrier solutions provide pharmacodynamic advantages for intraperitoneal instillation chemotherapy.

A better understanding of the pharmacodynamics of carrier solutions may increase the effectiveness of intraperitoneal chemotherapy. It appears that high-molecular-weight solutions offer a number of advantages. The use of carrier solutions of varying tonicity requires further investigation. Although the selection of an appropriate carrier solution seems to be of major importance in intraperitoneal instillation chemotherapy, in HIPEC this issue is less significant because of its short treatment duration, the continuous ability to adjust intra-abdominal fluid volume and the achievement of optimal exposure of the entire seroperitoneal surface to the cytotoxic drug by various techniques as mentioned above.

4.8 Duration of Hyperthermic Chemoperfusion

While in pre- or postoperative instillation peritoneal chemotherapy the drug solution is usually left in the peritoneal cavity for 4 to more than 24 h, the duration of HIPEC has been arbitrary and varies from 30 min to 2 h in different centres. No definite data are available to support a particular time period, but some results from pharmacokinetic and experimental studies should be considered in an attempt to define the optimal treatment duration. In some clinical studies drug loss from the peritoneal drug solution has been measured. The drug loss from the perfusate can be explained by the intended attachment and penetration of the peritoneal surface and its tumour deposits, the attachment to other organs and structures as well as the absorption from the peritoneal cavity to the systemic compartment. In such studies, approximately 70% of the administered mitomycin C was eliminated from the perfusate after 2 h of HIPEC (Jacquet et al. 1998b; Fernandez-Trigo et al. 1996). Others demonstrated a mitomycin C absorption rate of only 40% after 60 min (Koga et al. 1988; Panteix et al. 1993; Carretani et al. 2005), while approximately half the irinotecan or oxaliplatin dose was absorbed from the peritoneal fluid after 30 min of HIPEC (Elias et al. 2003, 2004), leaving the opportunity for further improvement of treatment efficacy by prolonged perfusion unexploited. In a study from the Netherlands Cancer Institute, approximately 75% of the cisplatin dose was lost from the perfusion fluid after a dwelling time of 90 min (van der Vaart 1998). Similar results were reported in another study (Panteix et al. 2002). After a perfusion time of 90 min, the average percentage of cisplatin absorbed was 65% (42%–85%). They estimated that only approximately 20% of the cisplatin had reached the systemic circulation, implying that a high proportion of the drug was absorbed by target tumour cells after these 90 min of HIPEC. Other investigators found the mean amount of drug cleared from the perfusion fluid during a 90-min hyperthermic perfusion to be approximately 75% for cisplatin and doxorubicin (Cho et al. 1999; Rossi et al. 2002). In a pharmacokinetic study of high dose carboplatin during HIPEC, up to 77% of carboplatin was absorbed after 90 min (Steller et al. 1999). However, a great inter-individual variation was observed and at the higher dose considerable haematological toxicity was observed, making prolonged time for drug absorption unwarranted. In the case of docetaxel, an average of 80% of the initially administered total amount is lost from the perfusate after 2 h of HIPEC (de Bree et al. 2003b). In conclusion, a HIPEC duration of 30–60 min is probably too short for optimal absorption of cytotoxic agents by tumour nodules, while it seems unlikely that prolonged perfusion duration of more than 90 or 120 min will add substantially more to the efficacy of this treatment modality, because after this period only a small amount of drug is still available in the perfusate for absorption. However, Elias and associates aim with very high intraperitoneal drug doses for a short period (30 min) to obtain an optimal peritoneal fluid AUC (Elias et al. 2003). With an intentionally short treatment time, they attempt to avoid significant toxic systemic drug exposure by allowing only half of the drug dose to be absorbed. Shortening of operation time and decreasing costs are additional reasons. Furthermore, higher intraperitoneal temperatures can be tolerated for such a short time. However, whether this duration of hyperthermia is enough to allow thermal enhancement of the drug's cytotoxicity is unclear.

Regarding the duration of heat, in a mouse model a 30-min period of 41.5°C was insufficient to enhance the cytotoxic effect of intraperitoneally administered docetaxel, while mild hyperthermic conditions for 90 min resulted in significantly increased mean tumour growth time (Mohamed et al. 2004). Sequencing of hyperthermia by applying heat for two 30-min periods, immediately and 90 min after drug administration, was also effective in enhancing docetaxel cytotoxicity. By analyzing various experimental studies on the synergistic effect of hyperthermia and paclitaxel similar conclusions were made (de Bree et al. 2006; Michalakis et al. 2006). Hyperthermia for 30 min is inadequate to increase paclitaxel cytotoxicity, while treatment efficacy appears to be improved when hyperthermia is administered for 2 h.

These studies suggest that the duration of HIPEC should exceed at least 90 min to take advantage of thermal enhancement of drug cytotoxicity. In conclusion, perfusion duration of 90–120 min seems most adequate, taking into account the above-mentioned pharmacokinetic and hyperthermia studies.

References

Averbach AM, Sugarbaker PH (1996) Methodologic considerations in treatment using intraperitoneal chemotherapy. Cancer Treat Res 82:289–309

Benoit L, Duvillard C, Rat P, Chauffert B (1999) Effects de la temperature intra-abdominale sur la diffuion tissulaire et tumorale du cisplatine intraperitoneal dans un modele de carcinose peritoneale chez le rat. Chirurgie 124:375–379

de Bree E, Romanos J, Tsiftsis DD (2002a) Hyperthermia in anticancer treatment. Eur J Surg Oncol 28:95

de Bree E, Witkamp AJ, Zoetmulder FAN (2002b) Intraperitoneal chemotherapy for colorectal cancer. J Surg Oncol 79:46–61

de Bree E, Romanos J, Michalakis J et al. (2003a) Intraoperative hyperthermic intraperitoneal chemotherapy with docetaxel as second-line treatment for peritoneal carcinomatosis of gynaecological origin. Anticancer Res 23:3019–3028

de Bree E, Rosing H, Beijnen JH et al. (2003b) Pharmacokinetic study of docetaxel in intraoperative hyperthermic i.p. chemotherapy for ovarian cancer. Anti-Cancer Drugs 14:103–110

de Bree E, Theodoropoulos PA, Rosing H et al. (2006) Treatment of ovarian cancer using intraperitoneal chemotherapy with taxanes: From laboratory bench to bedside. Cancer Treat Rev (in press)

Cavaliere R, Ciocatto EC, Giovanella BC et al. (1967) Selective heat sensitivity of cancer cells. Biochemical and clinical studies. Cancer 20:1351–1381

Carretani D, Nencini C, Urso R et al. (2005) Pharmacokinetics of mitomycin C after resection of peritoneal carcinomatosis and intraperitoneal chemohyperthermic perfusion. J Chemother 17:668–673

Chauffert B, Favoulet P, Polycarpe E et al. (2003) Rationale supporting the use of vasoconstrictors for intraperitoneal chemotherapy with platinum derivates. Surg Oncol Clin N Am 12:835–848

Cho HK, Lush RM, Bartlett DL et al. (1999) Pharmacokinetics of cisplatin administered by continuous hyperthermic peritoneal perfusion (CHPP) to patients with peritoneal carcinomatosis. J Clin Pharmacol 39:394–401

diZerega GS, Verco SJ, Young P et al. (2002) A randomized, controlled pilot study of the safety and efficacy of 4% icodextrin solution in the reduction of adhesions following laparoscopic gynaecological surgery. Hum Reprod 17:1031–1038

Dudar TE, Jain RK (1984) Differential response of normal and tumor microcirculation to hyperthermia. Cancer Res 44:605–612

Elias D, El Otmany A, Bonnay M et al. (2002) Human pharmacokinetic study of heated intraperitoneal oxaliplatin in increasingly hypotonic solutions after complete resection of peritoneal carcinomatosis. Oncology 63:346–352

Elias DM, Sideris L (2003) Pharmacokinetics of heated intraoperative intraperitoneal oxaliplatin after complete resection of peritoneal carcinomatosis. Surg Oncol Clin N Am 12:755–769

Elias D, Matsuhisa T, Sideris L et al. (2004) Heated intraoperative intraperitoneal oxaliplatin plus irinotecan after complete resection of peritoneal carcinomatosis: pharmacokinetics, tissue distribution and tolerance. Ann Oncol 15:1558–1565

Fernandez-Trigo V, Stuart OA, Stephens A, Hoover LD, Sugarbaker PH (1996) Surgically directed chemotherapy: heated intraperitoneal lavage with mitomycin C. Cancer Treat Res 81:51–56

Flessner MF (2005) The transport barrier in intraperitoneal therapy. Am J Physiol Renal Physiol 288: F433–F442

Fujimoto S, Takahashi M, Kobayashi K et al. (1992) Cytohistologic assessment of antitumor effects of intraperitoneal hyperthermic perfusion with mitomycin C for patients with gastric cancer with peritoneal metastasis. Cancer 1992 70:2754–2760

Grantah R, Sivananthan S, Tannock IF (2006) The penetration of anticancer drugs through tumor tissue as a function of cellular adhesion and packing density of tumor cells. Cancer Res 66:1033–1039

Groos E, Masters JR (1986) Intravesical chemotherapy: studies on the relation between osmolality and cytotoxicity. J Urol 136:399–402

Hofstra LS, Bos AME, de Vries EGE et al. (2002) Kinetic modelling and efficacy of intraperitoneal paclitaxel combined with intravenous cyclophosphamide and carboplatin as first-line treatment in ovarian cancer. Gynecol Oncol 85:517–523

Jacquet P, Sugarbaker PH (1996) Peritoneal-plasma barrier. Cancer Treat Res 82:53–63

Jacquet P, Averbach A, Stuart OA et al. (1998a) Hyperthermic intraperitoneal doxorubicin: pharmacokinetics, metabolism, and tissue distribution in a rat model. Cancer Chemother Pharmacol 41:147–154

Jacquet P, Averbach A, Stephens AD et al. (1998b) Heated intraoperative intraperitoneal mitomycin C and early postoperative intraperitoneal 5-fluorouracil: pharmacokinetic studies. Oncology 55:130–138

Koga S, Hamazoe R, Maeta M et al. (1988) Prophylactic therapy for peritoneal recurrence of gastric cancer by continuous hyperthermic peritoneal perfusion with mitomycin-C. Cancer 61:232–237

Kondo A, Maeta M, Oka A et al. (1996) Hypotonic intraperitoneal cisplatin chemotherapy for peritoneal carcinomatosis in mice. Br J Cancer 73:1166–1170

Kyle AH, Huxham LA, Chiam ASJ et al. (2004) Direct assessment of drug penetration into tissue using a novel application of three-dimensional cell culture. Cancer Res 64:6304–6309

de Lima Vazquez V, Stuart OA, Mohamed F, Sugarbaker PH (2003) Extent of parietal peritonectomy does not change intraperitoneal chemotherapy pharmacokinetics. Cancer Chemother Pharmacol 52:108–112

Lindner P, Heath DD, Shalinsky DR et al. (1993) regional lymphatic drug exposure following intraperitoneal administration of 5-fluorouracil, carboplatin, and etoposide. Surg Oncol 2:105–112

Litterst CL, Torres IJ, Arnold S et al. (1982) Adsorption of antineoplastic drugs following large-volume ip administration to rats. Cancer Treat Rep 66:147–155

Los G, Verdegaal EM, Mutsaers PH, McVie JG (1991) Penetration of carboplatin and cisplatin into rat peritoneal tumor nodules after intraperitoneal chemotherapy. Cancer Chemother Pharmacol 28:159–165

Markman M, Kulp B, Peterson G, Kennedy A, Belinson J (2002) Second-line therapy of ovarian cancer with paclitaxel administered by both the intravenous and intraperitoneal routes: Rationale and case reports. Gynecol Oncol 86:95–98

McVie JG, Dikhoff T, Van der Heide J et al. (1985) Tissue concentration of platinum after intraperitoneal cisplatinum administration in patients. Proc Am Assoc Cancer Res 26:162

Michalakis J, Georgatos SD, de Bree E et al. (2006) Short term exposure of cancer cells to micromolar doses of paclitaxel, with or without hyperthermia, induces long term inhibition of cell proliferation and cell death in vitro. Ann Surg Oncol (in press)

Mohamed F, Sugarbaker PH (2003) Carrier solutions for intraperitoneal chemotherapy. Surg Oncol Clin N Am 12:813–824

Mohamed F, Marchettini P, Stuart OA, Sugarbaker PH (2003a) Pharmacokinetics and tissue distribution of intraperitoneal docetaxel with different carrier solutions. J Surg Res 113:114–120

Mohamed F, Marchettini P, Stuart OA et al. (2003b) A comparison of hetastarch and peritoneal dialysis solution for intraperitoneal chemotherapy delivery. Eur J Surg Oncol 29:261–265

Mohamed F, Marchetti P, Stuart OA, Sugarbaker PH (2003c) Pharmacokinetics and tissue distribution of intraperitoneal paclitaxel with different carrier solutions. Cancer Chemother Pharmacol 52:405–410

Mohamed F, Stuart OA, Glehen O et al. (2004) Docetaxel and hyperthermia: factors that modify thermal enhancement. J Surg Oncol 88:14–20

Overgaard J (1977) Effects of hyperthermia on malignant cells in-vivo, a review and hypothesis. Cancer 39:2637–2646

Ozols RF, Locker GY, Doroshow JH et al. (1979) Pharmacokinetics of adriamycin and tissue penetration in murine ovarian cancer. Cancer Res 39:3209–3214

Panteix G, Guillaumont M, Cherpin L et al. (1993) Study of the pharmacokinetics of mitomycin C in humans during intraperitoneal chemohyperthermia with special mention of the concentration in local tissues. Oncology 50:366–370

Panteix G, Beaujard A, Garbit F et al. (2002) Population pharmacokinetics of cisplatin in patients with advanced ovarian cancer during intraperitoneal hyperthermia chemotherapy. Anticancer Res 22:1329–1336

Pestieau SR, Schnake KJ, Stuart OA, Sugarbaker PH (2001) Impact of carrier solutions on pharmacokinetics of intraperitoneal chemotherapy. Cancer Chemother Pharmacol 47:269–276

Rossi C, Foletto M, Mocellin S et al. (2002) Hyperthermic intraoperative intraperitoneal chemotherapy with cisplatin and doxorubicin in patients who undergo cytoreductive surgery for carcinomatosis and sarcomatosis. Cancer 94:492–499

Rothenberg ML, Liu PY, Braly PS et al. (2003) Combined intraperitoneal and intravenous chemotherapy for women with optimally debulked ovarian cancer: Results from an Intergroup Phase II trial. J Clin Oncol 21:1313–1319

Rubin J, Jones Q, Planch A, Bowder JD (1988) The minimal importance of hollow viscera to peritoneal transport during peritoneal dialysis in rats. Am Soc Artif Intern Organs Transact 42:912–915

van Ruth S, Verwaal VJ, Hart AA, van Slooten GW, Zoetmulder FAN (2003) Heat penetration in locally applied hyperthermia in the abdomen during intraoperative hyperthermic intraperitoneal chemotherapy. Anticancer Res 23:1501–1508

Speyer JL, Sugarbaker PH, Collins JM et al. (1981) Portal levels and hepatic clearance of 5-fluorouracil after intraperitoneal administration in humans. Cancer Res 41:1916–1922

Steller MA, Egorin MJ, Trimble EL et al. (1999) A pilot phase I trial of continuous hyperthermic peritoneal perfusion with high-dose carboplatin as primary treatment of patients with small-volume residual ovarian cancer. Cancer Chemother Pharmacol 43:106–114

Sticca RP, Dach BW (2003) Rationale for hyperthermia with intraoperative intraperitoneal chemotherapy agents. Surg Oncol Clin N Am 12:689–701

Storm FK (1989) Clinical hyperthermia and chemotherapy. Radiol Clin N Am 27:621–627

Sugarbaker PH, Stuart OA, Vidal-Jove J et al. (1996) Pharmacokinetics of the peritoneal-plasma barrier after systemic mitomycin C administration. Cancer Treat Res 82:41–52

Sugarbaker PH, Stuart OA, Carmignani CP (2006) Pharmacokinetic changes induced by the volume of chemotherapy solution in patients treated with hyperthermic intraperitoneal mitomycin C. Cancer Chemother Pharmacol 57:703–708

Takemoto M, Kuroda M, Urano M et al. (2003) The effect of various chemotherapeutic agents given at mild hyperthermia on different types of tumours. Int J Hyperthermia 19:193–203

Tannock IF, Lee CM, Tunggal JK et al. (2002) Limited penetration of anticancer drugs through tumor tissue: a potential cause of resistance of solid tumors to chemotherapy. Clin Cancer Res 8:878–884

Tsiftsis D, de Bree E, Romanos J et al. (1999) Peritoneal expansion by artificially produced ascites during perfusion chemotherapy. Arch Surg 134:545–549

Tsujitani S, Oka A, Kondo A et al. (1999) Administration in a hypotonic solution is preferable to dose escalation in intraperitoneal cisplatin chemotherapy for peritoneal carcinomatosis in rats. Oncology 57:77–82

Tsujitani S, Fukuda K, Saito H et al. (2002) The administration of hypotonic intraperitoneal cisplatin during operation as a treatment for the peritoneal dissemination of gastric cancer. Surgery 131 [1 Suppl]: S98–S104

Tunggual JK, Cowan DSM, Shaikh H, Tannock IF (1999) Penetration of anticancer drugs through solid tissue: a factor that limits the effectiveness of chemotherapy for solid tumors. Clin Cancer Res 5:1583–1586

Urano M, Kuroda M, Nishimura Y (1999) For the clinical application of thermochemotherapy given at mild temperatures. Int J Hyperthermia 15:79–107

van der Vaart PJM, van der Vange N, Zoetmulder FAN et al. (1998) Intraperitoneal cisplatin with regional hyperthermia in advanced ovarian cancer: Pharmokinetics and cisplatin-DNA adduct formation in patients and ovarian cancer cell lines. Eur J Cancer 34:148–154

Weisberger AS, Levine B, Storaasli JP (1955) Use of nitrogen mustard in treatment of serous effusions of neoplastic origin. J Am Med Assoc 159:1704–1707

Wondergem J, Stephens LC, Strebel FR et al. (1991) Effect of adriamycin combined with whole body on tumor and normal tissue. Cancer Res 51:3559–3567

5 Experimental and Pharmacokinetic Studies in Intraperitoneal Chemotherapy: From Laboratory Bench to Bedside

Eelco de Bree and Dimitris D. Tsiftsis

Recent Results in Cancer Research, Vol. 169
© Springer-Verlag Berlin Heidelberg 2007

Extrapolation of experimental results to clinical practice should be done very carefully, because of the differences between the conditions on the laboratory bench and those in the human body. In the clinical setting, circumstances are much more complicated and drug activity is moderated by many physiological factors. On the other hand, the possibility of creating standardized conditions may be of great help for interpretation of treatment efficacy since great inter-individual differences may encumber this process. Furthermore, experimental studies provide indicative information that may be very valuable since it is practically impossible to study each treatment parameter in comparative clinical studies. The relatively small number of patients available for intraperitoneal chemotherapy trials complicates clinical evaluation of optimal treatment.

Before continuing on to a detailed description of the properties of different drugs, we should be aware of the fact that results of in vitro and in vivo experimental studies often differ, with factors such as tumour physiology, microcirculation, pH and hypoxia playing an essential role in the activity of drugs and their interaction with hyperthermia. In addition, the use of different cell lines and treatment protocols further confuses interpretation of these studies.

Most experimental hyperthermic chemotherapy studies were designed to answer questions concerning the combination of systemic chemotherapy and external regional or whole body hyperthermia. Consequently, in almost all studies the cells or tumours were exposed to relatively low drug doses for a prolonged period of time in combination with a short time (30–60 min) of hyperthermia. During hyperthermic intraperitoneal chemotherapy (HIPEC), however, the local drug concentrations are considerably higher and hyperthermic conditions are maintained usually for 1.5–2 h. Major investigators on this issue have stated that the drug concentration on the target must be high enough to allow sufficient thermal enhancement (Urano et al. 1999; Takemoto et al. 2003). Therefore, lack of thermal enhancement of a drug's cytotoxicity in some studies with conventional drug concentrations and short heating time does definitely not exclude the existence of such an effect under HIPEC conditions.

Because of the considerable inter-individual variations in pharmacokinetics and significant differences in the treatment protocols that are used worldwide, results of pharmacokinetic studies (Table 5.1) should be considered indicative rather than exact data. The great variation in mean concentration and exposure ratios among studies are probably due to differences in treatment duration, techniques and regimens. Some reported ratios may be overestimated because areas under the curve (AUCs) were calculated only over intraperitoneal treatment time, while in fact drug levels may be still detectable, especially in plasma, for a prolonged time after treatment termination.

Table 5.1 Results of pharmacokinetic studies on intraperitoneal administration of various drugs, indicative for their pharmacokinetic advantage[a]

Drug	$C_{max\ i.p.}/C_{max\ plasma}$	$AUC_{i.p.}/AUC_{plasma}$
Melphalan	93	17–63
Cisplatin	10–36	12–22
Carboplatin		15–20
Oxaliplatin	25	16
Mitomycin C	100	13–80
Adriamycin	249–474	162–230
Mitoxantrone		100–1400
Methotrexate	72	
5-Fluorouracil	1,000	117–1,400
Floxuridine		1,000–2,700
Gemcitabine		791
Irinotecan (SN-38)		15 (4)
Topotecan		54
Etoposide		2–9
Paclitaxel	800–1,000	550–2,300
Docetaxel	45–200	150–3,000

[a] Mean ratios of studies are shown
C, concentration; max, maximal; i.p., intraperitoneal; AUC, area under concentration versus time curve

AUC ratios are often higher after instillation chemotherapy than after HIPEC, especially for agents with slow peritoneal clearance. These significant differences may be explained by the short duration of HIPEC compared to the longer treatment time for instillation intraperitoneal chemotherapy. Increased systemic drug absorption due to better exposure of the agent to the seroperitoneal surface and heat-induced vasodilatation during HIPEC may also play an important role.

5.1 Alkylating Agents

5.1.1 Melphalan

Melphalan, an alkylating agent, is one of the conventional drugs active in ovarian cancer that has been used for intraperitoneal chemotherapy. After intraperitoneal melphalan administration the mean peritoneal fluid AUC was 17 to 63 times higher than for plasma, while the peak peritoneal concentration averaged 93-fold greater (Howell et al. 1984; Piccart et al. 1988). There are no data published regarding its depth of penetration into tumour noduli, but high drug concentrations have been measured in intra-abdominal tissue in a rat model (Glehen et al. 2004). Since higher drug concentrations are clearly associated with increased tumour cell kill (Alberts et al. 1985), it appears to be an attractive agent for intraperitoneal chemotherapy.

Hyperthermia seems to alter the pharmacokinetics and tissue distribution of intraperitoneally administered melphalan (Glehen et al. 2004). While the peritoneal fluid AUC was lower and the time to reach maximal plasma concentration shorter under hyperthermic conditions, no difference in plasma AUC was observed compared with normothermic intraperitoneal perfusion chemotherapy in a rat model. Concurrent hyperthermia resulted in increased intra-abdominal tissue concentrations of melphalan after intraperitoneal perfusion chemotherapy.

In various experimental in vitro and in vivo models with different cancer cell types, a remarkable thermal enhancement has been observed for melphalan (Honess and Bleehen 1985; Urano et al. 1995; Takemoto et al. 2003). In the large collective experience of the Urano group, melphalan exhibited the highest increase in cytotoxicity of many drugs tested in the same experimental animal model when combined with hyperthermia (Urano et al. 1999). In clinical practice this has led to melphalan being one of the most commonly used drugs in hyperthermic isolated limb perfusion for locoregional advanced melanoma and sarcoma.

5.1.2 Cyclophosphamide and Ifosfamide

The alkylating agents ifosfamide and cyclophosphamide cannot be studied for thermal enhancement in vitro because these agents must be converted into their active form in vivo. Several in vivo studies have demonstrated a significantly increased cytotoxic effect of cyclophosphamide and ifosfamide under hyperthermic conditions (Hazen et al. 1981; Honess and Bleehen 1982; Urano et al. 1985; Monge et al. 1988; Kuroda et al. 1997; Stojkovic et al. 2002; Takemoto et al. 2003). It seems that prolonged (90 instead of 30 min) or delayed hyperthermia may be necessary to obtain optimal thermal enhancement for ifosfamide because of the time required for conversion in its active form (Kuroda et al. 1997; Urano et al. 1999). Despite this synergistic effect with heat, the need for their activation by hepatic microsomal enzymes makes them unsuitable for intraperitoneal administration during HIPEC. Nevertheless, because of their remarkable heat sensitization, they might be recommended for intravenous delivery during HIPEC with other heat-synergized drugs (Sugarbaker et al. 2005).

Ifosfamide derivates that do not require activation have been tested for their synergistic effect with heat. The significant observed increase in cytotoxicity of such an agent caused by hyperthermia, taken together with its known preclinical toxicity profile, encourages its further preclinical and, ultimately, clinical testing for regional hyperthermic chemotherapy (Kutz et al. 1997).

5.1.3 Mitomycin C

Mitomycin C is an antitumour antibiotic that belongs to the group of alkylating agents and is used against gastrointestinal malignancies. During intraperitoneal chemotherapy with 10–35 mg/m2 mitomycin C, drug concentrations are approximately 100 times those in serum, while the mean peritoneal fluid-to-plasma AUC ratio is 13–80 for mitomycin C in human pharmacokinetic studies (Fujimoto et al. 1989; Sugarbaker et al. 1990; Kuzuya et al. 1994; Jacquet et al. 1998b; Chang et al. 2001; de Lima Vazquez 2003; van Ruth et al. 2003b). Since a single-dose administration of mitomycin C at the start of HIPEC has the disadvantage of rapid decrease of intraperitoneal drug concentrations, administration of a totally higher drug amount (35 mg/m2) in three divided doses is advocated in the Netherlands Cancer Institute (van Ruth et al. 2003b). Because of its proven concentration-dependent responses, mitomycin C is an attractive drug for intraperitoneal use (Alberts et al. 1985; Link et al. 1998).

In an attempt to improve its pharmacokinetic profile by retaining mitomycin for a prolonged time in the peritoneal cavity, activated carbon particles absorbing mitomycin C have been administered intraperitoneally. Delayed release of mitomycin C allowed a higher total dose to be delivered and resulted in prolonged high peritoneal fluid concentrations (Hagiwara et al. 1992). Extended survival time was observed when compared with administration of aqueous mitomycin C solution in a rabbit model (Hagiwara et al. 1988).

The penetration depth of mitomycin C into the bladder wall after intravesical drug delivery is estimated to be approximately 2 mm (Wientjes et al. 1991). After HIPEC with mitomycin C high local tumour tissue drug concentrations have been detected (Panteix et al. 1993), while histological assessment of tumour noduli suggested its cytotoxic effect to be approximately 5 mm of depth from the seroperitoneal surface (Fujimoto et al. 1992).

Research on thermal enhancement of mitomycin C, the currently most commonly used chemotherapeutic drug for HIPEC, began decades ago. In an in vitro study, significant enhancement of drug-induced cytotoxicity was observed at 42°C with mitomycin C in a colon adenocarcinoma cell line (Barlogie et al. 1980). Cell death occurred regardless of tumour cell proliferative activity, which indicates that mitomycin C and hyperthermia should also be effective against tumours with a low mitotic rate such as pseudomyxoma peritonei. Similar increased cytotoxicity of mitomycin C was observed in vitro for other cell lines at a temperature of 42–43°C (Ohnoshi et al. 1985; van der Heijden et al. 2005). In some in vivo studies such an effect has been observed at 41.5–42.5°C (Monge et al. 1988; Takemoto et al. 2003). Others were unable to demonstrate a significant thermal enhancement for mitomycin C at temperatures below 42°C in in vitro and in vivo studies (Urano et al. 1994, 1999; Takemoto et al. 2003) From these experimental studies there is some indication that significant thermal enhancement is consistently obtained only at temperatures of 42°C and higher, a temperature range that is not routinely reached in tumour tissue during HIPEC.

5.2 Platinum Derivatives

5.2.1 Cisplatin

Cisplatin has been used widely over the last decades for intraperitoneal chemotherapy, mostly because of its significant cytotoxic effect against gastric cancer, ovarian cancer and mesothelioma and not because of its pharmacokinetic profile, which is not as favourable as that of many other drugs. The mean peritoneal-to-plasma AUC ratio varies from 12 to 22 in different clinical studies, whereas the maximal concentration of cisplatin measured in intraperitoneal fluid has been measured to be an average of 10–36 times higher than in plasma (Howell et al. 1982; Zakris et al. 1987; Piccart et al. 1988; Canal et al. 1989; O'Dwyer et al. 1991a; Ma et al. 1997; Bartlett et al. 1998; van der Vaart et al. 1998; Cho et al. 1999; Rossi et al. 2002). Its significantly increased efficacy at higher drug concentrations makes it an attractive drug for intraperitoneal use (Alberts et al. 1985; Link et al. 1998). It seems that with intraperitoneal temperature elevation there is an increased rate of generation and retention of reactive metabolites of cisplatin in the peritoneal cavity (Zakris et al. 1987).

In an effort to increase exposure of the peritoneal cavity to cisplatin, this drug has been incorporated in microspheres that were designed to release incorporated cisplatin slowly over several weeks. In mice, higher local tissue concentrations for a longer period and lower systemic drug levels were measured after intraperitoneal delivery of these microspheres than after administration of the conventional cisplatin aqueous solution. Additionally, a higher total cisplatin dose could be administered, resulting in an enhanced therapeutic effect (Hagiwara et al. 1993a). These observations were confirmed in a clinical pilot study (Hagiwara et al. 1993b)

In an animal model, the penetration depth of cisplatin in tumour noduli was estimated to be 1–2 mm during instillation intraperitoneal chemotherapy. The cisplatin concentration in the periphery of peritoneal tumours was 2–3 times higher after intraperitoneal than after intravenous administration, whereas in the centre of the tumour no significant concentration difference could be detected (Los et al. 1990a). In a clinical HIPEC study, most pronounced cisplatin activity was observed at 0–3 mm from the tumour border, but increased activity was also found at a depth of 3–5 mm (van der Vaart et al. 1998).

Dose and treatment duration are important for effective intraperitoneal chemotherapy. An intraperitoneal cisplatin exposure sufficient for ovarian cancer cell death, as defined in in vitro studies, is not reached with a relatively low dose of 50 mg/m2 for 2 h (Royer et al. 2005), while a dose of 110 mg/m2 for 2 h seems adequate (Furukawa et al. 1993). Usually 60–120 mg/m2 cisplatin is administered; the lower doses for prolonged instillation intraperitoneal chemotherapy and the higher doses for short-term intraoperative use. Concomitant intravenous administration of thiosulfate protects renal function and may allow higher cisplatin doses of 200–400 mg/m2 without the development of renal insufficiency (Howell et al. 1982; Markman et al. 1985; Canal et al. 1989; Furukawa et al. 1993; Ma et al. 1997; Bartlett et al. 1998). Cisplatin is compatible with many other agents and hence it can be used in combination with other drugs in a multidrug intraperitoneal chemotherapy regimen.

Synergism between cisplatin and hyperthermia apparently has been shown in multiple studies. In 1980, Barlogie et al. were the first to report thermal enhancement for cisplatin in vitro in a human colon cancer cell line. Subsequently, other studies confirmed those findings in more detail. Important experimental studies were conducted by Los and co-investigators. Increased intracellular drug uptake and cytotoxicity seemed to be temperature dependent in in vitro experiments (Los et al. 1991b). They observed that heat increases primarily cellular uptake of cisplatin and secondarily DNA adduct formation (Los et al. 1993). In vivo, tumour cisplatin concentrations were three times higher under hyperthermic than normothermic conditions in colon carcinoma-bearing rats (Los et al. 1994). This resulted in a significantly increased cytotoxic effect. This effect is selective for malignant cells, as the tumour cells were twice more likely to take up cisplatin than cells of surrounding tissues (Los et al. 1991a). Gradually, increase of cisplatin cytotoxicity at temperatures above 37°C has been as well demonstrated by Urano and associates in in vitro and in vivo studies using a fibrosarcoma tumour cell line (Urano et al. 1990, 1999). Many other investigators have also reported the existence of thermal enhancement of cisplatin cytotoxicity in vivo using other tumour models (Douple et al. 1982; Mella 1985; Herman et al. 1988; Baba et al. 1989; Nishimura et al. 1990; Lindegaard et al. 1992; Schem et al. 1992; Kusumoto et al. 1995; van Bree et al. 1996a; Stojkovic et al. 2002). Hence, cisplatin is an attractive agent for HIPEC.

Cisplatin has also been combined with tumour necrosis factor (TNF) during HIPEC. TNF increases the cellular uptake of cisplatin and improves cisplatin-DNA adduct formation under hyperthermic conditions in vitro (Buell et al. 1997). Intraperitoneally delivered TNF is hardly absorbed from the peritoneal cavity and consequently no lethal TNF-induced systemic toxicity is anticipated. In a phase I trial (Bartlett et al. 1998), the AUC for TNF in the perfusate was an average of 4,854 times higher than its AUC in the plasma. The recommended doses were 250 mg/m2 cisplatin and 0.1 mg/l TNF at 42–43°C, when sodium thiosulfate was administered systemically. The dose-limiting toxicity was renal insufficiency.

In a recent experimental study (Zeamari et al. 2003), instillation intraperitoneal chemotherapy with cisplatin was compared with normothermic and hyperthermic intraperitoneal perfusion chemotherapy in a rat model. With equal drug doses, higher maximal concentrations and AUCs in plasma and peritoneal fluid were observed after perfusion than after instillation intraperitoneal chemotherapy, but peritoneal fluid-to-plasma AUC ratios were similar. High cisplatin concentrations were measured in small peritoneal tumours after instillation intraperitoneal chemotherapy, but equal tissue concentrations of cisplatin were achieved with perfusion chemotherapy by using only less than half the dose used for instillation chemotherapy. Heating the perfusate to 40°C did not alter significantly pharmacokinetics or tumour tissue concentrations. The latter is in contradiction with the previously mentioned observations by Los and associates. Unfortunately, cytotoxicity of the regimens was not evaluated in this study.

5.2.2 Carboplatin

Carboplatin is a second platinum agent active against ovarian cancer that has been used for intraperitoneal chemotherapy. It also exhibits a significant dose-effect relation. The mean peritoneal-to-plasma AUC ratio is approximately 15–20 after intraperitoneal instillation of carboplatin (McClay et al. 1993; Miyagi et al. 2005). In a pharmacokinetic study, the platinum AUC in serum was the same regardless of intraperitoneal or intravenous administration of carboplatin, but platinum AUC in the peritoneal cavity was 17 times higher when carboplatin was administered by the intraperitoneal route (Miyagi et al. 2005). This study suggests that, although the AUC ratio is not considerably high, intraperitoneal delivery of carboplatin may be more favourable than intravenous administration. Reduction of splanchnic blood flow by intravenous administration of vasopressin further increased its pharmacokinetic advantage in a pig model (Lindner et al. 1996).

Compared with intraperitoneal administration of an equimolar dose of cisplatin in a rat model, carboplatin has a more favourable pharmacokinetic profile with slower clearance from the peritoneal cavity resulting in a 3 times higher peritoneal fluid AUC (Los et al. 1991a). However, the highly limited penetration depth of carboplatin of only 0.5 mm makes this platinum compound less suitable for intraperitoneal treatment of peritoneal carcinomatosis. Moreover, a 7 times higher amount of platinum was detected after cisplatin treatment than after equimolar carboplatin treatment, while 10 times more carboplatin than cisplatin had to be injected intraperitoneally to obtain comparable platinum concentrations in the peritoneal tumours.

Observations similar to those for cisplatin have been reported for carboplatin in combination with hyperthermia by Los and co-workers, although enhancement of carboplatin cytotoxicity seems to occur at higher temperature levels. While gradual increase of intracellular cisplatin uptake was already seen at temperatures above 38.5°C, for carboplatin temperatures equal to or above 41.5°C were required to observe such an effect (Los et al. 1993). In an intraperitoneal tumour animal model, the addition of hyperthermia led to a 4 times higher tumour concentration of carboplatin and consequently to a significantly increased cytotoxicity (Los et al. 1994). Various other studies have also demonstrated potentiation of carboplatin cytotoxicity by hyperthermia (Xu and Alberts 1988; Schem et al. 1992; Kusumoto et al. 1995; Murray et al. 1997; Choi et al. 2003).

5.2.3 Oxaliplatin

Oxaliplatin is a third-generation platinum complex highly active against gastrointestinal malignancies, especially colorectal cancer. The peritoneal fluid versus plasma AUC ratio was 16 after intraperitoneal oxaliplatin administration in a rat model, while high intra-abdominal tissue drug concentrations were measured (Pestieau et al. 2001). In an experimental animal model, early postoperative intraperitoneal chemotherapy with oxaliplatin was effective in prevention of peritoneal carcinomatosis and treatment of small volume peritoneal seeding of colon cancer (Hribaschek et al. 2002). The clinical use of oxaliplatin for HIPEC has been pioneered by Elias and colleagues (Elias et al. 2002, 2003, 2004), who simultaneously administered 5-fluorouracil and leucovorin intravenously. These drugs potentiate the activity of oxaliplatin but cannot be mixed with it because of pH incompatibility. During HIPEC with a high dose (460 mg/m2) of oxaliplatin for 30 min, high peritoneal fluid concentrations were obtained with a maximal drug concentration 25 times higher in peritoneal fluid than in plasma. Despite the rapid absorption from the peritoneal cavity, the short treatment time resulted in a mean plasma AUC of ultrafiltrated platinum that was slightly smaller than that obtained with intravenous oxaliplatin over 2 h at 130 mg/m2. Drug concentrations were approximately 18 times higher in peritoneal tumour noduli than in non-bathed muscle tissue, while platinum concentrations were similar in thin tumour tissue and peritoneum. Addition of irinotecan to oxaliplatin intraperitoneally during HIPEC did not alter its pharmacokinetics.

Compared with the classic cisplatin in a rat model, the AUC in the peritoneal cavity for both total and unfiltrated drug was almost 2 times higher for oxaliplatin than cisplatin after intraperitoneal administration of equimolar doses, while the AUC for oxaliplatin in plasma was a factor of 4 higher than for cisplatin (Los et al. 1990b). These results indicate that peritoneal tumours received a higher exposure from oxaliplatin than cisplatin directly in the peritoneal cavity and indirectly via the systemic circulation. Despite these pharmacological advantages, no significant differences in total platinum concentrations and distribution of platinum in peritoneal tumours were observed. These results suggest a drug penetration depth of 1–2 mm under normothermic conditions, similar to cisplatin. When tumour cells were incubated in vitro with equimolar concentrations of both platinum compounds, 2 to 4 times less platinum uptake was found in cells treated with oxaliplatin. Oxaliplatin was not cross-resistant for cisplatin when tested in a cisplatin-resistant cell line, which may indicate its value in ovarian cancer patients who did not respond to earlier cisplatin treatment (Los et al. 1990b).

In vitro, thermal enhancement of the cytotoxicity and platinum-DNA adduct formation has been observed for oxaliplatin at 41–43°C (Rietbroek et al. 1997a; Urano and Ling 2002; Atallah et al. 2004). In a rat model, hyperthermia at 40–42°C seemed to cause a minor increase in oxaliplatin tissue concentrations (Pestieau et al. 2001). Hyperthermia at 41.5°C significantly increased the tumour growth time in vivo in mice treated with high-dose oxaliplatin. This was not observed for low-dose oxaliplatin (Mohamed et al. 2003a).

5.3 Anthracyclins

5.3.1 Adriamycin

The anthracycline adriamycin, also an antitumour antibiotic, is an attractive agent for intraperitoneal delivery because of its definite activity in ovarian, pancreas and gastric carcinoma, mesothelioma and sarcoma as well as its concentration-effect relation (Alberts et al. 1985). Pharmacokinetics for intraperitoneal adriamycin administration are highly favourable, with a mean or median peritoneal fluid-to-plasma AUC ratio of 162–230 and maximal intraperitoneal drug concentrations an average of 249–474 times higher than in plasma (Ozols et al. 1982; Sugarbaker et al. 1991; Rossi et al. 2002). In a rat model, plasma and peritoneal fluid AUCs under hyperthermic conditions (43°C) were comparable to those under normothermic conditions, but drug concentrations in intra-abdominal tissues were significantly increased by hyperthermia (Jacquet et al. 1998a). In a murine ovarian cancer model, the penetration depth of adriamycin after intraperitoneal administration has been estimated to be only 4–6 cell layers, while drug concentration in free ascites tumour cells was 50 times higher than after intravenous use (Ozols et al. 1979).

In in vitro studies, the intracellular concentration of adriamycin is increased by elevated temperature as the overall result of increase in drug influx with unchanged efflux (Nagaoka et al. 1986; Sakaguchi et al. 1992). A good correlation has been found in vitro between intracellular adriamycin uptake and its cytotoxic effect. Both intracellular uptake and cytotoxicity increased with increasing temperature (39–43°C) and the degree of synergistic effect of the combination of adriamycin and hyperthermia was temperature dependent (Hahn et al. 1975; Nagaoka et al. 1986). Timing of hyperthermia seems of potential importance to the design of optimal schedules for thermochemotherapy. While plasma membrane permeability to adriamycin initially increases during hyperthermia, a decreased permeability has been observed in vitro when duration of hyperthermia exceeds 30 min. This phenomenon was also seen when heat was applied before exposure to adriamycin and lasted for at least 2 to 24 h (Hahn and Strande 1976; Osborne and MacKillop 1987). Another in vitro study supports the concept that adriamycin cytotoxicity may be enhanced at elevated temperatures only when tumours are treated for prolonged time with a large drug dose (Urano et al. 1994). The data from in vivo studies remain inconsistent. Significant thermal enhancement of adriamycin has been demonstrated in some animal models (Hahn et al. 1975; Overgaard 1976; Dahl 1983; Haas et al. 1984; Sakaguchi et al. 1992) but could not be confirmed in other studies (Monge et al. 1988; Urano et al 1994). In one study (Rotstein et al. 1983), a single exposure to adriamycin and hyperthermia (41°C for 30 min) was not effective in decreasing the rate of tumour growth in rat tumour models, while thermal enhancement of adriamycin cytotoxicity was observed after repeated weekly treatments.

In in vitro and in vivo studies on liposome-encapsulated adriamycin, hyperthermia enhanced adriamycin release, increased tumour uptake of liposome-encapsulated adriamycin but did not do so for free adriamycin and enhanced its antitumour efficacy (Ning et al. 1994).

5.3.2 Mitoxantrone

On the basis of its high degree of cytotoxicity against human ovarian cancer, its relative lack of vesicant activity and its in vitro-proven remarkable concentration-response behaviour (Alberts et al. 1985; Link et al. 1998), intraperitoneal chemotherapy with mitoxantrone seems a most promising option for treatment of ovarian cancer. High intraperitoneal and concurrently low plasma drug levels have been measured after intraperitoneal administration of 20–40 mg/m2 mitoxantrone, with a very high mean AUC peritoneal fluid versus plasma ratio of 1,100–1,400 (Alberts et al. 1988; Blochl-Daum et al. 1988; Nagel et al. 1992; Nicoletto et al. 2000). With lower doses the mean pharmacokinetic advantage decreased to 115 (Civalleri et al. 2002). Mitoxantrone is an agent that causes chemical peritonitis at higher dose levels, with abdominal pain being the dose-limiting toxicity. The incidence of sclerosing peritonitis at the long term makes it an attractive agent for palliative treatment of malignant ascites (Link et al. 2003).

Promising data have been reported for intraperitoneal administration of mitoxantrone-loaded microspheres in animal studies (Jameela et al. 1996; Luftensteiner et al. 1999). Lower maximal intraperitoneal and plasma drug concentrations were measured after intraperitoneal administration of microspheres containing mitoxantrone when compared with equal doses of free mitoxantrone, while after 4 h similar drug concentration curves were observed. The intraperitoneal-to-plasma AUC ratios were high (148–211), but lower than for equal doses of conventional mitoxantrone (223–370). However, the maximal tolerable dose was higher, probably because of lower peak concentrations. Slow release of mitoxantrone from the microspheres was associated with higher efficacy and less toxicity (i.e. especially chemical peritonitis) compared with intraperitoneal administration of free mitoxantrone.

Decades ago, significantly increased cytotoxicity of mitoxantrone was observed at an elevated temperature of 42°C for different cell lines in in vitro studies (Herman 1983; Ohnoshi et al. 1985; Juvekar et al. 1986; Wang et al. 1987). More recently, such a thermal enhancement at 42–43°C has been confirmed in vivo in animal models (Wiedemann et al. 1992; Schopman et al. 1996). No data are available for a synergistic effect between mitoxantrone and heat at temperatures lower than 42°C. Interestingly, hyperthermia did not enhance mitoxantrone effectiveness in tumour regrowing after irradiation in a rat model (van Bree et al. 1996b).

5.4 Antimetabolites

5.4.1 Methotrexate

Methotrexate, an antimetabolite, is an older drug effective against colorectal and ovarian cancer. Intraperitoneal infusion results in a mean intraperitoneal-to-plasma concentration ratio of approximately 72 (Goel et al. 1989). In a rat model, while methotrexate pharmacokinetics were relatively independent of dose and dosing mode (i.e. intraperitoneal bolus or infusion drug administration), methotrexate-induced toxicity appeared to be highly dependent on the dosing mode used, with the highest maximal tolerable doses observed for bolus administration (Lobo and Balthasar 2003). Intraperitoneal delivery of a slow-release methotrexate formulation exhibited prolonged intraperitoneal drug levels and increased therapeutic efficacy compared with intraperitoneal administration of the conventional methotrexate (Chatelut et al 1994).

Concomitant systemic administration of anti-methotrexate antibodies has been suggested in an attempt to avoid systemic dose-limiting toxicity. Pharmacokinetic studies in a rat model demonstrated decreased free methotrexate AUC in plasma after intraperitoneal methotrexate administration and concurrent intravenous anti-methotrexate antibody administration, while intraperitoneal drug concentrations and AUC as well as methotrexate absorption from the peritoneal cavity were not altered (Balthasar and Fung 1996). Systemic administration of anti-methotrexate antibodies allowed increases in the maximally tolerated dose of intraperitoneal methotrexate and consequently enhanced the therapeutic efficacy of intraperitoneal methotrexate chemotherapy in a murine model of peritoneal cancer (Lobo and Balthasar 2005). Remarkably, when a very high dose of these antibodies is concurrently systemically administered for a shorter period, its effect is rather agonistic than antagonistic, resulting in enhanced systemic cytotoxicity (Lobo et al. 2003).

Dipyridamole, which enhances the cytotoxicity of many drugs mainly by inhibiting cellular drug efflux, has been simultaneously administered intraperitoneally to obtain selective intraperitoneal biochemical modulation of methotrexate (Goel et al. 1989). Pharmacokinetics of intraperitoneally administered dipyridamole is considerably favourable, with a mean peritoneal-to-plasma concentration ratio of non-protein-bound dipyridamole of more than 2,300. The dose-limiting toxicity of this combination was chemical peritonitis.

Methotrexate is one of the classic agents that exhibits hyperthermic enhancement of its cytotoxicity. In various experimental in vitro and in vivo studies such an effect has evidently been demonstrated (Herman et al. 1981; Monge et al. 1988; Kosmidis et al. 1988; Schopman et al. 1995; Maskaleris et al. 1998). However, as an antimetabolite, methotrexate is not indicated for HIPEC because of the short treatment duration.

5.4.2 5-Fluorouracil and Floxuridine

One of the traditional intraperitoneal agents for gastrointestinal tract cancer is the antimetabolite 5-fluorouracil (5-FU). It has also been used in combination with cisplatin in patients with peritoneal carcinomatosis of gynaecological origin. It is a valuable drug for intraperitoneal use because of its significant cytotoxic effect, which is evidently concentration dependent (Alberts et al. 1985; Link et al. 1998; Jakobsen et al. 2002). Its high rate of metabolism during its passage through the liver after intraperitoneal delivery allows high doses to be administered and results in a most favourable pharmacokinetic profile. After intraperitoneal administration of 5-FU, intraperitoneal drug concentrations were 1,000 times those in serum, while its mean peritoneal fluid-to-plasma AUC ratio was 117–1,400 in human pharmacokinetic studies (Arbuck et al. 1986; Campora et al. 1987; Sugarbaker et al. 1990; Schilsky et al. 1990; Kuzuya et al. 1994; Kerr et al. 1996; Jacquet et al. 1998b). The wide range of mean AUC ratios in the above-mentioned studies are the result of major differences in treatment protocols. These high intraperitoneal drug exposures seem to cause high peritoneal tumour drug uptake, which was much higher than after intravenous administration of 5-FU in a rat model (Mahteme et al. 2004). The very high portal vein 5-FU concentrations after intraperitoneal administration make it also suitable to treat occult or evident liver metastases (Speyer et al. 1981). In a pig model, AUC of 5-FU was almost 6 times higher for regional lymph than for plasma (Lindner et al. 1993), making the intraperitoneal route also attractive for additional treatment of lymphatic spread. When 5-FU was incorporated in microspheres, higher intraperitoneal and local tissue concentrations were obtained in rats than when aqueous 5-FU was administered intraperitoneally (Hagiwara et al. 1996). More importantly, less toxicity and an enhanced therapeutic effect were observed.

Floxuridine (FUDR), an active metabolite of 5-FU, is a unique drug since it is nearly completely absorbed from plasma after a single pass through the liver, suggesting even more advantageous pharmacokinetics than for 5-FU. Mean peritoneal fluid-to-plasma AUC ratios as high as 1,000–2,700 have been reported (Muggia et al. 1991; Israel et al. 1995). Although in a gastric peritoneal carcinomatosis animal model continuous intraperitoneal infusion of FUDR resulted in prolonged high intraperitoneal drug concentrations and appeared to be more effective than bolus administration at equivalent doses, increased toxicity necessitated significant dose reduction and consequently overall no advantage in inhibiting tumour growth could be achieved by continuous infusion (Inoue et al. 2004).

Concurrent reduction of splanchnic blood flow by intravenous administration of vasopressin in an attempt to diminish drug absorption did not increase the pharmacological advantage in an animal model, contrary to its beneficial effect on carboplatin and etoposide pharmacokinetics (Lindner et al. 1996). Leucovorin analogues have been added to the intraperitoneal drug solution to enhance the effect of 5-FU and FUDR. Although their pharmacological advantage was considerable (AUC ratios of 11–39), it is doubtful whether very high intraperitoneal FUDR concentrations require such modulation for optimal cytotoxicity (Israel et al. 1995). Preclinical data suggest that the action of fluoropyrimidines may also be enhanced by the addition of hydroxyurea. Concomitant intravenous administration of hydroxyurea resulted in adequate intraperitoneal concentrations and was well tolerated (Garcia et al. 2001).

In initial reports no thermal enhancement could be demonstrated for 5-FU in vitro and in vivo (Rose et al. 1979; Mini et al. 1986; Monge et al. 1988; Urano et al. 1991; Harada et al. 1995), but recently some synergism between 5-FU and its active metabolite FUDR has been detected in in vivo studies (Maehera et al. 1992; Takemoto et al. 2003). Others examined the effects of hyperthermia (38–42°C) on the metabolism of 5-FU in vitro and observed the highest intracellular concentrations of its active as well as inactive catabolic metabolites at a temperature of 39°C (Maeta et al. 1993). They concluded that the optimal temperature for potentiating the intracellular metabolism of 5-FU is 39°C in vitro. Nevertheless, antimetabolites like 5-FU and FUDR are not indicated for HIPEC because of the short chemotherapy duration time. As discussed above, only direct cytotoxic agents are effective for this treatment modality.

5.4.3 Gemcitabine

Gemcitabine has been shown to possess a broad spectrum of antitumour activity against various malignancies, particularly pancreatic and ovarian cancer. In in vitro studies greater drug exposure is associated with increased cytotoxicity (Ruiz van Haperen et al. 1993). The mean intraperitoneal versus plasma AUC ratio for gemcitabine after intraperitoneal drug administration was only 13–27 in a rat model, while in women with ovarian cancer a mean factor of 791 has been calculated (Pestieau et al. 1998; Sabbatini et al. 2004). Although the combination with hyperthermia did not alter pharmacokinetics, higher intra-abdominal tissue concentrations were obtained under hyperthermic than under normothermic conditions in a rat model (Pestieau et al. 1998). Intraperitoneal chemotherapy with gemcitabine has demonstrated to be effective in a peritoneal carcinomatosis rat model (Ridwelski et al. 2002). An essential adverse effect of this administration route is the cause of significant intra-abdominal adhesions and fibrosis, requiring frequently laparotomy and making its intraperitoneal application in a curative setting less attractive (Sabbatini et al. 2004). However, similar to the case for mitoxantrone, this side-effect may be beneficial for palliative treatment of malignant ascites.

Conflicting results have been reported regarding the combination of gemcitabine and hyperthermia. The timing of hyperthermia may be of importance for gemcitabine. It has been shown both in vitro and in vivo that simultaneous application may result in decreased cytotoxicity of gemcitabine, whereas delayed hyperthermia resulted in significant thermal enhancement (Haveman et al. 1995; van Bree et al. 1999). In another study, cytotoxicity of gemcitabine did not alter under hyperthermic conditions (Hermisson and Weller 2000). However, others demonstrated minor to significant synergism of low and high dose gemcitabine with concomitant hyperthermia, both in vitro and in vivo (Mohamed et al. 2003a; van der Heijden et al. 2005; Vertrees et al. 2005). Nevertheless, being an antimetabolite, it cannot be used for intraoperative chemotherapy.

5.5 Topoisomerase Inhibitors

5.5.1 Irinotecan

Its high activity against gastrointestinal cancer, especially when used in combination with 5-FU, and the fact that dose intensification leads to an increased efficacy (Houghton et al. 1996; Ducreux et al. 2003) make the camptothecin derivate irinotecan a promising drug to be tested for intraperitoneal chemotherapy. Irinotecan is a prodrug that needs to be converted by carboxylesterase to SN-38 to exert its cytotoxic effect as a topoisomerase I inhibitor. The active metabolite is 100- to 1,000-fold more cytotoxic than irinotecan. In malignant ascites converting enzymes seemed to be nearly absent. High concentrations of this enzyme are detectable in the liver, in the gastrointestinal tract as well as locally in human tumours, the latter making it theoretically suitable for intraperitoneal use. Irinotecan has a complicated pharmacologic profile in vivo and one should be aware of a variety of possible interactions (Matsui et al. 2003). Pharmacokinetics of intraperitoneal irinotecan delivery were initially studied in mice (Guichard et al. 1998). The peritoneal-to-plasma drug exposure ratio was 15 for irinotecan and 4 for its active metabolite SN-38. Peritoneal fluid AUC values were significantly higher after intraperitoneal administration than after intravenous injection. It has also been demonstrated that administration by the intraperitoneal route is not only more effective in treating colonic peritoneal carcinomatosis but also less toxic than intravenous administration in animal models (Guichard et al. 1998; Maruyama et al. 1999; Hribaschek et al. 2002, 2006). One must approach these promising data carefully because of the great variability in carboxylesterase activity among species and consequently pharmacokinetics are significantly different in the laboratory animal from that in humans. In one small pharmacokinetic study, only a minor fraction of irinotecan was metabolized in its active form SN-38 intraperitoneally and no pharmacokinetic advantage was observed for simple intraperitoneal delivery of 40–60 mg, suggesting inability of this bio-transformation by cancer cells on peritoneal surfaces (Matsui et al. 2003). On the contrary, others demonstrated SN-38 in the peritoneal fluid immediately after the beginning of a HIPEC procedure with 300-700 mg/m2 irinotecan, suggesting the presence of carboxylesterase in the peritoneal cavity of patients with peritoneal carcinomatosis (Elias et al. 2004). High intraperitoneal irinotecan and SN-38 concentrations were measured during the 30 min of this procedure. Although rapidly absorbed from the peritoneal cavity, the plasma AUC of irinotecan was quite similar to that obtained with intravenous systemic intravenous administration of 350 mg/m2 irinotecan over 30 min. More importantly, the irinotecan concentration in tumour bathed in the perfusate was 16–23 higher than that in non-bathed muscle tissue. Among bathed tissues, drug concentrations in tumour tissue were generally higher than in peritoneum. Tissue concentrations did not increase for doses higher than 400 mg/m2, despite higher peritoneal fluid and plasma concentrations.

Contradicting results regarding synergism between irinotecan and heat have been reported in experimental studies. Absence of a synergetic effect with heat (60 min, 42–43°C) in vitro has been reported (Teicher et al. 1993). Thermal enhancement has been observed by others for low doses of this topoisomerase I inhibitor at 44°C, but impaired cytotoxicity was observed for high dose irinotecan at the same temperature (Kondo et al. 1995). In another in vitro study on the combination of SN-38, the active metabolite of irinotecan, and heat, cytotoxicity was increased at 41.8°C, but not at 40.5°C and 42.5°C (Katschinski and Robins 1999). In vivo, thermal enhancement of irinotecan cytotoxicity has been demonstrated for low and high drug doses at 41.5°C (Mohamed et al. 2003a).

5.5.2 Topotecan

Topotecan, a topoisomerase I inhibitor, is active against ovarian cancer and modulates cytotoxic activity of drugs like melphalan and cisplatin. Intraperitoneal instillation chemotherapy with 5–30 mg/m2 topotecan resulted in a mean peritoneal fluid-to-plasma AUC ratio for total topotecan of 54 (Hofstra et al. 2001). Increased efficacy is anticipated after intraperitoneal delivery because of its dose-effect relation (Houghton et al. 1996).

Published data regarding the combination of heat and topotecan are sparse and conflicting. While topotecan cytotoxicity was not enhanced by hyperthermia (60 min, 42–43°C) in one in vitro study (Teicher et al. 1993), thermal enhancement was demonstrated for some cell lines in another (Hermisson and Weller 2000). No in vivo study on this issue has yet been reported.

5.5.3 Etoposide

Etoposide is a topoisomerase II inhibitor used against many tumours, including gastrointestinal and ovarian cancer. Maximal tolerable doses of up to 700 mg/m2 have been reported in dose-finding studies on intraperitoneal chemotherapy with etoposide, but when administered intraperitoneally in combination with platinum compounds lower doses have been used. Although the mean total etoposide exposure for the peritoneal cavity is reported to be only 1.5–8.8 times greater than that of plasma, the mean peritoneal-to-plasma exposure ratio of unbound etoposide has been calculated to be 35–65 after a single intraperitoneal administration (Zimm et al. 1987; O'Dwyer et al. 1991a, b; McClay et al. 1993). Additionally, AUC in regional lymph has been demonstrated to be twice that of plasma after intraperitoneal administration of etoposide in an animal model (Lindner et al. 1993). In a mouse model, etoposide suspended in oil demonstrated more favourable pharmacokinetics and tissue distribution than an aqueous solution of etoposide after intraperitoneal injection (Lee et al. 1995). Since in vitro studies demonstrated increased cytotoxicity with higher drug concentration and exposure (Wolff et al. 1987), improved efficacy is to be expected after intraperitoneal administration.

Concurrent reduction of splanchnic blood flow by intravenous administration of vasopressin increased the pharmacokinetic advantage of etoposide almost 3 to 5 times in a pig model (Lindner et al. 1996). Dipyridamole is an agent that enhanced etoposide cytotoxicity by a factor of 5.5 in an ovarian carcinoma cell culture model, by increasing intracellular drug concentrations through efflux inhibition (Howell et al. 1989). In a phase I trial dipyridamole has been administered intraperitoneally concurrently with etoposide to achieve selective intraperitoneal cytotoxic enhancement (Isonishi et al. 1991). A 72-h continuous intraperitoneal infusion of maximal 175 mg/m2 etoposide per day in combination with 24 mg/m2 dipyridamole per day was tolerable and led to a constant 30 times higher total etoposide concentration in peritoneal fluid than in plasma. This difference was by a factor of 47–440 for total dipyridamole. While free drug concentrations were high in the peritoneal cavity, neither free etoposide nor free dipyridamole could be detected in plasma.

Thermal enhancement of etoposide cytotoxicity was absent when heat was added simultaneously in in vitro studies, whereas heating the cells many hours before or after drug exposure enhanced cell death (Cohen et al. 1989; Pantazis et al. 1999; van Heek-Romanowski et al. 2001). Since the latter is not achievable intraoperatively, etoposide seems not to be indicated as a chemotherapeutic drug for HIPEC.

5.6 Taxanes

5.6.1 Paclitaxel

The taxanes paclitaxel and docetaxel are novel agents active against ovarian and gastric cancer and mesothelioma that seem to be fascinating drugs for intraperitoneal chemotherapy (de Bree et al. 2006a,b). Several animal and clinical studies have demonstrated highly favourable pharmacokinetics of paclitaxel during intraperitoneal instillation chemotherapy and HIPEC (Markman et al. 1992; Markman 1996; Francis et al. 1995; Hofstra et al. 2001; Fushida et al. 2002a; Mohamed and Sugarbaker 2003a; Mohamed et al. 2003c, d). The maximal paclitaxel concentration is approximately 800–1,000 times higher in the peritoneal cavity than in plasma after intraperitoneal administration. Peak intraperitoneal drug levels are in the micromolar range rather than the nanomolar range as for intravenous administration, while cytotoxic drug levels are generally maintained in the peritoneal cavity for several days. The intraperitoneal-to-plasma AUC ratio varies from 550 to 2,300 in these studies. Since the response to taxanes seems to be dose dependent for systemic chemotherapy (Kohn et al. 1994; Reed et al. 1996; Takimoto and Rowinsky 2003; Omura et al. 2003) increased efficacy is anticipated during intraperitoneal chemotherapy. Moreover, it has been demonstrated that synchronous intravenous administration of drugs suchas cyclophosphamide and carboplatin does not influence pharmacokinetics of intraperitoneally administered paclitaxel (Hofstra et al. 2001).

A recent clinical study (Gelderblom et al. 2002) stressed the importance of the surfactant vehicle Cremophor EL, in which paclitaxel has to be dissolved before its use. Cremophor EL appeared to be largely responsible for the pharmacokinetic advantage of intraperitoneal over intravenous administration of paclitaxel. At high local concentrations, paclitaxel is entrapped in Cremophor EL micelles, leading to prolonged intraperitoneal activity (Sparreboom et al. 1999).

As mentioned previously, besides having high intraperitoneal drug concentrations for a prolonged period of time, it is important to obtain adequate tissue penetration and high target tissue concentrations. Paclitaxel penetrated approximately 40 cell layers in 4 h and more than 80 cell layers in 24 h in an in vitro model (Kuh et al. 1999). In animal models high paclitaxel concentrations were measured in peritoneal tumour nodules and free cancer cells after intraperitoneal drug administration (Innocenti et al. 1995; Mohamed et al 2003d; Ohashi et al. 2005). This resulted in a remarkably high complete remission rate in mice with peritoneal carcinomatosis.

Conflicting results have been reported regarding the interaction of heat and taxanes (de Bree et al. 2006b). Four in vitro studies (Knox et al. 1993; Rietbroek et al. 1997b; Leal et al. 1999; van Bree et al. 2000) and one in vivo experiment (Mohamed et al. 2003a) demonstrated the lack of thermal enhancement at 41.5–43°C for conventional doses of paclitaxel. Results of two of those in vitro studies (Rietbroek et al. 1997b; Leal et al. 1999) indicated that hyperthermia may even exert an adverse effect by inhibiting paclitaxel-related cell cycle effects and cytotoxicity, despite producing higher drug concentrations in heated cells. In the Medical School of Crete we studied the effect of heat on the efficacy of paclitaxel under condition mimicking those during HIPEC (Michalakis et al. 2005, 2006). We observed a synergistic effect in some cell lines after exposing them in vitro to higher drug concentrations (micromolar in stead of nanomolar) at 41.5°C and 43°C for a longer period of time (2 h instead of 30–60 min). Short exposure with micromolar drug concentrations was highly effective to kill tumour cells. Remarkably, while apoptosis is considered to be responsible for cell death at nanomolar concentrations, necrosis was the main cause of cell death in this study with micromolar drug concentrations. Additionally, one other in vitro (Othman et al. 2001) and three in vivo investigations (Sharma et al. 1998; Cividalli et al. 1999, 2000) showed increased cytotoxicity of paclitaxel at a temperature of 43°C when increased local drug concentrations were provided.

5.6.2 Docetaxel

Animal and human studies also revealed very favourable pharmacokinetics for the second taxane, docetaxel (Fushida et al. 2002b; de Bree et al. 2003; Morgan et al. 2003; Mohamed et al. 2003b; Marchetti et al. 2002; Shimada et al. 2003). Similar to paclitaxel, maximal docetaxel concentrations are in the micromolar range after intraperitoneal delivery rather than the nanomolar range as measured after intravenous administration. The peak drug concentration is 45–200 times higher intraperitoneally than in plasma, while the intraperitoneal docetaxel AUC is 150–3,000 higher than that of plasma. Its dose-effect relation in clinical systemic chemotherapy studies makes it an attractive agent for intraperitoneal use (Rowinsky 1997).

As mentioned above, the surfactant vehicles seem to be of significant importance to the pharmacokinetics of taxanes. The taxanes need to be dissolved in these vehicles to overcome their low solubility. The solvent vehicle of paclitaxel is traditionally 4.2% Cremophor EL, while 1.5% Polysorbate-80 is conventionally used for docetaxel. In a rat model, the absorption rate of taxanes after peritoneal administration was strongly influenced, in a concentration-dependent manner, by the surfactant vehicle used (Yokogawa et al. 2004). The intraperitoneal-to-plasma AUC ratio was 3 times lower for docetaxel than for paclitaxel when the conventional vehicles were used. AUC ratios similar to those of paclitaxel were obtained when docetaxel was dissolved in 4.2% Cremophor EL or 7.5% Polysorbate-80.

Most importantly, high tumour tissue concentrations were measured after intraperitoneal docetaxel administration in animal models, resulting in a remarkable response rate especially at higher dose levels (Marchetti et al. 2002; Mohamed et al. 2003b; Yonemura et al. 2004; Shimada et al. 2005).

Two in vitro studies (Rietbroek et al. 1997b; Dumontet et al. 1998) failed to demonstrate increased efficacy of docetaxel at a temperature of 43°C. Recently, thermal enhancement of intraperitoneally administered docetaxel was studied in a murine model for different doses at temperatures of 41.5°C and 43.5°C (Mohamed et al. 2003a, 2004). In the first study, 30 min of moderate hyperthermia increased significantly the cytotoxicity of docetaxel both at low and high doses. Greater heat enhancement was observed when a high dose of docetaxel was administered. In the second study by the same investigators, thermal enhancement was only observed after 90 min of mild hyperthermia. In contrast to their first study, no difference in mean tumour growth time was observed when hyperthermia was applied for 30 min in comparison to administration of docetaxel under normothermic conditions.

5.7 Conclusions and Future Directions

While the rationale for intraperitoneal chemotherapy is well established and its pharmacokinetic advantage is evident, many aspects remain to be investigated, including issues regarding optimal drug choice and dose, the role and degree of hyperthermia, the most adequate carrier solution, appropriate treatment duration and the most favourable type and technique of intraperitoneal chemotherapy. Laboratory studies may be very helpful in solving these issues, since it is practically impossible to study all these parameters in humans. However, extrapolation from results of in vitro studies and animal models to the clinical practice must be done cautiously.

The drug of choice for intravenous administration is not necessarily the one that is most optimal for intraperitoneal chemotherapy. More favourable pharmacokinetics and hyperthermic enhancement may make a systemically less effective drug highly advantageous for intraperitoneal chemotherapy. Furthermore, pharmacological modifications may improve its efficacy, although their definite effectiveness has still to be confirmed in proper studies. Different dissolution of drugs (i.e. in microspheres or surfactant vehicles) and simultaneous intraperitoneal administration of modulators like TNF, vasoconstrictors, vasopressin and dipyridamole may improve drug pharmacokinetics and pharmacodynamics. Concurrent intravenous administration of anti-drug antibodies may allow administration of higher drug doses intraperitoneally, while simultaneous intravenous administration of agents that enhance a certain drug's cytotoxicity may improve treatment efficacy. Moreover, combining intraperitoneal with intravenous chemotherapy may be more effective, the drug penetrating from both the site of the peritoneal surface as well as through the capillary wall into the peritoneal tumour nodules.

Although the classic agents as cisplatin, 5-FU and mitomycin C are still most frequently used for intraperitoneal chemotherapy, newer chemotherapeutic drugs are being administered more and more often. Taxanes, paclitaxel and docetaxel, seem to be extremely promising because of their highly advantageous pharmacokinetic profile and their significant activity against ovarian and gastric cancer and mesothelioma, while oxaliplatin and irinotecan seem to be attractive agents for patients with peritoneal carcinomatosis of gastrointestinal origin.

In conclusion, although intraperitoneal chemotherapy has proven to be effective, as discussed in the following chapters, there seems to be a long way to go to optimize this treatment modality. Research at the laboratory bench with in vitro studies and animal models appears to be of significant importance to success in improving the clinical results at the bedside.

References

Alberts DS, Young L, Mason N, Salmon SE (1985) In vitro evaluation of anticancer drugs against ovarian cancer at concentrations achieved by intraperitoneal administration. Semin Oncol 3 [Suppl 4]:38–42

Alberts DS, Surwit EA, Peng YM et al. (1988) Phase I clinical and pharmacokinetic study of mitoxantrone given to patients by intraperitoneal administration. Cancer Res 48:5874–5877

Atallah D, Marsaud V, Radanyi C et al. (2004) Thermal enhancement of oxaliplatin-induced inhibition of cell proliferation and cell cycle progression in human carcinoma cell lines. Int J Hyperthermia 20:405–419

Baba H, Siddik ZH, Strebel FR et al. (1989) Increased therapeutic gain of combined cis-diamminedichloroplatinum(II) and whole body hyperthermia therapy by optimal heat/drug scheduling. Cancer Res 49:7041–7044

Balthasar JP, Fung H-L (1996) Inverse targeting of peritoneal tumors: selective alteration of the disposition of methotrexate through the use of anti-methotrexate antibodies and antibody fragments. J Pharm Sci 85:1035–1043

Barlogie B, Corry PM, Drewinko B. In vitro thermochemotherapy of human colon cancer cells with cis-dichlordiammineplatinum(II) and Mitomycin C. Cancer Res 40:1165–1168

Bartlett DL, Buell JF, Libutti SK et al. (1998) A phase I trial of continuous hyperthermic peritoneal perfusion with tumor necrosis factor and cisplatin in the treatment of peritoneal carcinomatosis. Cancer 83:1251–1261

Blochl-Daum B, Eichler HG, Rainer H et al. (1988) Escalating dose regimen of intraperitoneal mitoxantrone: phase I study – clinical and pharmacokinetic evaluation. Eur J Cancer Clin Oncol 24:1133–1138

van Bree C, Rietbroek R, Schopman EM et al. (1996a) Local hyperthermia enhances the effect of cis-diamminedichloro-platinum(II) on non-irradiated and pre-irradiated rat solid tumors. Int J Radiat Oncol Biol Phys 36:135–140

van Bree C, Schopman EM, Bakker PJ et al. (1996b) Local hyperthermic treatment does not enhance mitoxantrone effectiveness for responses of a rat model tumour regrowing after irradiation. J Cancer Res Clin Oncol 122:147–153

van Bree C, Beumer C, Rodermond HM et al. (1999) Effectiveness of 2',2'difluorodeoxycytidine (Gemcitabine) combined with hyperthermia in rat R-1 rhabdomyosarcoma in vitro and in vivo. Int J Hyperthermia 15:549–556

van Bree C, Savoneije JH, Franken NA et al. (2000) The effect of p53-function on the sensitivity to paclitaxel with or without hyperthermia in human colorectal carcinoma cells. Int J Oncol 16:739–744

de Bree E, Rosing H, Beijnen JH et al. (2003) Pharmacokinetic study of docetaxel in intraoperative hyperthermic i.p. chemotherapy for ovarian cancer. Anti-Cancer Drugs 14:103–110

de Bree E, Rosing H, Michalakis J et al. (2006a) Intraperitoneal chemotherapy with taxanes for ovarian cancer with peritoneal dissemination. Eur J Surg Oncol (in press)

de Bree E, Theodoropoulos PA, Rosing H et al. (2006b) Treatment of ovarian cancer using intraperitoneal chemotherapy with taxanes: From laboratory bench to bedside. Cancer Treat Rev (in press)

Buell JF, Reed E, Lee KB et al. (1997) Synergistic effect and possible mechanisms of tumor necrosis factor and cisplatin cytotoxicity under moderate hyperthermia against gastric cancer cells. Ann Surg Oncol 4:141–148

Camora E, Esposito M, Civalleri D et al. (1987) Serum, urine and peritoneal fluid levels of 5-FU following intraperitoneal administration. Anticancer Res 7:829–832

Canal P, de Forni M, Chatelut E et al. (1989) Clinical and pharmacokinetic study of intraperitoneal cisplatin at two dose levels: 100 mg/m2 alone or 200 mg/m2 with i.v. thiosulfate. Acta Med Austriaca 16:84–86

Chang E, Alexander HR, Libutti SK et al. (2001) Laparoscopic continuous hyperthermic peritoneal perfusion. J Am Coll Surg 193:225–229

Chatelut E, Suh P, Kim S (1994) Sustained-release methotrexate for intracavitary chemotherapy. J Pharm Sci 83:429–432

Cho HK, Lush RM, Bartlett DL et al. (1999) Pharmacokinetics of cisplatin administered by continuous hyperthermic peritoneal perfusion (CHPP) to patients with peritoneal carcinomatosis. J Clin Pharmacol 39:394–401

Choi EK, Park SR, Lee JH et al. (2003) Induction of apoptosis by carboplatin and hyperthermia alone or combined in WERI human retinoblastoma cells. Int J Hyperthermia 19:431–443

Civalleri D, Vannozzi MO, DeCian F et al. (2002) Intraperitoneal mitoxantrone: a feasibility and pharmacokinetic study. Eur J Surg Oncol 28:172–179

Cividalli A, Cruciani G, Livdi E et al. (1999) Hyperthermia enhances the response of paclitaxel and radiation in a mouse adenocarcinoma. Int J Radiat Oncol Biol Phys 44:407–412

Cividalli A, Livdi E, Ceciarelli F et al. (2000) Hyperthermia and paclitaxel-epirubicin chemotherapy: enhanced cytotoxic effect in a murine mammary adenocarcinoma. Int J Hyperthermia 16:61–71

Cohen JD, Robins HI, Schmitt CL (1989) Tumoricidal interactions of hyperthermia with carboplatin, cisplatin and etoposide. Cancer Lett 44:205–210

Coley WB (1893) The treatment of malignant tumors by repeated inoculations of erysipelas – with a report of ten original cases. Am J Med Sci 105:487–511

Dahl O (1983) Hyperthermic potentiation of doxorubicin and 4'-epi-doxorubicin in a transplantable neurogenic rat tumor (BT4A) in BD IX rats. Int J Radiat Oncol Biol Phys 9:203–207

Douple EB, Strohbehn JW, de Sieyes DC et al. (1982) Therapeutic potentiation of cis-dichlorodiamminep latinum(II) and radiation by interstitial microwave hyperthermia in a mouse tumor. Nat Cancer Inst Monogr 61:259–262

Ducreux M, Kohne CH, Schwartz GK, Vanhoefer U (2003) Irinotecan in metastatic colorectal cancer: dose intensification and combination with new agents, including biological response modifiers. Ann Oncol 14 [Suppl 2]:ii17–ii23

Dumontet C, Bodin F, Michal Y (1998) Potential interactions between antitubulin agents and temperature: implications for modulation of multidrug resistance. Clin Cancer Res 4:1563–1566

Elias D, Bonnay M, Puizillou JM et al. (2002) Heated intraoperative intraperitoneal oxaliplatin after complete resection of peritoneal carcinomatosis: pharmacokinetics and tissue distribution. Ann Oncol 13:267–272

Elias DM, Sideris L (2003) Pharmacokinetics of heated intraoperative intraperitoneal oxaliplatin after complete resection of peritoneal carcinomatosis. Surg Oncol Clin N Am 12:755–769

Elias D, Matsuhisa T, Sideris L et al. (2004) Heated intraoperative intraperitoneal oxaliplatin plus irinotecan after complete resection of peritoneal carcinomatosis: pharmacokinetics, tissue distribution and tolerance. Ann Oncol 1558–1565

Francis P, Rowinsky E, Schneider J et al. (1995) Phase I feasibility and pharmacologic study of weekly paclitaxel: a Gynecologic Oncology Group pilot study. J Clin Oncol 13:2961–2967

Fujimoto S, Shresta RD, Kokubum M et al. (1989) Pharmacokinetic analysis of mitomycin C for intraperitoneal hyperthermic perfusion in patients with far-advanced or recurrent gastric cancer. Reg Cancer Treat 2:198–202

Furukawa T, Kumai K, Kubota T et al. Experimental and clinical studies on the intraperitoneal administration of cis-diamminedichloroplatinum (II) for peritoneal carcinomatosis caused by gastric cancers. Surg Today 23:298–306

Fushida S, Furui N, Kinami S et al. (2002a) [Pharmacologic study of intraperitoneal paclitaxel in gastric cancer with peritoneal dissemination]. Gan To Kagaku Ryoho 29:2164–2167

Fushida S, Nao F, Kinami S et al. (2002b) [Pharmacologic study of intraperitoneal docetaxel in gastric cancer with peritoneal dissemination]. Gan To Kagaku Ryoho 29:1759–1763

Garcia AA, Mugia FM, Spears CP et al. (2001) Phase I and pharmacological study of i.v. hydroxyurea infusion given with i.p. 5-fluoro-2'-deoxyuridine and leucovorin. Anticancer Drugs 12:505–511

Gelderblom H, Verweij J, van Zomeren DM et al. (2002) Influence of Cremophor EL on the bioavailability of intraperitoneal paclitaxel. Clin Cancer Res 8:1237–1241

Glehen O, Stuart OA, Mohamed F, Sugarbaker PH (2004) Hyperthermia modifies pharmacokinetics and tissue distribution of intraperitoneal melphalan in a rat model. Cancer Chemother Pharmacol 54:79–84

Goel R, Cleary SM, Horton C et al. (1989) selective intraperitoneal biochemical modulation of methotrexate by dipyridamole. J Clin Oncol 7:262–269

Guichard S, Chatelut E, Lochon I et al. (1998) Comparison of the pharmacokinetics and efficacy of irinotecan after administration by the intravenous versus intraperitoneal route in mice. Cancer Chemother Pharmacol 42:165–170

Haas GP, Klugo RC, Hetzel FW et al. (1984) The synergistic effect of hyperthermia and chemotherapy on murine transitional cell carcinoma. J Urol 132:828–833

Hagiwara A, Takahashi T, Ueda T et al. (1988) Intraoperative chemotherapy with carbon particles absorbing mitomycin C for gastric cancer with peritoneal dissemination in rabbits. Surgery 104:874–881

Hagiwara A, Takahashi T, Kojima O et al. (1992) Prophylaxis with carbon-absorbed mitomycin against recurrence of gastric cancer. Lancet 339:629–631

Hagiwara A, Takahashi T, Kojima O et al. (1993a) Pharmacologic effects of cisplatin microspheres on peritoneal carcinomatosis in rodents. Cancer 71:844–850

Hagiwara A, Takahashi T, Sawai K et al. (1993b) Clinical trials with intraperitoneal cisplatin microspheres for malignant ascites – a pilot study. Anticancer Drug Des 8:463–470

Hagiwara A, Takahashi T, Sawai K et al. (1996) Pharmacological effects of 5-fluorouracil microspheres on peritoneal carcinomatosis in animals. Br J Cancer 74:1392–1396

Hahn GM, Braun J, Har-Kedar I (1975) Thermochemotherapy: synergism between hyperthermia (42–43°) and adriamycin (or bleomycin) in mammalian cell inactivation. Proc Natl Acad Sci USA 72:937–940

Hahn GM, Strande DP (1976) Cytotoxic effects of hyperthermia and adriamycin on Chinese hamster cells. J Natl Cancer Inst 57:1063–1067

Harada S, Ping L, Obara T et al. (1995) The antitumor effect of hyperthermia combined with fluorouracil and its analogues. Radiat Res 142:232–241

Haveman J, Rietbroek RC, Geerdink A et al. (1995) effect of hyperthermia on the cytotoxicity of 2',2'-difluorodeoxycytidine (gemcitabine) in cultured SW1573 cells. Int J Cancer 62:627–630

Hazen G, Ben-Hur E, Yerushalmi A (1981) Synergism between hyperthermia and cyclophosphamide in vivo: the effect of dose fractionation. Eur J Cancer 17:681–684

van Heek-Romanowski R, Putter S, Trarbach T, Kremens B (2001) Etoposide toxicity on human neuroblastoma cells in vitro is enhanced by preceding hyperthermia. Med Pediatr Oncol 36:197–198

van der Heijden AG, Verhaegh G, Jansen CFJ et al. (2005) Effect of hyperthermia on the cytotoxicity of 4 chemotherapeutic agents currently used for the treatment of transitional cell carcinoma of the bladder: an in vitro study. J Urol 173:1375–1380

Herman TS, Cress AE, Sweets C, Gerner EW (1981) Reversal of resistance to methotrexate by hyperthermia in Chinese hamster ovary cells. Cancer Res 41:3840–3843

Herman TS (1983) Effect of temperature on the cytoxicity of videstine, amsarcina, and mitoxantrone. Cancer Treat Rep 67:1019–1022

Herman TS, Teicher BA, Chan V et al. (1988) Effect of hyperthermia on the action of cis-diamminidichloroplatinum (II), Rhodamine 1232 [tetrachloroplatinum (II)], Rhodamine 123, and potassium tetrachloroplatinate in vitro and in vivo. Cancer Res 48:2335–2341

Hermisson M, Weller M (2000) Hyperthermia enhanced chemosensitivity of human malignant glioma cells. Anticancer Res 20:1819–1823

Hofstra LS, Bos AM, Vries EG et al. (2001) A phase I and pharmacokinetic study of intraperitoneal topotecan. Br J Cancer 85:1627–1633

Honess DJ, Bleehen NM (1982) Sensitivity on normal mouse marrow and RIF-1 tumor to hyperthermia combined with cyclophosphamide or BCNU: a lack of therapeutic gain. Br J Cancer 46:236–248

Honess DJ, Bleehen NM (1985) Thermochemotherapy with cisplatinum, CCNU, BCNU, clorambucil and melphalan on murine marrow and two tumours: therapeutic gain for melphalan only. Br J Radiol 58:63–72

Houghton PJ, Stewart CF, Zamboni WC et al. (1996) Schedule-dependent efficacy of camptothecins in models of human cancer. Ann NY Acad Sci 803:188–201

Howell SB, Pfeifle CL, Wung WE et al. (1982) Intraperitoneal cisplatin with systemic thiosulfate protection. Ann Intern Med 97:845–851

Howell SB, Pfeifle CE, Olshen RA (1984) Intraperitoneal chemotherapy with melphalan. Ann Intern Med 101:14–18

Howell SB, Hom DK, Sanga R et al. (1989) Dipyridamole enhancement of etoposide sensitivity. Cancer Res 49:3178–3183

Hribaschek A, Pross M, Kuhn R et al. (2002) Prevention and treatment of peritoneal carcinomatosis in experimental investigations with CPT-11 and oxaliplatin. Anti-Cancer Drugs 13:605–614

Hribaschek A, Kuhn R, Pross M et al. (2006) Intraperitoneal versus intravenous CPT-11 given intra- and postoperatively for peritoneal carcinomatosis in a rat model. Surg Today 36:57–62

Inoue K, Onishi H, Kato Y et al. (2004) Comparison of intraperitoneal continuous infusion of Floxuridine and bolus administration in a peritoneal gastric cancer xenograft model. Cancer Chemother Pharmacol 53:415–422

Innocenti F, Danesi R, Di Paolo A et al. (1995) Plasma and tissue disposition of paclitaxel (taxol) after intraperitoneal administration in mice. Drug Metab Dispos 23:713–717

Israel VK, Jiang C, Muggia FM et al. (1995) Intraperitoneal 5-fluoro-2'-deoxyuridine (FUDR) and (S)-leucovorin for disease predominantly confined to the peritoneal cavity: a pharmacokinetic and toxicity study. Cancer Chemother Pharmacol 37:32–38

Isonishi S, Kirmani S, Kim S et al. (1991) Phase I and pharmacokinetic trial of intraperitoneal etoposide in combination with the multi-drug-resistance-modulating agent dipyridamole. J Natl Cancer Inst 83:621–626

Jacquet P, Averbach A, Stuart OA et al. (1998a) Hyperthermic intraperitoneal doxorubicin: pharmacokinetics, metabolism, and tissue distribution in a rat model. Cancer Chemother Pharmacol 41:147–154

Jacquet P, Averbach A, Stephens AD et al. (1998b) Heated intraoperative intraperitoneal mitomycin C and early postoperative intraperitoneal 5-fluorouracil: pharmacokinetic studies. Oncology 55:130–138

Jakobsen A, Berglund A, Glimelius B et al. (2002) Dose-effect relationship of bolus 5-fluorouracil in the treatment of advanced colorectal cancer. Acta Oncol 41:525–531

Jameela SR, Latha PG, Subramoniam A, Jayakrishnan A (1996) Antitumour activity of mitoxantrone-loaded chitosan microspheres against Ehrlich carcinoma. J Pharm Pharmacol 48:658–688

Juvekar AS, Chitnis MP, Adwankar MK, Advani SH (1986) Effect of mitoxantrone on human chronic myeloid leukemia cells in vitro, combined with hyperthermia. Neoplasma 33:477–482

Katschinski DM, Robins HI (1999) Hyperthermic modulation of SN-38 induced topoisomerase 1 DNA crosslinking and SN-38 cytotoxicity through altered topoisomerase I activity. Int J Cancer 80:104–109

Kerr DJ, Young AM, Neoptolemos JP et al. (1996) Prolonged intraperitoneal infusion of 5-fluoruracil using a novel carrier solution. Br J Cancer 74:2032–2035

Knox JD, Mitchel RE, Brown DL (1993) Effects of taxol and taxol/hyperthermia treatments on the functional polarization of cytotoxic T lymphocytes. Cell Motil Cytoskeleton 24:129–138

Kohn EC, Sarosy G, Bicher A et al. (1994) Dose-intense taxol: high response rate in patients with platinum-resistant recurrent ovarian cancer. J Natl Cancer Inst 86:18–24

Kondo T, Ueda K, Kano E (1995) Combined effects of hyperthermia and CPT-11 on DNA strand breaks in mouse mammary carcinoma FM3A cells. Anticancer Res 15:83–86

Kosmidis PA, Uzunoglou N, Elemenoglou J, Kottaridis S (1988) Combination of hyperthermia and methotrexate in the treatment of transplanted Walker sarcoma. Chemioterapia 7:184–188

Kuh H-J, Jang S, Wientjes JM et al. (1999) Determinants of paclitaxel penetration and accumulation in human solid tumor. J Pharmacol Exper Ther 290:871–880

Kuroda M, Urano M, Reynolds R (1997) Thermal enhancement of the effect of ifosfamide against a spontaneous murine fibrosarcoma, FSa-II. Int J Hyperthermia 13:125–131

Kusumoto T, Holden SA, Ara G, Teicher BA (1995) Hyperthermia and platinum complexes: time between treatments and synergy in vitro and in vivo. Int J Hyperthermia 11:575–586

Kutz ME, Mulkerin DL, Wiedemann GJ et al. (1997) In vitro studies of the hyperthermic enhancement of activated ifosfamide (4-hydroperoxy-ifosfamide) and glucose isophosphoramide mustard. Cancer Chemother Pharmacol 40: 167–171

Kuzuya T, Yamauchi M, Ito A et al. (1994) Pharmacokinetic characteristics of 5-fluorouracil and mitomycin C in intraperitoneal chemotherapy. J Pharm Pharmacol 46:685–689

Leal BZ, Meltz ML, Mohan N, Kuhn J, Prihoda TJ, Herman TS (1999) Interaction of hyperthermia with Taxol in human MCF-7 breast adenocarcinoma cells. Int J Hyperthermia 15:225–236

Lee JS, Takahashi T, Hagiwara A et al. (1995) Safety and efficacy of intraperitoneal injection of etoposide in oil suspension in mice with peritoneal carcinomatosis. Cancer Chemother Pharmacol 36:211–216

de Lima Vazquez V, Stuart OA, Mohamed F, Sugarbaker PH (2003) Extent of parietal peritonectomy does not change intraperitoneal chemotherapy pharmacokinetics. Cancer Chemother Pharmacol 52:108–112

Lindegaard J, Radacic M, Khalil AA et al. (1992) Cisplatin and hyperthermia treatment of a CH3 mammary carcinoma in vivo. Acta Oncol 31:347–351

Lindner P, Heath DD, Shalinsky DR et al. (1993) regional lymphatic drug exposure following intraperitoneal administration of 5-fluorouracil, carboplatin, and etoposide. Surg Oncol 2:105–112

Lindner P, Heath DD, Howell SB et al. (1996) Vasopressin modulation of peritoneal, lymphatic, and plasma drug exposure following intraperitoneal administration. Clin Cancer Res 2:311–317

Link KH, Leder G, Pillasch J et al. (1998) In vitro concentration response studies and in vitro phase II tests as the experimental basis for regional chemotherapeutic protocols. Semin Surg Oncol 14:189–201

Link KH, Roitman M, Holtappels M et al. (2003) Intraperitoneal chemotherapy with mitoxantrone in malignant ascites. Surg Oncol Clin N Am 12:865–872

Lobo ED, Balthasar JP (2003) Pharmacokinetic-pharmacodynamic modelling of methotrexate-induced toxicity in mice. J Pharm Sci 92:1654–1664

Lobo ED, Soda DM, Balthasar JP (2003) Application of pharmacokinetic-pharmacodynamic modelling to predict the kinetic and dynamic effects of anti-methotrexate antibodies in mice. J Pharm Sci 92:1665–1672

Lobo ED, Balthasar JP (2005) Application of anti-methotrexate Fab fragments for the optimization of intraperitoneal methotrexate therapy in a murine model of peritoneal cancer. J Pharm Sci 94:1957–1964

Los G, Mutsaerts PH, Lenglet WJ et al. (1990a) Platinum distribution in intraperitoneal tumors after intraperitoneal cisplatin treatment. Cancer Chemother Pharmacol 25:389–394

Los G, Mutsaerts PH, Ruevekamp M, McVie JG (1990b) The use of oxaliplatin versus cisplatin in intraperitoneal chemotherapy in cancers restricted to the peritoneal cavity in the rat. Cancer Lett 51:109–117

Los G, Verdegaal EM, Mutsaers PH, McVie JG (1991a) Penetration of carboplatin and cisplatin into rat peritoneal tumor nodules after intraperitoneal chemotherapy. Cancer Chemother Pharmacol 28:159–165

Los G, Sminia P, Wondergem J et al. (1991b) Optimisation of intraperitoneal cisplatin therapy with regional hyperthermia in rats. Eur J Cancer 27:472–477

Los G, van Vugt MJH, den Engelse L, Pinedo HM (1993) Effects of temperature on the interaction of cisplatin and carboplatin with cellular DNA. Biochem Pharmacol 46:1229–1237

Los G, van Vugt MJH, Pinedo HM (1994) Response of peritoneal solid tumours after intraperitoneal chemohyperthermia treatment with cisplatin and carboplatin. Br J Cancer 69:235–241

Luftensteiner CP, Schwendenwein I, Paul B et al. (1999) Evaluation of mitoxantrone-loaded albumin microspheres following intraperitoneal administration to rats. J Control Release 57:35–44

Ma GY, Bartlett DL, Reed E et al. (1997) Continuous hyperthermic peritoneal perfusion with cisplatin for the treatment of peritoneal mesothelioma. Cancer J Sci Am 3:174–179

Maehera Y, Sakaguchi Y, Takahashi I et al. (1992) 5-Fluorouracil's cytotoxicity is enhanced both in vitro and in vivo by concomitant treatment with hyperthermia and dipyridamole. Cancer Chemother Pharmacol 29:257–260

Maeta M, Sawata T, Kaibara N (1993) Effects of hyperthermia on the metabolism of 5-fluorouracil in vitro. Int J Hyperthermia 9:105–113

Mahteme H, Larsson B, Sundin A et al. (2004) Uptake of 5-fluorouracil (5-FU) in peritoneal metastases in relation to the route of drug administration and tumour debulking surgery. An autoradiography study in the rat. Eur J Cancer 40:142–147

Marchetti P, Stuart OA, Mohamed F et al. (2002) Docetaxel: pharmacokinetics and tissue levels after intraperitoneal and intravenous administration in a rat model. Cancer Chemother Pharmacol 49:499–503

Markman M, Cleary S, Howell SB (1985) Nephrotoxicity of high-dose intracavitary cisplatin with intravenous thiosulphate protection. Eur J Cancer Clin Oncol 21:1015–1018

Markman M, Rowinsky E, Hakes T et al. (1992) Phase I trial of intraperitoneal taxol: a Gynecologic Oncology Group study. J Clin Oncol 10:1485–1491

Markman M (1996) Intraperitoneal Taxol. Cancer Treat Res 81:1–5

Maruyama M, Nagahama T, Yuasa Y (1999) Intraperitoneal versus intravenous CPT-11 for peritoneal seeding and liver metastasis. Anticancer Res 19:4187–4191

Maskaleris T, Lialiaris T, Triantaphyllidis C (1998) Induction of cytogenetic damage in human lymphocytes in vitro and of antineoplastic effects in Ehrlich ascites tumor cells in vivo treated by methotrexate, hyperthermia and/or caffeine. Mutat Res 422:229–236

Matsui A, Okuda M, Tsujitsuka K et al. (2003) Pharmacology of intraperitoneal CPT-11. Surg Oncol Clin N Am 12:795–811

McClay EF, Goel R, Andrews P et al. (1993) A phase I and pharmacokinetic study on intraperitoneal carboplatin and etoposide. Br J Cancer 68:783–788

Mella O (1985) Combined hyperthermia and cis-diamminedichloroplatinum in BD IX rats with transplanted BT4A tumours. Int J Hyperthermia 1:171–184

Michalakis J, Georgatos SD, Romanos J et al. (2005) Micromolar taxol, with or without hyperthermia, induces mitotic catastrophe and cell necrosis in HeLa cells. Cancer Chemother Pharmacol 56:615–622

Michalakis J, Georgatos SD, de Bree E et al. (2006) Short term exposure of cancer cells to micromolar doses of paclitaxel, with or without hyperthermia, induces long term inhibition of cell proliferation and cell death in vitro. Ann Surg Oncol (in press)

Mini E, Dombrowski J, Moroson BA, Bertino JR (1986) Cytotoxic effects of hyperthermia, 5-fluorouracil and their combination on a human leukemia T-lymphoblast cell line, CCRF-CEM. Eur J Cancer Clin Oncol 22:927–934

Miyagi Y, Fujiwara K, Kigawa J et al. (2005) Intraperitoneal carboplatin infusion may be a pharmacologically more reasonable route than intravenous administration as a systemic chemotherapy. A comparative pharmacokinetic analysis of platinum using a new mathematical model after intraperitoneal vs. intravenous infusion of carboplatin – a Sankai Gynecology Study Group (SGSG) study. Gynecol Oncol 99:591–596

Mohamed F, Sugarbaker PH (2003a) Intraperitoneal taxanes. Surg Oncol Clin N Am 12: 825–833

Mohamed F, Marchettini P, Stuart OA et al. (2003a) Thermal enhancement of new chemotherapeutic agents at moderate hyperthermia. Ann Surg Oncol 10:463–468

Mohamed F, Marchettini P, Stuart OA, Sugarbaker PH (2003b) Pharmacokinetics and tissue distribution of intraperitoneal docetaxel with different carrier solutions. J Surg Res 113:114–120

Mohamed F, Marchettini P, Stuart OA et al. (2003c) A comparison of hetastarch and peritoneal dialysis solution for intraperitoneal chemotherapy delivery. Eur J Surg Oncol 29:261–265

Mohamed F, Marchetti P, Stuart OA, Sugarbaker PH (2003d) Pharmacokinetics and tissue distribution of intraperitoneal paclitaxel with different carrier solutions. Cancer Chemother Pharmacol 52:405–410

Mohamed F, Stuart OA, Glehen O et al. (2004) Docetaxel and hyperthermia: factors that modify thermal enhancement. J Surg Oncol 88:14–20

Monge OR, Rofstad EK, Kaalhus O (1988) Thermochemotherapy in vivo of a C3H mouse mammary carcinoma: single fraction heat and drug treatment. Eur J Cancer Clin Oncol 24:1661–1669

Morgan RJ, Doroshow JH, Synold T et al. (2003) Phase I trial of intraperitoneal docetaxel in the treatment of advanced malignancies primarily confined to the peritoneal cavity. Clin Cancer Res 9:5896–5901

Muggia FM, Chan KK, Russell C et al. (1991) Phase\I and pharmacological evaluation of intraperitoneal 5-fluoro-2'-deoxyuridine. Cancer Chemother Pharmacol 28:241

Murray TG, Cicciarelli N, McCabe CM et al. (1997) In vitro efficacy of carboplatin and hyperthermia in a murine retinoblastoma cell line. Invest Ophtahalmol Vis Sci 38:2516–2522

Nagaoka S, Kawasaki S, Sasaki K, Nakanishi T (1986) Intracellular uptake, retention and cytotoxic effect of adriamycin combined with hyperthermia in vitro. Jpn J Cancer Res 77:205–211

Nagel JD, Varossieau FJ, Dubbelman R et al. (1992) Clinical pharmacokinetics of mitoxantrone after intraperitoneal administration. Cancer Chemother Pharmacol 29:480–484

Nicoletto MO, Padrini R, Galeotti F et al. (2000) Pharmacokinetics of intraperitoneal hyperthermic perfusion with mitoxantrone in ovarian cancer. Cancer Chemother Pharmacol 45:457–462

Ning S, Macleod K, Abra RM et al. (1994) Hyperthermia induces doxorubicin release from long-circulating liposomes and enhances their anti-tumor efficacy. Int J Radiat Oncol Biol Phys 29:827–834

Nishimura Y, Ono K, Hiraoka M et al. (1990) Treatment of murine SCC VII tumors with localized hyperthermia and temperature-sensitive liposomes containing cisplatin. Radiat Res 122:161–167

O'Dwyer PJ, LaCreta F, Hogan M et al. (1991a) Pharmacokinetic study of etoposide and cisplatin by the intraperitoneal route. J Clin Pharmacol 31:253–258

O'Dwyer PJ, LaCreta F, Daugherty JP et al. (1991b) Phase I pharmacokinetic study of intraperitoneal etoposide. Cancer Res 51:2041–2046

Ohashi N, Kodera Y, Nakanishi H et al. (2005) Efficacy of intraperitoneal chemotherapy with paclitaxel targeting peritoneal micrometastases as revealed by GFP-tagged human gastric cancer cell lines in nude mice. Int J Oncol 27:637–644

Ohnoshi T, Ohnuma T, Beranek JT, Holland JF (1985) Combined cytotoxicity effect of hyperthermia and anthracycline antibiotics on human tumor cells. J Natl Cancer Inst 74:275–281

Omura GA, Brady MF, Look KY et al. (2003) Phase III trial of paclitaxel at two dose levels, the higher dose accompanied by filgrastim at two dose levels in platinum-pretreated epithelial ovarian cancer: an Intergroup study. J Clin Oncol 21:2843–2848

Osborne EJ, MacKillop WJ (1987) The effect of exposure to elevated temperatures on membrane permeability to adriamycin in Chinese hamster ovary cells in vitro. Cancer Lett 37:213–224

Othman T, Goto S, Lee JB, Taimura A et al. (2001) Hyperthermic enhancement of the apoptotic and antiproliferative activities of paclitaxel. Pharmacology 62:208–212

Overgaard J (1976) Combined adriamycin and hyperthermia treatment of a murine mammary carcinoma in vivo. Cancer Res 36:3077–3081

Ozols RF, Young RC, Speyer JL et al. (1982) Phase I and pharmacological studies of adriamycin administered intraperitoneally to patients with ovarian cancer. Cancer Res 42:4265–4269

Ozols RF, Locker GY, Doroshow JH et al. (1979) Pharmacokinetics of adriamycin and tissue penetration in murine ovarian cancer. Cancer Res 39:3209–3214

Pantazis P, Han Z, Wyche J (1999) Schedule-dependent efficiency of thermochemotherapy in vitro with etoposide and heating at 43 degree C. Anticancer Res 19:995–998

Panteix G, Guillaumont M, Cherpin L et al. (1993) Study of the pharmacokinetics of mitomycin C in humans during intraperitoneal chemohyperthermia with special mention of the concentration in local tissues. Oncology 50:366–370

Pestieau SR, Stuart OA, Chang D et al. (1998) Pharmacokinetics of intraperitoneal gemcitabine in a rat model. Tumori 84:706–711

Pestieau SR, Belliveau JF, Griffin H et al. (2001) Pharmacokinetics of intraperitoneal oxaliplatin: experimental studies. J Surg Oncol 76:106–114

Piccart MJ, Abrams J, Dodion PF et al. (1988) Intraperitoneal chemotherapy with cisplatin and melphalan. J Natl Cancer Inst 80:1118–1124

Reed E, Bitton R, Sarosy G, Kohn E (1996) Paclitaxel dose intensity. J Infus Chemother 6:59–63

Ridwelski K, Meyer F, Hribaschek A et al. (2002) Intraoperative and early postoperative chemotherapy into the abdominal cavity using gemcitabine may prevent postoperative occurrence of peritoneal carcinomatosis. J Surg Oncol 79:10–16

Rietbroek RC, van der Vaart PJ, Haveman J et al. (1997a) Hyperthermia enhances the cytotoxicity and platinum-DNA adduct formation of lobaplatin and oxaliplatin in cultured SW 1573 cells. J Cancer Res Clin Oncol 123:6–12

Rietbroek RC, Katschinski DM, Reijers MH et al. (1997b) Lack of thermal enhancement for taxanes in vitro. Int J Hyperthermia 13:525–533

Rose WC, Veras GH, Laster WR, Schabel FM Jr (1979) Evaluation of whole-body hyperthermia as an adjunct to chemotherapy in murine tumors. Cancer Treat Rep 63:1311–1325

Rossi C, Foletto M, Mocellin S et al. (2002) Hyperthermic intraoperative intraperitoneal chemotherapy with cisplatin and doxorubicin in patients who undergo cytoreductive surgery for carcinomatosis and sarcomatosis. Cancer 94:492–499

Rotstein LE, Daly J, Rozsa P (1983) Systemic thermochemotherapy in a rat model. Can J Surg 26:113–116

Rowinsky EK (1997) The taxanes: dosing and schedule considerations. Oncology 11:7–19

Royer B, Guardiola E, Polycarpe E et al. (2005) Serum and intraperitoneal pharmacokinetics of cisplatin within intraoperative intraperitoneal chemotherapy: influence of protein binding. Anti-Cancer Drugs 16:1009–1016

Ruiz van Haperen VW, Veerman G, Vermorken JB, Peters GJ (1993) 2',2'-Difluoro-deoxycytidine (gemcitabine) incorporation into RNA and DNA of tumour cell lines. Biochem Pharmacol 46:762–766

van Ruth S, Verwaal VJ, Zoetmulder FAN (2003b) Pharmacokinetics of intraperitoneal mitomycin C. Surg Oncol Clin N Am 12:771–780

Sabbatini P, Aghajanian C, Leitao M et al. (2004) Intraperitoneal cisplatin with intraperitoneal gemcitabine in patients with epithelial ovarian cancer: results of a phase I/II trial. Clin Cancer Res 10:2962–2967

Sakaguchi Y, Maehera Y, Emi Y et al. (1992) Adriamycin combined with hyperthermia and dipyridamole is cytotoxic both in vitro and in vivo. Eur Surg Res 24:249–256

Schem BC, Mella O, Dahl O (1992) Thermochemotherapy with cisplatin or carboplatin in the BT4 rat glioma in vitro and in vivo. Int J Radiat Biol Phys 23:109–114

Schilsky RL, Choi KE, Grimmer D et al. (1990) Phase I clinical and pharmacologic study of intraperitoneal cisplatin and fluorouracil in patients with advanced intraabdominal cancer. J Clin Oncol 8:2054–2061

Schopman EM, van Bree C, Kipp JB, Barendsen GW (1995) Enhancement of the effectiveness of methotrexate for the treatment of solid tumours by application of local hyperthermia. Int J Hyperthermia 11:561–573

Schopman EM, van Bree C, Bakker PJ et al. (1996) Hyperthermia-enhanced effectiveness of mitoxantrone in an experimental rat model. Int J Hyperthermia 12:241–254

Sharma D, Chelvi TP, Kaur J, Ralhan R (1998) Thermosensitive liposomal taxol formulation: heat-mediated targeted drug delivery in murine melanoma. Melanoma Res 8:240–244

Shimada T, Nomura M, Yokogawa K et al. (2005) Pharmacokinetic advantage of intraperitoneal injection of docetaxel in the treatment for peritoneal dissemination of cancer in mice. J Pharm Pharmacol 57:177–181

Sparreboom A, van Zuylen L, Brouwer E et al. (1999) CremophorEL-mediated alteration of paclitaxel distribution in human blood: clinical pharmacokinetic implications. Cancer Res 59:1454–1457

Speyer JL, Sugarbaker PH, Collins JM et al. (1981) Portal levels and hepatic clearance of 5-fluorouracil after intraperitoneal administration in humans. Cancer Res 41:1916–1922

Stojkovic R, Radacic M (2002) Cell killing of melanoma B16 in vivo by hyperthermia and cytotoxins. Int J Hyperthermia 18:62–71

Storm FK (1989) Clinical hyperthermia and chemotherapy. Radiol Clin N Am 27:621–627

Sugarbaker PH, Graves T, DeBruijn EA et al. (1990) Early postoperative intraperitoneal chemotherapy as an adjuvant therapy to surgery for peritoneal carcinomastosis from gastrointestinal cancer: pharmacological studies. Cancer Res 50:5790–5794

Sugarbaker PH, Sweatman TW, Graves T et al. (1991) Early postoperative intraperitoneal adriamycin. Pharmacological studies and preliminary clinical report. Reg Cancer Treat 4:127–131

Sugarbaker PH, Torres Mora J, Carmignani P et al. (2005) Update on chemotherapeutic agents utilized for perioperative intraperitoneal chemotherapy. Oncologist 10:112–122

Takemoto M, Kuroda M, Urano M et al. (2003) The effect of various chemotherapeutic agents given at mild hyperthermia on different types of tumours. Int J Hyperthermia 19:193–203

Takimoto CH, Rowinsky EK (2003) Dose-intense paclitaxel: déjà vu all over again? J Clin Oncol 21:2810–2814

Teicher BA, Holden SA, Khanadakar V, Herman TS (1993) Addition of topoisomerase I inhibitor to trimodality therapy [cis-diamminedichloroplatinum(II)/heat/radiation] in a murine tumor. J Cancer Res Clin Oncol 119:645–651

Urano M, Begley J, Reynolds R (1994) Interaction between adriamycin cytotoxicity and hyperthermia: growth-phase-dependent thermal sensitization. Int J Hyperthermia 10:817–826

Urano M, Kim M, Kahn J et al. (1985) Effect of thermochemotherapy (combined cyclophosphamide and hyperthermia) given at various temperatures with or without glucose administration on a murine fibrosarcoma. Cancer Res 45:4162–4166

Urano M, Kahn J, Kenton LA (1990) The effect of cisd iamminedichloroplatinum(II) treatment at elevated temperatures on murine fibrosarcoma, FSa-II. Int J Hyperthermia 6:563–570

Urano M, Kahn J, Reynolds R (1991) The effect of 5-fluorouracil at elevated temperatures on a spontaneous mouse tumour: Arrhenius analysis and tumour response. Int J Radiat Biol 59:239–249

Urano M, Wong K-H, Reynolds R, Begley J (1995) The advantageous use of hypoxic tumor cells in cancer therapy: identical chemosensitization by metronidazole and misonidazole at moderately elevated temperatures. Int J Hyperthermia 11:379–388

Urano M, Kuroda M, Nishimura Y (1999) For the clinical application of thermochemotherapy given at mild temperatures. Int J Hyperthermia 15:79–107

Urano M, Ling CC (2002) Thermal enhancement of melphalan and oxaliplatin cytotoxicity in vitro. Int J Hyperthermia 18:307–315

van der Vaart PJM, van der Vange N, Zoetmulder FAN et al. (1998) Intraperitoneal cisplatin with regional hyperthermia in advanced ovarian cancer: pharmokinetics and cisplatin-DNA adduct formation in patients and ovarian cancer cell lines. Eur J Cancer 34:148–154

Vertrees RA, Das GC, Popov VL et al. PJ (2005) Synergistic interaction of hyperthermia and gemcitabine in lung cancer. Cancer Biol Ther 4:1144–1153

Wang BS, Lumanglas AL, Silva J et al. (1987) Cancer Treat Rep 71:831–836

Wiedemann G, Mella O, Roszinski S et al. (1992) Hyperthermia enhances mitoxantrone cytotoxicity on human breast carcinoma and sarcoma xenografts in nude mice. Int J Radiat Oncol Biol Phys 24:669–673

Wientjes MG, Dalton JT, Badalament RA et al. (1991) Bladder wall penetration of intravesical mitomycin C in dogs. Cancer Res 51:4347–4354

Wolff SN, Grosh WW, Prater K, Hande KR (1987) In vitro pharmacodynamic evaluation of VP-16–213 and implications for chemotherapy. Cancer Chemother Pharmacol 19:246–249

Xu MJ, Alberts DS (1988) Potentiation of platinum analogue cytotoxicity by hyperthermia. Cancer Chemother Pharmacol 21:191–196

Yokogawa K, Jin M, Furui N et al. (2004) Disposition kinetics of taxanes after intraperitoneal administration in rats and influence of surfactant vehicles. J Pharm Pharmacol 56:629–634

Yonemura Y, Endou Y, Bando E et al. (2004) Effect of intraperitoneal administration of docetaxel on peritoneal dissemination of gastric cancer. Cancer Lett 210:189–196

Zakris EL, Dewhirst MW, Riviere JE et al. (1987) Pharmacokinetics and toxicity of intraperitoneal cisplatin combined with regional hyperthermia. J Clin Oncol 5:1613–1620

Zeamari S, Floot B, van der Vange N, Stewart FA (2003) Pharmacokinetics and pharmacodynamics of cisplatin after intraoperative hyperthermic intraperitoneal chemoperfusion (HIPEC). Anticancer Res 23:1643–1648

Zimm S, Cleary SM, Lucas WE et al. (1987) Phase I/pharmacokinetic study of intraperitoneal cisplatin and etoposide. Cancer Res 47:1712–1716

6 Technology for the Delivery of Hyperthermic Intraoperative Intraperitoneal Chemotherapy: A Survey of Techniques

Amod A. Sarnaik, Jeffrey J. Sussman, Syed A. Ahmad, Benjamin C. McIntyre, Andrew M. Lowy

Recent Results in Cancer Research, Vol. 169
© Springer-Verlag Berlin Heidelberg 2007

6.1 Introduction

The management of peritoneal metastases remains one of the most challenging problems in clinical oncology. Over the last decade, interest in the use of aggressive cytoreductive surgery combined with intraoperative hyperthermic intraperitoneal chemotherapy (HIPEC) has increased. This interest has been fueled by data from single institutions and collected series demonstrating long-term survival for selected patients with peritoneal surface metastases treated with this combined modality approach. Along with the availability of new cytotoxic and biological therapies for gastrointestinal cancers, recent data demonstrating the value of intraperitoneal therapy for ovarian cancer have provided new energy to investigations of HIPEC. Despite the proliferation of single-institution studies, there has been only a single large randomized study of HIPEC in colon carcinoma.

There are theoretical advantages to the administration of intraperitoneal over systemic chemotherapy. Because of the peritoneal-plasma barrier, intraperitoneal administration of chemotherapy results in intraperitoneal levels that are 20–600 times higher than plasma levels (Elias et al. 1994). The resulting increased therapeutic index theoretically enhances tumoricidal activity with a resulting toxicity profile that cannot be achieved with systemic chemotherapy. Hyperthermia acts synergistically to augment the effects of cytotoxic chemotherapy. Tumor cells are intrinsically sensitive to temperatures greater than 42°C. This is due to several factors including increased tumor cell hypoxia, acidosis, and inadequate compensatory vasodilation in tumors relative to normal tissue. Hyperthermia causes increased tumor cell permeability and induces metabolic stress, both of which augment the effect of chemotherapy. Hyperthermia exhibits a direct activating effect on certain chemotherapeutic agents, including mitomycin C, a commonly used drug in HIPEC. Finally, chemotherapy given in the operating room after cytoreductive surgery allows for maximal removal of microscopic disease. This is essential for treatment success, as chemotherapy agents are unable to completely penetrate tumors greater than 5 mm in size.

Although the use of HIPEC has gained wider acceptance, the specifics of its administration lack uniformity. HIPEC has been administered intraoperatively via the open abdomen, the closed abdomen, or with a peritoneal cavity expansion device. In this review, the methodology, risks, and benefits associated with each technique are discussed, including data regarding morbidity and mortality.

6.2 Technique of Intraperitoneal Hyperthermic Chemoperfusion

To take advantage of the synergistic effect of chemotherapy and hyperthermia, several techniques to enable intraoperative perfusion of the peritoneal cavity with hyperthermic chemotherapy have been developed. Regardless of the specific technology that is employed, the procedure proceeds after cytoreduction. Core temperatures can be monitored by a Swan-Ganz thermister, bladder and esophageal or rectal temperature probes. During the perfusion procedure, the patient's core temperature rises rapidly and must be controlled to avoid systemic hyperthermia. We prefer to precool the patient to approximately 35°C before hyperthermic perfusion and to use body warmers set to ambient air temperature during the perfusion. Precooling is accomplished simply by limiting the use of body warming during the period of cytoreduction with exposure of the abdominal viscera. Other methods of maintaining an acceptable core temperature include packing the patient in ice around the head and axillae and the use of cooling blankets. With the use of precooling, we have not found this to be necessary in a majority of cases. Intraperitoneal temperature monitors are placed to monitor liver temperature, peritoneal surface temperature, and inflow/outflow perfusate temperature. The perfusion is performed with a roller pump that can regulate flow rate, such the pump used for cardiopulmonary bypass. The roller pump is connected to a heat exchanger modified to allow for heating of the perfusate to as high as 47°C (Cincinnati Subzero, Cincinnati, OH). A single inflow and two outflow catheters are used in our particular system. At the University of Cincinnati, a perfusion team trained in cardiopulmonary bypass staffs each HIPEC procedure and monitors flow rates, volumes, and intraperitoneal temperatures. Flow rates generally are in the range of 1–1.5 l/min. Chemotherapy is added to the perfusate when the in-flow target temperature is reached. In the literature, different authors have reported a target in-flow temperature that varies from 41 to 56°C; however, the target intraperitoneal temperature is 41–44°C (Elias et al. 1994). HIPEC is continued for 45 to 120 min; the optimal timing is unknown, but drug half-life must be taken into account if longer perfusion periods are utilized. Our standard is a 90-min period of HIPEC. After completion of HIPEC, virtually all chemotherapy is removed by open abdominal lavage, which terminates further systemic absorption.

6.3 Closed Technique

The closed technique is a commonly used method to deliver HIPEC. Typically, after macroscopic cytoreduction, one inflow catheter and two outflow catheters are placed. The outflow catheters are placed in dependent positions, such as the pelvis and under the right hemidiaphragm. Temperature probes are placed in the abdomen proximal to and remote from the catheter tips to monitor in-flow and out-flow temperatures (Fig. 6.1). After temporary closure of the abdominal skin, heated chemotherapy perfusate is infused. The abdominal cavity is manually agitated externally during the perfusion period to promote uniform distribution of the heated chemotherapy perfusate. After completion of perfusion, the abdomen is reopened, and the perfusate is evacuated. The catheters may be left in place if postoperative intraperitoneal chemotherapy is planned. Appropriate anastomoses are performed, and the patient is closed in the standard fashion. Increased interest in HIPEC has led to the commercial development of heated intraoperative perfusion systems that contain a roller pump and a heat exchanger in a single unit. The units are commercially available from different vendors.

A major advantage of the closed technique is the ability to rapidly achieve and maintain hyperthermia, because there is minimal heat loss from the closed abdomen. In addition, there is minimal direct contact or aerosolized exposure of the operating room staff to the chemotherapy. The main disadvantage of the closed technique is the lack of uniform distribution of the heated intraperitoneal chemotherapy, which theoretically could result in significant morbidity. When methylene blue was instilled with the closed technique, uneven distribution was observed (Stephens et al. 1999). Elias et al. observed poor thermal distribution during the closed technique by the use

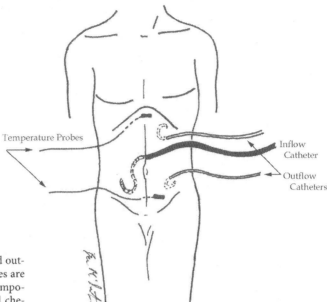

Fig. 6.1 Closed technique: inflow and outflow catheters and temperature probes are inserted after cytoreduction. After temporary closure of the abdomen, heated chemotherapy is perfused

of six thermal probes placed in different positions (Elias et al. 2000). Uneven distribution in HIPEC is problematic, because intraperitoneal hyperthermia has a narrow therapeutic index. The tumoricidal effect of hyperthermia is manifested at 41–43°C (Elias et al. 1994). Rats exposed to intraperitoneal temperatures of 45°C suffered 90% mortality, while intraperitoneal temperatures of 44 °C resulted in 0% mortality (Shimizu et al. 1991). Inadequate circulation of heated intraperitoneal perfusate leads to pooling and accumulation of heat and chemotherapy in dependent parts of the abdomen. Undesirable pooling may result in increased systemic absorption as well instigating foci of hyperthermic injury that could contribute to postoperative ileus, bowel perforation, and fistula.

Jacquet et al reported on the morbidity and mortality following the use of cytoreduction and closed intraoperative HIPEC followed by one cycle of postoperative intraperitoneal chemotherapy in the treatment of 60 patients with peritoneal metastases from colon or appendiceal adenocarcinoma. The overall morbidity rate was 35%. Complications included prolonged ileus, anastomotic leak, bowel perforation, bile leak, pancreatitis, and hematologic toxicities. These complications were associated in patients with higher intra-abdominal temperatures during HIPEC and in patients with a higher number of peritonectomy procedures and a longer operative duration (Jacquet et al. 1996).

Multiple small trials have indicated that cytoreduction and intraoperative closed abdominal HIPEC can be performed safely and may be more efficacious than surgery alone. Inadequate intraperitoneal circulation during HIPEC using the closed abdomen technique may increase the rate of intra-abdominal complications.

6.4 Open Abdomen (Coliseum) Technique

The open abdomen technique has also been referred to as the „coliseum technique." Cytoreduction and placement of temperature probes and inflow and outflow catheters are performed as described above. A Silastic sheet is sutured over a Thompson retractor and to the patient's skin over the abdominal incision (Fig. 6.2a). This suspends the abdominal wall, creating a "coliseum" or "soup bowl-like" container for the instillation of the peritoneal perfusate. An incision is made in the middle of the sheet to allow manual manipulation of the intra-abdominal contents to prevent stasis of the heated perfusate. A smoke evacuator is used to clear the aerosolized chemotherapy liberated during the procedure. HIPEC is performed for 1–2 h, as in the closed technique. Similarly, appropriate anastomoses are per-

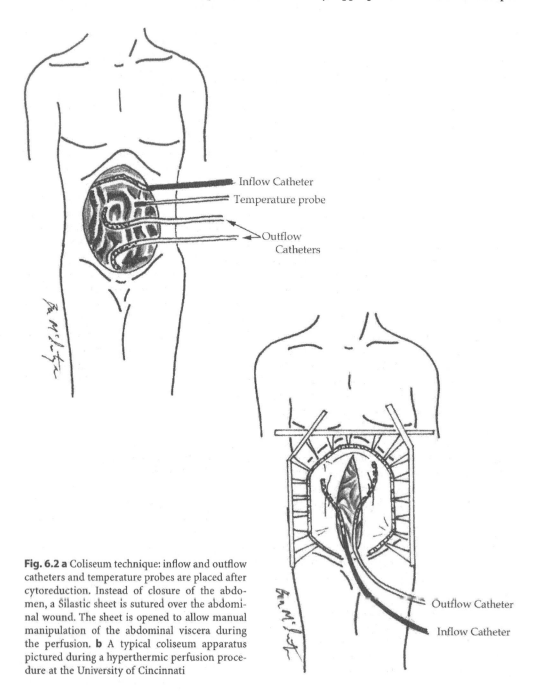

Fig. 6.2 a Coliseum technique: inflow and outflow catheters and temperature probes are placed after cytoreduction. Instead of closure of the abdomen, a Silastic sheet is sutured over the abdominal wound. The sheet is opened to allow manual manipulation of the abdominal viscera during the perfusion. **b** A typical coliseum apparatus pictured during a hyperthermic perfusion procedure at the University of Cincinnati

formed after drainage and lavage of the peritoneal cavity.

The principal benefit of the coliseum technique is the assurance that heated chemotherapy is adequately distributed throughout the abdominal cavity. Because of the direct manipulation of the intra-abdominal viscera during perfusion, all peritoneal surfaces are equally exposed to the therapy. This limits pooling of the heated perfusate and thereby theoretically reduces systemic absorption of chemotherapy, postoperative ileus, perforation, or fistula formation (Stephens et al. 1999).

One disadvantage of the coliseum technique is that the open abdomen naturally leads to heat dissipation. This can make it more difficult to achieve hyperthermia, particularly if higher temperatures are desired. Next, because the abdominal wall is suspended, it may be inadequately exposed to the perfusate. Another possible disadvantage of the coliseum technique when compared with the closed technique is the theoretical increased exposure of operating room personnel to chemotherapy. Because the surgeon is required to manually manipulate the viscera, there is increased potential for contact exposure. Because the abdomen is open during perfusion, heated chemotherapy can aerosolize, creating inhalational exposure. Stuart et al evaluated the issue of safety during the coliseum technique (Stuart et al. 2002). Urine from members of the operating team was assayed for chemotherapy levels. Air was sampled proximal to the operative field, and levels were measured. Finally, sterile gloves commonly used in the operating room were examined for permeability to chemotherapy. All assessments of potential exposures were found to be in compliance with established safety standards. Thus the theoretically increased risk of exposure of the operative team to chemotherapy during the coliseum technique has not been substantiated (Stuart et al. 2002).

Cavaliere et al. reported the treatment of 40 patients with low-grade peritoneal carcinomatosis. After peritonectomy, patients were given open HIPEC or early postoperative unheated intraperitoneal chemotherapy if the patient's condition warranted a shorter operative time. Perioperative mortality was 5%, with a complication rate of 35%. Morbidity and mortality directly corresponded to duration of the procedure. The authors observed a learning curve of 18 months, after which the complication rate significantly reduced. The overall treatment was effective compared with historical controls, as the 2-year survival rate was 61%, and the median survival was 30 months (Cavaliere et al. 2000).

Stephens et al. reported their experience treating 183 patients with peritoneal metastases arising from primary tumors of the appendix, colon, or stomach. The overall complication rate was 27%. The most frequent complications were pancreatitis (6%), fistula (4.5%), postoperative bleeding (4.5%), and hematologic side effects (4.5%). While none of the HIPEC variables was associated with major morbidity, higher temperatures were associated with bile leaks, ileus, and deep vein thrombosis. Additionally, the number of peritonectomy procedures was generally associated with increased postoperative morbidity.

The coliseum technique provides even heat distribution during HIPEC, which in theory could reduce morbidity as compared to the closed technique. However, this has yet to be definitively proven in the context of a prospective clinical trial. Side effects from HIPEC using the coliseum technique appear to be principally related to the magnitude of the peritonectomy.

6.5 Peritoneal Cavity Expander Technique

An alternative method to increase the distribution of heated chemotherapy involves the use of a peritoneal cavity expander (PCE), first reported by Fujimura et al (Fujimura et al. 1990). Before deployment of the PCE, cytoreduction is performed in a standard fashion. The PCE is an acrylic cylinder containing inflow and outflow catheters that are secured over the wound. When filled with heated perfusate, the PCE can accommodate the small intestine, allowing the small intestine to float freely and be manually manipulated in the perfusate (Fig. 6.2b). After HIPEC is complete, the perfusate is drained, and the PCE is removed. By temporarily increasing the volume of the peritoneal cavity, a more uniform distribution is theoretically achieved compared with the closed technique. The main disadvantage of the PCE technique is the risk of exposure to the operating room personnel as discussed for the open technique.

Fujimura et al. reported the treatment of 25 patients with "severe" peritoneal dissemination using PCE HIPEC. Complications included one case of intra-abdominal hemorrhage and one case of intra-abdominal abscess. No perioperative deaths were noted. The treatment resulted in a median survival time of 2 years. The median survival of historical controls ranged from 2 to 2 months, suggesting that HIPEC utilizing PCE may be effective (Fujimura et al. 1999).

Hirose et al. studied the use of PCE HIPEC for the treatment of gastric cancer-related carcinomatosis. Patients treated for existing carcinomatosis with PCE HIPEC had a higher survival rate than control subjects, but the results were not statistically significant. Interestingly, all the patients who were completely resected were alive at the conclusion of the study, while those patients who had retained macroscopic disease died within 1 year. Overall perioperative morbidity and mortality were similar in the HIPEC and control groups (Hirose et al. 1999).

Tsiftsis et al. reported on the expansion of the peritoneal cavity without the use of a device by intentionally creating artificial ascites. Using a closed technique, they infused 4–9 l of heated chemotherapy perfusate, keeping intra-abdominal pressure between 12 and 26 mmHg. This allows for expansion of the peritoneal cavity but avoids evaporative losses and the inevitable leakage around the peritoneal cavity expander device. In 23 cases, they reported 14 minor complications and one death due to an anastomotic leak. They reported intraoperative hemodynamic data that demonstrated the artificial ascites was well tolerated (Tsiftsis et al. 1999).

PCE is a viable option for the open abdominal technique of HIPEC. Although there are no studies directly comparing PCE to the coliseum or closed techniques, the reported results appear to be similar. The main drawback of PCE is the need to become familiar with the apparatus as well as the theoretical risk to operating room personnel of chemotherapy exposure. A summary of the advantages and disadvantages of the above techniques is provided in Table 6.1.

6.6 Developing a HIPEC Program

As interest in intraperitoneal therapies has increased, the development of HIPEC programs

Table 6.1 Techniques of hyperthermic intraperitoneal chemotherapy administration

Technique	Advantages	Disadvantages
Early postoperative	Multiple cycles of chemotherapy	More systemic toxicity
		Uneven distribution of chemotherapy
		No hyperthermia
Closed intraoperative	Less exposure of OR staff to chemotherapy	Uneven distribution of chemotherapy
Open intraoperative	Uniform distribution of chemotherapy	More exposure of OR staff to chemotherapy
	Less hospital time	
Peritoneal cavity expander	Uniform distribution of chemotherapy	More exposure of OR staff to chemotherapy
		More complex apparatus

OR, operating room

has become of interest to an increasing number of surgeons. It is critical that several facts be taken into account by physicians and institutions interested in such program development. First, operative and perioperative training in cytoreductive surgery and HIPEC at a major center is essential. Ideally such training should be in the form of a surgical oncology fellowship or its equivalent, or an extended apprenticeship. Because of the labor-intensive nature of the operations, it is best if programs consist of more than one physician trained in HIPEC. The surgeon comprises only part of the necessary team. It is essential that skilled perfusionists or their equivalent be available to monitor flow rates and intraperitoneal temperatures during the procedure. Anesthesiologists should be educated regarding the physiological changes that take place during HIPEC and should understand the need for ongoing communication with the operating surgeon during the procedure. The operating room team needs to be familiar with the specialized equipment used during HIPEC and educated regarding the proper care and disposal of materials exposed to chemotherapeutic agents. Standard operating procedures should be developed, taking into account local hospital by-laws and in accordance with the requirement of government regulatory agencies. The major equipment used to perform HIPEC includes a roller pump and a heat exchanger. Minor equipment needs include temperature probes and perfusion tubing. As previously mentioned, different approved devices are currently available that comprise both a heat exchanger and a roller pump.

Preoperative care at our institution involves extensive patient education with a clinical nurse specialist to ensure that patients have realistic expectations regarding the procedure, the hospitalization, and aftercare associated with cytoreductive surgery and HIPEC. We also have established a patient-to-patient network that allows preoperative counseling by persons who have previously undergone cytoreductive surgery and HIPEC. We have found this to be an extremely valuable component of our program. Postoperative care requires a surgical intensive care unit and physicians familiar with the common issues related to care of the HIPEC patient. Finally, because cytoreductive surgery and HIPEC remain a treatment in evolution, every attempt should be made to treat patients under the auspices of prospective clinical trials. Data should be collected and maintained such that outcomes can be studied and reported. The ideal program will combine the clinical treatment program with more basic investigations allowing for the genesis of translational research.

6.7 Summary

Peritoneal metastases are common sequelae of gastrointestinal malignancy. The treatment of peritoneal metastases through use of aggressive surgical cytoreduction including peritonectomy coupled with HIPEC has now been reported in several large single-institution series. The available literature suggests that in experienced hands and with appropriate patient selection cytoreduction and HIPEC can be an effective therapy, particularly when all macroscopic tumor deposits are removed. Different techniques involving the administration of intraperitoneal chemotherapy have been reported, including the closed intraoperative technique, the open or coliseum technique, and the open technique using a PCE device. All techniques have been associated with mortality and morbidity that is significant, but generally consistent with other major surgical procedures. In theory, the coliseum and PCE techniques may have less associated morbidity because of improved heat distribution; however, this remains to be definitively proven in a controlled clinical trial. Such controlled studies are critical to defining the best techniques for HIPEC administration and the appropriate role for this treatment regimen in patients with peritoneal metastases. The development of a program in cytoreductive surgery and HIPEC requires a comprehensive patient care team led by appropriately trained surgeons. Such teams are best suited to provide the highest-quality care to patients with peritoneal surface malignancy.

References

Ahmad SA, Sussman JJ, Kim J, Soldano DA, Pennington LJ, James LE, Lowy AM (2004) Reduced morbidity following cytoreductive surgery and intraperitoneal hyperthermic perfusion. Ann Surg Oncol 11:387–392

Cavaliere F, Perri P, Di Filippo F, Giannarelli D, Botti C, Cosimelli M et al. (2000) Treatment of peritoneal carcinomatosis with intent to cure. J Surg Oncol 74:41–44

Ceelen WP, Hesse U, de Hemptinne B, Pattyn P (2000) Hyperthermic intraperitoneal chemoperfusion in the treatment of locally advanced intra-abdominal cancer. Br J Surg 87:1006–1015

Elias D, Detroz B, Debaene B, Damia E, Leclerq B, Rougier P et al. (1994) Treatment of peritoneal carcinomatosis by intraperitoneal chemo-hyperthermia: reliable and unreliable concepts. Hepatogastroenterology 41:207–213

Fujimura T, Yonemura Y, Fujita H, Michiwa Y, Kawamura T, Nojima N et al. (1999) Chemohyperthermic peritoneal perfusion for peritoneal dissemination in various intraabdominal malignancies. Int Surg 84:60–66

Fujimura T, Yonemura Y, Fushida S, Urade M, Takegawa S, Kamata T et al. (1990) Continuous hyperthermic peritoneal perfusion for the treatment of peritoneal dissemination in gastric cancers and subsequent second-look operation. Cancer 65:65–71

Fugimoto S, Takahashi M, Kobayashi K, Kasanuki J, Ohkubo H (1996) Heated intraperitoneal mitomycin C infusion treatment for patients with gastric cancer and peritoneal metastasis. Cancer Treat Res 81:239–245

Hirose K, Katayama K, Iida A, Yamaguchi A, Nakagawara G, Umeda S et al. (1999) Efficacy of continuous hyperthermic peritoneal perfusion for the prophylaxis and treatment of peritoneal metastasis of advanced gastric cancer: evaluation by multivariate regression analysis. Oncology 57:106–114

Jacquet P, Stephens AD, Averback AM, Chang D, Ettinghausen SE, Dalton RR, Steves MA, Sugarbaker PH (1996) Analysis of morbidity and mortality in 60 patients with peritoneal carcinomatosis treated by cytoreductive surgery and heated intraoperative intraperitoneal chemotherapy. Cancer 77:2622–2629

Gilly FN, Carry PY, Sayag AC, Brachet A, Panteix G, Salle B, Bienvenu J, Burgard G, Guibert B, Banssillon V, Braillon G (1994) Regional chemotherapy and intraoperative hyperthermia for digestive cancers with peritoneal carcinomatosis. Hepatogastroenterology 41:124–129

Park BJ, Alexander RH, Libutti SK, Wu P, Royalty D, Kranda KC et al. (1999) Treatment of primary peritoneal mesothelioma by continuous hyperthermic peritoneal perfusion. Ann Surg Oncol 6:582–590

Shimizu T, Maeta M, Koga S (1991) Influence of local hyperthermia on the healing of small intestinal anastomoses in the rat. Br J Surg 78:57–59

Stephens AD, Alderman R, Chang D, Edwards GD, Esquivel J, Sebbag G et al. (1999) Morbidity and mortality analysis of 200 treatments with cytoreductive surgery and hyperthermic intraoperative intraperitoneal chemotherapy using the Coliseum technique. Ann Surg Oncol 6:790–796

Stuart OA, Stephens AD, Welch L, Sugarbaker PH (2002) Safety monitoring of the Coliseum technique for heated intraoperative chemotherapy with Mitomycin C. Ann Surg Oncol 9:186–191

Sugarbaker PH (1999) Management of peritoneal-surface malignancy: the surgeon's role. Langenbeck's Arch Surg 384:576–587

Tsiftsis D, de Bree E, Romanos J, Petrou A, Sanidas E, Askoxylakis J, Zervos K, Michaloudis D (1999) Peritoneal expansion by artificially produced ascites during perfusion chemotherapy. Arch Surg 134:545–549

Witkamp AJ, de Bree E, Kaag MM, van Slooten GW, van Coevorden, Zoetmulder FAN (2001) Extensive surgical cytoreduction and intraoperative hyperthermic intraperitoneal chemotherapy in patients with pseudomyxoma peritonei. Br J Surg 88:459–463

Yonemura Y, Ninomiya I, Kaji M, Sugiyama K, Fugimura K, Sawa T et al. (1995) Prophylaxis with intraoperative chemohyperthermia against peritoneal recurrence of serosal invasion-positive gastric cancer. World J Surg 19:450–455

7 Adjuvant Intraperitoneal Chemotherapy: A Review

Paul H. Sugarbaker

7.1 Introduction

The rationale for adding perioperative chemotherapy to the management of gastrointestinal and ovarian cancer was developed by Cunliffe and Sugarbaker in 1989. They based the rationale for this novel approach on the patterns of recurrence of both gastrointestinal and ovarian cancer [1]. Their literature review established that the resection site recurrence and peritoneal carcinomatosis occurred in a majority of patients who failed the surgical treatment of primary gastric cancer. Even a higher resection site and peritoneal carcinomatosis failure rate was noted with the surgical removal of primary pancreas cancer. In colorectal cancer patients rectal cancer presented a higher incidence of local regional recurrence than colon cancer, but local-regional recurrence was a definite cause of death in both colon and rectal cancer patients. These authors suggested a novel treatment, early postoperative intraperitoneal chemotherapy with 5-fluorouracil, doxorubicin, and/or cisplatin.

The pharmacological rationale for this direct instillation of chemotherapy into the peritoneal cavity after a potentially curative gastrointestinal cancer resection was further developed by Sugarbaker and colleagues with pharmacological studies [2]. High local-regional concentrations of intraperitoneal chemotherapy, prolonged exposure of the peritoneal surfaces, and a minimum of systemic toxicity was demonstrated. 5-Fluorouracil was thought to not only protect the peritoneal surfaces but also act as an adjuvant to prevent the development of liver metastases. Mitomycin C was suggested as a chemotherapy agent with a wide range of responses in both gastrointestinal and gynecologic malignancy that was pharmacologically appropriate for perioperative intraperitoneal administration.

The addition of heat to the intraperitoneal chemotherapy treatments was first explored by Spratt et al. [3]. They treated a single patient with pseudomyxoma peritonei and established that both heat and chemotherapy were well tolerated in this single patient and promised to develop into an effective treatment strategy for patients with the dissemination of cancer on peritoneal surfaces. Koga and colleagues performed pharmacological studies with heated intraperitoneal chemotherapy in experimental animals and then went on to perform an early trial in patients with primary gastric cancer to test the efficacy of heated intraoperative intraperitoneal chemotherapy in patients with resected gastric cancer [4, 5].

7.2 Gastric Cancer

The gastrointestinal cancer that can be most effectively treated by adjuvant intraperitoneal chemotherapy with significant benefit is gastric malignancy. Sugarbaker summarized the surgical approach that would incorporate peritonectomy into the management of gastric cancer with peritoneal seeding. He also developed the concept of centripetal gastrectomy, which would minimize the contamination of the resection site by cancer cells traumatically disrupted from the primary tumor as a result of the cancer resection [6].

In 1988 Koga and colleagues from Tottori University, Yonago, Japan published promising results in a historically controlled study of 38 patients and in a randomized controlled study of 47 patients [5]. Their results showed a statistically significant improvement in survival in the historical control group (p=0.04). In the randomized study, considered to be grossly statistically underpowered, there was no significant improvement in survival. However, it should be mentioned that the 3-year survival of the treated group was 83%, compared to 67% in those patients who had gastrectomy alone. The incidence of anastomotic leak in the two groups of patients was similar. This group is to be credited with providing us with the first promising results from adjuvant treatment of gastric cancer with perioperative intraperitoneal chemotherapy.

Fujimura and colleagues from Kanazawa University, Kanazawa, Japan used cisplatin and mitomycin C in a randomized controlled study of hyperthermic and normothermic intraoperative chemotherapy [7]. The group receiving heated intraoperative intraperitoneal chemotherapy had a 68% 3-year survival, the group receiving normothermic intraperitoneal chemotherapy had a 51% 3-year survival, and the group having surgery alone had a 23% 3-year survival. These three curves were significantly different by the log-rank test (p<0.01). The Kanazawa group should be credited with a sound pharmacological study of their patients, with data that strongly suggested the benefits of hyperthermia, and with the provision of data that further support the perioperative use of intraperitoneal chemotherapy for gastric cancer. Hamazoe and coworkers from Tottori University in Yonago, Japan published in 1993 a randomized controlled study of hyperthermic peritoneal irrigation with mitomycin C [8]. Forty-two patients were in the experimental arm, and 40 patients had gastrectomy only. The 5-year survival rate was 64.2% for the treated patients and 52.5% for the control group. This was statistically insignificant, with a p-value of 0.243. However, the mortality rate from peritoneal recurrence was less in the treated group, and this result approached statistical significance (p=0.085).

Yonemura and colleagues in 1995 published a second study of 79 patients who had the prophylactic treatment for peritoneal recurrence with heated intraoperative intraperitoneal chemotherapy using mitomycin C and cisplatin compared to 81 patients who underwent potentially curative surgery during the same period [9]. These important data showed that there was no difference in survival in patients with histologically proven, serosal invasion-negative tumors. However, if there was histologically proven invasion by tumor, there was a 5-year survival of 50% in the treated group as compared to 30% in the control. This was statistically significant, with a p-value of 0.016. Also, surprisingly, those patients with stage IV disease showed a 45% survival with heated intraperitoneal chemotherapy treatment as compared to 5% at 5 years in the control group. This was statistically significant, with a p-value <0.001. Yonemura and colleagues suggested that hyperthermic intraperitoneal irrigation intraoperatively was an important adjunct to the treatment of patients with serosal invasion-positive gastric cancer.

Ikeguchi and colleagues in 1995 reported on 174 randomized patients treated with gastrectomy plus heated intraperitoneal chemotherapy versus gastrectomy and standard systemic chemotherapy [10]. In the group of patients with one to nine lymph node metastases there was a trend toward increased 5-year survival. Sixty-six percent in the treated group survived 5 years as compared to 44% in the control group (p=0.084). In the group with no lymph nodes positive or patients with 10 or more lymph nodes positive, the beneficial effects of heated intraperitoneal chemotherapy were not evident. These authors noted that the incidence of free cancer cells in the peritoneal cavity was 6% in patients without positive lymph nodes, 17% in patients with one to nine lymph nodes positive, and 38% in patients with 10 or more positive nodes. These authors suggest that patients with lymph node positivity should be expected to have a high rate of local-regional recurrence and peritoneal metastases in the absence of a local-regional adjuvant treatment.

In 1999 Fujimoto and colleagues from Funabashi, Japan treated 141 gastric cancer patients with macroscopic serosal invasion and randomly assigned these patients to two groups [11]. Seventy-one patients underwent hyperthermic intraoperative intraperitoneal chemotherapy, and the other group underwent gastric resection alone. The peritoneal recurrence rate in the treated group was significantly decreased (p 0.0001). The 8-year survival was 62% in the treated group and 49% in the control group. This was a significant benefit with a p-value of 0.036. This group concluded that heated intraoperative intraperitoneal chemotherapy reduced the local recurrence rate and improved the long-term survival in patients with gastric cancer who had macroscopic serosal invasion.

Yu and colleagues from Kyungpook University, Taegu, Korea published a randomized controlled study of 248 patients with advanced gastric cancer. These patients were treated with early postoperative intraperitoneal chemotherapy using mitomycin C and 5-fluorouracil in addition to gastrectomy or gastrectomy alone. The 5-year survival rate in patients with stage III disease was 18% for the surgery-only group and 49% for the group that had surgery plus intraperitoneal chemotherapy (p=0.011) [12]. In a follow-up of these data 3 years later the overall survival was improved in the treated group, with a 5-year overall survival of 54% in the treated group and 38% in the gastrectomy-only group (p=0.0278). The patients who profited most were those who had gross serosal invasion [13]. In this study the survival was 52% in the treated group and 25% in the gastrectomy-alone group (p<0.0001). In patients with resectable stage IV cancer the survival was 28% in the treated group and 5% in the gastrectomy-only group (p=0.0098).

The morbidity and mortality of the early postoperative intraperitoneal chemotherapy was addressed by Yu and colleagues in further publications [14]. The overall morbidity was higher in the control group, 28.8% versus 20%. This difference was not significant. Intra-abdominal sepsis without anastomotic leak (p=0.008) and postoperative bleeding (p=0.002) occurred more often in the study group. Postoperative mortality was higher in the study group (5.6%) than in the control group (0.8%), but this was not significant (p=0.299). Yu and colleagues performed a period analysis of the morbidity, demonstrating that it followed a pattern of a learning curve.

Recently, a meta-analysis of adjuvant intraperitoneal chemotherapy for gastric cancer was reported by Xu and colleagues from Sun Yat-sen University in Guangzhou, China [15]. They pooled the data from 11 trials involving 1,161 cases. Their conclusion was that intraperitoneal chemotherapy benefits patients after a curative resection. The odds ratio was 0.51, with a 95% confidence interval of 0.40–0.65. Xu and colleagues suggested that intraperitoneal chemotherapy was of benefit but indicated that rigorously designed trials should be conducted to draw more definitive conclusions.

In summary, the natural history studies suggest that local-regional recurrence of gastric cancer is an important part of surgical treatment failure. Also, the pharmacology of intraperitoneal chemotherapy suggests that it should be able to eradicate microscopic residual disease and a very low volume of carcinomatosis. Phase II and phase III studies summarized in a meta-analysis suggest that intraperitoneal chemotherapy is of benefit in resectable gastric cancer. It appears to have its greatest benefit in patients who have invasion of the serosa. Also, in resectable stage IV gastric cancer patients, when the surgery is radical it is benefited by this approach.

A single study in the adjuvant treatment of gastric cancer is important in that it shows an absence of benefit. The multi-institutional study reported by Sautner and colleagues from Austria used multiple cycles of delayed intraperitoneal cisplatin as an adjuvant to gastric cancer resection [16]. This failed to show any benefit. This is understandable when one looks into the mechanism of action of early postoperative intraperitoneal chemotherapy in an adjuvant setting. It is used to prevent local-regional disease dissemination that occurs prior to or at the time of surgery. It is more likely to occur in patients who have serosal-positive disease or lymph node positivity. Starting the chemotherapy a month after surgery from this perspective is unlikely to be of any benefit. As expected, no benefit was observed in this study.

7.3 Colorectal Cancer

The earliest studies with adjuvant intraperitoneal chemotherapy for colorectal cancer were performed by Sugarbaker et al. at the National Institutes of Health, USA. This group randomized 66 patients with advanced primary or rectal cancer to receive 12 cycles of intraperitoneal or intravenous 5-fluorouracil [17]. This study showed that the maximum tolerable dose of 5-fluorouracil given by the intravenous route was 904 mg. For the intraperitoneal route it was 1,361 mg. This was statistically significant, with a p<0.001. Among the patients with recurrent disease after intravenous 5-fluorouracil, 10 of 11 patients on second look had peritoneal implants. Only of 2 of 10 patients who recurred after intraperitoneal 5-fluorouracil showed peritoneal implants (p=0.003). These authors concluded that the natural history of surgically treated colorectal cancer was changed through the use of intraperitoneal 5-fluorouracil. In these patients with advanced primary disease no survival differences were noted between the two groups.

A second randomized and controlled study of long-term intraperitoneal 5-fluorouracil was reported in 1998 by Scheithauer et al. from Vienna, Austria [18]. They randomized 241 patients with resected stage III or high-risk stage II (T4N0M0) colon cancer to receive standard therapy with 5-fluorouracil and levamisole given intravenously for 6 months. The investigational arm was 5-fluorouracil 300 mg/m2 and leucovorin 200 mg/m2 given intravenously on days 1 and 4 of a treatment cycle and intraperitoneally on days 1 and 3 every 4 weeks for a total of six courses. There was an improvement in survival with a p-value of 0.005 and an estimated 43% reduction in mortality in favor of the investigational arm. A lower rate of severe adverse reactions was noted in the patients receiving local-regional plus intravenous 5-fluorouracil (3% vs. 12%; p=0.01). These authors suggested that combined intraperitoneal plus systemic intravenous chemotherapy with 5-fluorouracil and leucovorin was an adjuvant treatment for patients with stage III colon cancer.

Vaillant and colleagues in a multi-institutional study from France tested adjuvant intraperitoneal 5-fluorouracil in patients with colon cancer at high risk for recurrence. Two hundred sixty-seven patients were randomized. One hundred thirty-three received intraperitoneal 5-fluorouracil on days 4–10 postoperatively. The control patient received resection only. Tolerance to treatment was excellent. Five-year survival rates were 74% in the experimental group and 69% in the control group. In patients who received the full treatment the 5-year disease-free survival rate was improved in the group of patients with stage II colon cancer but not in the group with stage III disease. These authors concluded that this short course of intraperitoneal 5-fluorouracil reduced the risk of recurrence in stage II cancers but was not of sufficient efficacy to reduce the death rate in stage III disease [19].

Pestieau and Sugarbaker reviewed 104 patients with carcinomatosis from colon or rectal carcinoma who were treated with cytoreductive surgery, heated intraoperative intraperitoneal chemotherapy with mitomycin C, and early postoperative intraperitoneal chemotherapy with 5-fluorouracil [20]. In this group were five patients who were diagnosed with peritoneal carcinomatosis at the time of resection of a primary colon cancer. These five patients were specially treated with wide resection of their colon cancer, peritonectomy of the surfaces involved by peritoneal seeding, and then heated intraperitoneal chemotherapy followed by early postoperative therapy. All five of these patients were long-term survivors, suggesting that early peritoneal seeding in patients with colon or rectal cancer can be treated very effectively with the combined treatment modality.

In a review of the management of microscopic residual disease in colorectal cancer, Sugarbaker listed the patients who are most likely to profit from adjuvant perioperative intraperitoneal chemotherapy [21]. These are patients who are at extremely high risk for local-regional recurrence; they should be recommended for treatment until the results of further clinical trials have been made available. These groups of patients are listed in Table 7.1.

Table 7.1 Patients with colorectal cancer recommended for perioperative intraperitoneal chemotherapy

Positive peritoneal cytology
Ovarian involvement
Peritoneal seeding on the serosal surface of the colon
Rupture of a necrotic tumor mass
Adjacent organ involvement
Intraoperative tumor spill
Perforation of the primary tumor
Involved lymph nodes at the margin of excision
Limited peritoneal seeding with a peritoneal cancer index of <20
Limited peritoneal seeding so that a complete cytoreduction can be achieved

7.4 Ovarian Cancer

Only recently have trials with adjuvant intraperitoneal chemotherapy for ovarian cancer been initiated. Ryu and colleagues from Seoul, Korea assessed the benefits of heated intraoperative intraperitoneal chemotherapy in patients being treated for primary ovarian cancer [22]. Fifty-seven patients underwent cytoreductive surgery with hyperthermic chemotherapy, and 60 patients underwent surgery only. The chemotherapy was carboplatin and á-interferon with an intraperitoneal temperature of 43°C. The overall 5-year survival was higher in the treated group (p=0.008). For stage III ovarian cancer patients whose tumor was reduced to less than 1 cm during a reoperative procure, the 5-year survival rate was 65.6% in the patients who underwent HIIC and 41% in the control patients (p=0.0046).

Zylberberg and colleagues from Paris, France initiated a bidirectional chemotherapy protocol for primary ovarian cancer [23]. This was a phase II trial of intraperitoneal cisplatin and paclitaxel combined with intravenous ifosfamide. All patients underwent second-look surgery. In the 26 patients treated, the median survival had not been reached at 53 months and the disease-free survival was 40 months. The remarkably beneficial effects of this bidirectional chemotherapy suggest the need to move this bidirectional chemotherapy combination into a prospective and randomized trial.

Alberts and colleagues published the first randomized controlled study using long-term intraperitoneal cisplatin in patients with ovarian cancer. This was reported in the New England Journal of Medicine in 1996 [24]. They randomized 654 patients. All patients received intravenous cyclophosphamide. Patients were randomized to receive either intravenous or intraperitoneal cisplatin at 100 mg/m2 at 3-weekly intervals. The risk of death was lower in the intraperitoneally treated group, with a hazard ratio of 0.76 and 95% confidence intervals of 0.61–0.96 (p=0.02). Neurotoxicities were significantly reduced in the group receiving intraperitoneal chemotherapy.

Markman and colleagues reported a phase III trial of intravenous and intraperitoneal chemotherapy for ovarian cancer patients [25]. Progression-free survival was superior for patients randomized to receive intraperitoneal cisplatin (p=0.01), and there was a borderline improvement in overall survival associated with the intraperitoneal cisplatin (p=0.05). Recently, a third trial of long-term combined intraperitoneal and intravenous chemotherapy was performed by Armstrong et al., also a member of the Gynecologic Oncology Group [26]. They randomized 429 patients. Although adverse side effects were more common in the intraperitoneal treatment group, the progression-free survival was improved from 18.3 to 23.8 months (p=0.05) by the addition of intraperitoneal cisplatin and paclitaxel. Also, the median duration of overall survival was improved from 49.7 to 65.6 months (p=0.03).

Although the quality of life was significantly worse during the intraperitoneal treatment, after the end of 1 year the quality of life in the two groups was the same.

This collection of data strongly suggests that intraperitoneal chemotherapy administration is of value in patients who are at high risk for disease progression on peritoneal surfaces. This includes gastric, colorectal, and ovarian cancer patients. The failure of the general oncologic community to move ahead with these results of treatment was discussed by Armstrong and her colleagues [26]. They called attention to the fact that there is prejudice against intraperitoneal chemotherapy treatments because it is an old idea that has not caught on over approximately two decades. Intraperitoneal administration is more complicated than intravenous administration. Also, it requires the combined efforts of surgeon and medical oncologist and asks from both a higher level of skill and experience in successfully completing the treatments.

Recently, Sugarbaker reviewed all of the agents that have been suggested for intraperitoneal chemotherapy delivery [27]. He suggested that some agents are ideal for use within the peritoneal cavity. These large molecules are cleared slowly from the peritoneal space and provide excellent prophylaxis against microscopic residual disease. Other agents are of less benefit intraperitoneally and may interfere with long-term intraperitoneal access by causing a sclerotic reaction and resulting nonuniform drug delivery to peritoneal surfaces. It seems safe to say that the failure of more general application of intraperitoneal chemotherapy comes about as a result of logistical problems with drug delivery.

7.5 Conclusion

These data suggest that intraperitoneal chemotherapy is of benefit in an adjuvant setting in those diseases at high likelihood of local-regional recurrence. The timing of this intraperitoneal chemotherapy can be perioperative as a planned part of the operative intervention. From a theoretical perspective this perioperative intraperitoneal chemotherapy may cause significant survival benefit. However, a one-time use of chemotherapy will not be sufficient with other diseases where it is not possible to clear all visible evidence of disease with surgery. An example would be the majority of patients with stage III ovarian cancer. In these patients adjuvant long-term intraperitoneal chemotherapy should be added to the benefits that are possible with the perioperative approach. Finally, a bidirectional approach both perioperatively and long term will likely result in the greatest improvement. Knowledgeable selection of drugs for intraperitoneal administration combined with intravenous chemotherapy to help control systemic microscopic disease is to be recommended. Certainly, many promising treatment modalities are available for patients with gastrointestinal and gynecologic malignancy.

Acknowledgements. The Foundation for Applied Research in Gastrointestinal Oncology is acknowledged.

References

1. Cunliffe WJ, Sugarbaker PH (1989) Gastrointestinal malignancy: Rationale for adjuvant therapy using early postoperative intraperitoneal chemotherapy (EPIC). Br J Surg 76:1082–1090
2. Sugarbaker PH, Graves T, DeBruijn EA, Cunliffe WJ, Mullins RE, Hull WE, Oliff L, Schlag P (1990) Rationale for early postoperative intraperitoneal chemotherapy (EPIC) in patients with advanced gastrointestinal cancer. Cancer Res 50:5790–5794
3. Spratt JS, Adcock RA, Muskovin M, Sherrill W, McKeown J (1980) Clinical delivery system for intraperitoneal hyperthermic chemotherapy. Cancer Res 40:256–260
4. Koga S, Hamazoe R, Maeta M, Shimizu M, Shimizu N, Kanayama H, Osaki Y (1984)Treatment of implanted peritoneal cancer in rats by continuous hyperthermic peritoneal perfusion in combination with an anticancer drug. Cancer Res 44:1840–1842
5. Koga S, Hamazoe R, Maeta M, Shimizu N, Murakami A, Wakatsuki T (1988) Prophylactic therapy for peritoneal recurrence of gastric cancer by continuous hyperthermic peritoneal perfusion with mitomycin C. Cancer 61:232–237

6. Sugarbaker PH, Yu W, Yonemura Y (2003) Gastrectomy, peritonectomy and perioperative intraperitoneal chemotherapy: The evolution of treatment strategies for advanced gastric cancer. Semin Surg Oncol 21:233–248
7. Fujimura T, Yonemura Y, Muraoka K, Takamura H, Hirono Y, Sahara H, Ninomiya I, Matsumoto H, Tsugawa K, Nishimura G, Sugiyama K, Miwa K, Miyazaki I (1994) Continuous hyperthermic peritoneal perfusion for the prevention of peritoneal recurrence of gastric cancer: randomized controlled study. World J Surg 18:150–155
8. Hamazoe R, Maeta M, Kaibara N (1994) Intraperitoneal thermochemotherapy for prevention of peritoneal recurrence of gastric cancer. Final results of a randomized controlled study. Cancer 73:2048–2051
9. Yonemura Y, Ninomiya I, Kaji M, Sugiyama K, Fujimura K, Sawa T, Katayama K, Tanaka S, Hirono Y, Miwa K, Miyazaki I (1995) Prophylaxis with intraoperative chemohyperthermia against peritoneal recurrence of serosal invasion-positive gastric cancer. World J Surg 19:450–454
10. Ikeguchi M, Kondou A, Oka A, Tsujitani S, Maeta M, Kaibara N (1995) Effects of continuous hyperthermic peritoneal perfusion on prognosis of gastric cancer with serosal invasion. Eur J Surg 161:581–586
11. Fujimoto S, Takahashi M, Mutou T, Kobayashi K, Toyosawa T (1999) Successful intraperitoneal hyperthermic chemoperfusion for the prevention of postoperative peritoneal recurrence in patients with advanced gastric carcinoma. Cancer 85:529–534
12. Yu W, Whang I, Suh I, Averbach A, Chang D, Sugarbaker PH (1998). Prospective randomized trial of early postoperative intraperitoneal chemotherapy as an adjuvant to resectable gastric cancer. Ann Surg 228:347–357
13. Yu W, Whang I, Chung HY, Averbach A, Sugarbaker PH (2001) Indications for early postoperative intraperitoneal chemotherapy of advanced gastric cancer: results of a prospective randomized trial. World J Surg 25:985–990
14. Yu W, Whang I, Averbach A, Chang D, Sugarbaker PH (1998) Morbidity and mortality of early postoperative intraperitoneal chemotherapy as adjuvant therapy for gastric cancer. Am Surg 64:1104–1108
15. Xu DZ, Zhan YQ, Sun XW, Cao SM, Geng QR (2004) Meta-analysis of intraperitoneal chemotherapy for gastric cancer. World J Gastroenterol 10:2727–2730
16. Sautner T, Hofbauer F, Depisch D, Schiessel R, Jakesz R (1994) Adjuvant intraperitoneal cisplatin chemotherapy does not improve long-term survival after surgery for advanced gastric cancer. J Clin Oncol 12:970–974
17. Sugarbaker PH, Gianola FJ, Speyer JL, Wesley R, Barofsky I, Meyers CE (1985). Prospective randomized trial of intravenous versus intraperitoneal 5-fluorouracil in patients with advanced primary colon or rectal cancer. Surgery 98:414-421
18. Scheithauer W, Kornek GV, Marczell A, Karner J, Salem G, Greiner R, Burger D, Stoger F, Ritschel J, Kovats E, Vischer HM, Schneeweiss B, Depisch D (1998) Combined intravenous and intraperitoneal chemotherapy with fluorouracil + leucovorin vs. fluorouracil + levamisole for adjuvant therapy of resected colon carcinoma. Br J Cancer 77:1349–1354
19. Vaillant JC, Nordlinger B, Deuffic S, Arnaud JP, Pelissier E, Favre JP, Jaeck D, Fourtanier G, Grandjean JP, Marre P, Letoublon C (2000) Adjuvant intraperitoneal 5-fluorouracil in high-risk colon cancer: a multicenter phase III trial. Ann Surg 231:449–456
20. Pestieau SR, Sugarbaker PH (2000) Treatment of primary colon cancer with peritoneal carcinomatosis: A comparison of concomitant versus delayed management. Dis Colon Rectum 43:1341–1348
21. Sugarbaker PH (1999) Successful management of microscopic residual disease in large bowel cancer. Cancer Chemother Pharmacol 43 [Suppl]:S15–S25
22. Ryu KS, Kim JH, Ko HS, Kim JW, Ahn WS, Park YG, Kim SJ, Lee JM (2004) Effects of intraperitoneal hyperthermic chemotherapy in ovarian cancer. Gynecol Oncol 94:325–332
23. Zylberberg B, Dormont D, Madelenat P, Darai E (2004) First-line intraperitoneal cisplatin-paclitaxel and intravenous ifosfamide in Stage IIIc ovarian epithelial cancer. Eur J Gynaecol Oncol 25:327–332
24. Alberts DS, Liu PY, Hannigan EV, O'Toole R, Williams SD, Young JA, Franklin EW, Clarke-Pearson DL, Malviya VK, DuBeshter B, Adelson MD, Hoskins WJ (1996) Intraperitoneal cisplatin plus intravenous cyclophosphamide versus intravenous cisplatin plus intravenous cyclophosphamide for stage III ovarian cancer. N Engl J Med 335:1950–1955
25. Markman M, Bundy BN, Alberts DS, Fowler JM, Clark-Pearson DL, Carson LF, Wadler S, Sickel J (2001) Phase III trial of standard-dose intravenous cisplatin plus paclitaxel versus moderately high-dose carboplatin followed by intravenous paclitaxel and intraperitoneal cisplatin in small-volume stage III ovarian carcinoma: an intergroup study of the Gynecologic Oncology Group, Southwestern Oncology Group, and Eastern Cooperative Oncology Group. J Clin Oncol 19:1001–1007
26. Armstrong DK, Bundy B, Wenzel L, Huang HQ, Baergen R, Lele S, Copeland LJ, Walker JL, Burger RA; Gynecologic Oncology Group (2006) Intraperitoneal cisplatin and paclitaxel in ovarian cancer. N Engl J Med 354:34–43
27. Sugarbaker PH, Mora JT, Carmignani P, Stuart OA, Yoo D (2005) Update on chemotherapeutic agents utilized for perioperative intraperitoneal chemotherapy. Oncologist 10:112–122

8 Clinical Research Methodology in Peritoneal Surface Oncology: A Difficult Challenge

François-Noël Gilly, Olivier Glehen, Annie C. Beaujard, Eddy Cotte

Since the 1980s there has been considerable renewed interest in peritoneal carcinomatosis (PC) of digestive and ovarian origins as well as in pseudomyxoma peritonei and peritoneal mesothelioma. This renewed interest is mainly due to the reported results from trials using cytoreductive surgery (CRS) and intraperitoneal chemohyperthermia (HIPEC). Except for the Dutch randomized study [1], only phase II studies have been reported in the literature. A good amount of knowledge has emerged from these numerous phase II studies, and many encouraging results have been reported from experienced multidisciplinary teams involved in peritoneal surface oncology [2, 3]. The time has probably come now for large randomized trials to definitively evaluate these aggressive combined therapies. Because of the complexity of peritoneal surface malignancies, such a large controlled trial will need to be a multi-institutional one. This point raises the need for a homogeneous clinical research methodology with a very precise description of all variables that could interact with results. Today, several PC staging systems are available as well as several completeness of cytoreduction scores and different ways of reporting survival, so that the hope for such a multi-institutional study could be considered a scientific utopia at present.

In this chapter, we try to approach what could be a nonexhaustive list of precise and defined variables for such a trial. This represents only our own contribution to this crucial work, and many other expert contributions will be necessary to improve this approach to clinical research methodology for peritoneal surface oncology. We review different variables that have been reported as significant prognostic factors as well as variables that appear to be important factors regarding morbidity and mortality rates following treatment by CRS combined with perioperative intraperitoneal chemotherapy.

8.1 Preoperative Variables

In a search of the literature on CRS combined with HIPEC, preoperative variables are rarely reported as significant prognostic factors. However, the exact past history of the disease must be detailed for each patient included in an aggressive way of treatment. Today, the most common variable used for PC is the status „synchronous" or „metachronous." Although this variable has never been demonstrated as a significant prognostic factor for survival [4], a large multi-institutional study may have to use it for a subgroup analysis, including for „metachronous patients" the exact time interval between the first diagnosis of disease and the date of PC diagnosis. This description can be an easy one for PC arising from colorectal or gastric cancer: One has to specify the initial location and the initial pTNM staging of the primary tumor combined with a synchronous or metachronous PC. Regarding ovarian cancers, such a description will be a difficult one: The variable „synchronous" or „metachronous" must be specified as well as the time interval between a first response to therapy and a peritoneal recurrence, the number of surgical looks performed, the number of recurrences, and the delay between these different recurrences.

Concerning the past history of the disease, all chemotherapy lines have to be reported as well as response (or absence of response) to systemic chemotherapy. In case of synchronous PC, the use of neoadjuvant systemic chemotherapy must be reported (type of chemotherapy and number of courses).

For of a large multicentric study dedicated to CRS and HIPEC, there is no doubt that numerous variables will be needed (those listed above as well as age, gender, WHO status, and differentiation of the primary tumor). And there is no doubt that they will define a heterogeneous population of patients treated by the same therapeutic approach, with a strong need for subgroup analysis.

8.2 Peroperative Variables

Peroperative variables are mainly represented by the precise description of PC (tumor volume, location of malignant nodules, number of involved intra-abdominal regions, presence or absence of ascites, presence or absence of free malignant cells within the abdominal cavity, presence or absence of extraperitoneal metastases) and by the precise description of CRS (completeness of cytoreduction, duration of surgery, extent and location of peritonectomy procedures performed, number of digestive anastomoses performed).

8.2.1 Concerning the Peroperative Description of PC

Concerning the peroperative description of PC, several PC staging systems are available: the Gilly PC staging system (GSS), Sugarbaker's Peritoneal Cancer Index (PCI), the Dutch simplified PCI, and the Japanese PC staging system.

The Gilly Staging System. This staging was first described in 1994 [5] and takes into account the size of malignant implants (<5 mm, 5 mm to 2 cm, >2 cm) and their distribution (localized or diffuse). The details of this staging system are summarized in Table 8.1. This staging system can be used in the preoperative period as well as in the posttherapeutic phase, allowing a downstaging index (for example, a patient with a stage 4 peritoneal carcinomatosis who underwent a complete macroscopic surgical cytoreduction can be described as a stage 4 DS 0 – DS meaning "downstaged").

The two principal advantages of the Gilly staging system are its simplicity and reproducibility. Its prognostic influence was demonstrated in the multicentric prospective study EVOCAPE 1 [6], which included 370 patients with peritoneal carcinomatosis from nongynecologic malignancies. This staging system has also been shown to be an important prognostic indicator in several clinical trials: Rey et al., in a prospective study of 35 patients with carcinomatosis treated by CRS and HIPEC, reported 1-year and 2-year actuarial survival rates that were 63% and 31% for stage 1 and 2 carcinomatosis and 31% and 12% for stage 3 and 4, respectively [7].

In the phase II prospective studies from Lyon on carcinomatosis treated by CRS and HIPEC, there were significant differences between the prognosis of stage 1 and 2 and stage 3 and 4 [8]. For resectable gastric cancers with stage 1 and

Table 8.1. The Gilly Peritoneal Carcinomatosis staging system (Gilly et al. 1994)

Stage	Peritoneal carcinomatosis description
Stage 1	Malignant tumor nodules less than 5 mm in diameter
	Localized in one part of the abdomen
Stage 2	Tumor nodules less than 5 mm in diameter
	Diffuse to the whole abdomen
Stage 3	Tumor nodules 5 mm to 2 cm in diameter
Stage 4	Large (more than 2 cm diameter) tumor deposits

2, the 1-year survival rate was 80%, whereas it was only 10% for stage 3 and 4 [9]. In a phase II study concerning 83 patients with peritoneal carcinomatosis of digestive origin there was a 16-month median survival time for stage 1 and 2 and a 6-month median survival time for stage 3 and 4 [10]. Routinely used by several surgical teams, this staging system is also used by medical oncologists and radiologists, who appreciate its simplicity and consider it a valuable guide to assist them in patient selection.

The Peritoneal Cancer Index (PCI). The PCI was reported by Jacquet and Sugarbaker [11]: It is a quantitative assessment of both cancer distribution and cancer implant size throughout the abdomen and the pelvis. This scoring system has been used to evaluate carcinomatosis, sarcomatosis, and peritoneal mesothelioma. Two components are involved in its calculation. One component is the distribution of tumor in the abdominopelvic regions, and the other component is the lesion size score. Distribution of the implants on abdominal and pelvic surfaces greatly influences the likelihood of a complete cytoreduction by visceral resections and peritonectomy procedures. The current delineation of the PCI uses 13 abdominal and pelvic regions, as described in Fig. 8.1.

Concerning the lesion size score included in the PCI, it refers to the greatest diameter of the implants that are distributed to the peritoneal surfaces. If there are many implants within an abdominopelvic region, the size of the greatest diameter of the largest implant is measured and recorded. Primary tumors or localized recurrences at the primary site that can be removed definitively en bloc are excluded from lesion size assessment. Implants are scored as lesion size 0 through 3 (LS-0 to LS-3). LS-0 means that no implants are seen throughout the region; this measurement is determined after a complete lysis of all adhesions and the complete inspection of all parietal and visceral peritoneal surfaces. LS-1 refers to implants that are visible up to 0.5 cm in greatest diameter. LS-2 identifies nodules greater than 0.5 cm and up to 5 cm. LS-3 refers to implants 5 cm or greater in diameter. Further, if there is a confluence of disease matting abdominal or pelvic structures together, this automatically is scored as LS-3. Even a thin confluence of cancerous implants is designated as LS-3. PCI is determined before and after cytoreductive

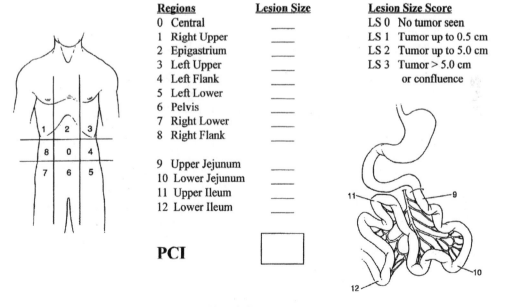

Fig. 8.1 Peritoneal Cancer Index (Jacquet and Sugarbaker 1996)

surgery, allowing scoring of the postoperative downstaging achieved.

The PCI is routinely used all over the world by surgical teams involved in PC. For carcinomatosis from colon cancer treated by CRS and HIPEC or early postoperative intraperitoneal chemotherapy (EPIC), Elias et al. [12] reported that the survival results were significantly better when the PCI was lower than 16. Sugarbaker reported from 100 patients with carcinomatosis from colon cancer a 5-year survival rate of 50% when the PCI was less than 10, a 5-year survival rate of 20% with a PCI of 11–20, and a 5-year survival rate of 0% with a PCI >20 [13]. Gomez Portilla et al. [14] also showed that the PCI could be used to predict long-term survival in patients with carcinomatosis from colon cancer treated by a second cytoreduction. Routinely used by surgeons involved in PC treatment, the PCI is rarely used by medical oncologists or radiologists.

The Japanese Research Society for Gastric Cancer (JRSGC) Carcinomatosis Staging System. In Japan, carcinomatosis from gastric cancer is classified by the JRSGC as follows: P0 means no implants to the peritoneum. P1 means cancerous implants directly adjacent to the stomach peritoneum, including the greater omentum. P2 means several scattered metastases to the distant peritoneum and ovarian metastasis alone. P3 means numerous metastases to the distant peritoneum. This classification has been used in Japanese studies as an accurate quantitative prognostic indicator [15].

The Dutch Simplified Peritoneal Carcinomatosis Index Assessment. At the Netherlands Cancer Institute, the extent of tumor is recorded on standardized forms indicating large (>5 cm), moderate (1–5 cm), small (<1 cm), or no involvement in seven abdominal regions. This assessment has been referred to as the "simplified PCI," or SPCI. The system is routinely used for colorectal and appendiceal cancer, and it has shown prognostic implications for outcome following CRS and HIPEC [16].

From our experience, we have already reported that a combination of the Gilly staging system and the PCI could probably be the most accurate method of PC description. The GSS and the PCI contribute to precise intraoperative description of carcinomatosis implants within the abdominopelvic cavity. Using both of them allows an accurate "map" of the lesions. For some instances of PC, GSS is the most accurate method (for an example of ovarian cancer with PC confined to the pelvic region with large confluence of implants, it will be scored as a GSS 4 – bad prognosis, while the PCI will only score 3 – favorable prognosis, mimicking small-size and limited peritoneal seeding). For other situations of PC, the PCI is more accurate (for an example of colorectal cancer with 2-mm implants under the right diaphragmatic cupula and large bulky malignant nodules in the right flank, it will be scored as a GSS 3 while PCI will only score 4). In Lyon, we systematically use both systems, GSS and PCI. A specific form is available in the operating room to allow a complete intraoperative description of lesions as well as a complete immediate post-CRS description of the remaining tumor volume.

8.2.2 Concerning the Completeness of Cytoreduction

Concerning the completeness of cytoreduction, using the UICC score for surgical resections in carcinomatosis could be correct. However, in patients with peritoneal carcinomatosis it is difficult or impossible to confirm a real R0 resection. The UICC score used is "R0-R1" for complete cytoreduction and R2 for incomplete cytoreduction. This has been used for the evaluation of cytoreductive surgery combined with HIPEC. In a trial of 56 patients with carcinomatosis from colon and ovarian cancer treated by CRS and HIPEC, Glehen et al. [3] reported a 2-year survival rate of 79% after R0-R1 resection, whereas it was 44.7% after R2 resection. In gastric cancer, Yonemura et al. [17] reported survival rates at 3 years of 40% in patients with R0-R1 cytoreduction combined with HIPEC, whereas it was 10% in patients with R2 cytoreduction.

To describe more precisely the completeness of cytoreduction performed, Sugarbaker and Chang [18] reported the CC Score (Completeness of Cytoreduction Score). For gastrointestinal cancers, the CC Score is defined as summarized in Fig. 8.2 and as follows: A CC-0 indicates that no peritoneal tumor nodules persist after CRS. A CC-1 indicates that tumor nodules persisting after cytoreduction are less than 2.5 mm in diameter (this is a nodule size thought to be penetrable by intracavitary chemotherapy). A CC-2 indicates residual tumor nodules 2.5 mm to 2.5 cm in diameter. A CC-3 indicates residual tumor nodules greater than 2.5 cm in diameter or a confluence of unresectable tumor nodules at any site within the abdomen and the pelvis. This CC Score has been evaluated through numerous prospective series, and a very similar staging system (named CCR-0, 1, or 2) has demonstrated its accuracy in an international registry reporting survival rates from 506 patients with colorectal cancer and PC treated by CRS and perioperative intraperitoneal chemotherapy (2).

Finally, to be exhaustive on peroperative variables, a special mention must be dedicated to the number of digestive anastomoses performed. This variable has been reported as a significant prognostic factor for postoperative morbidity [19, 20]. However, the number of anastomoses performed is probably not reported in the same way throughout the different reported series. For example, a right colectomy with an ileocolic anastomosis could represent "one" anastomosis. On the other hand, a total gastrectomy and a Roux-en-Y anastomosis could be reported as "one" anastomosis or "three" anastomoses (esophagojejunal anastomosis, duodenal stump closure, and jejuno-jejunal anastomosis). The definition of "digestive anastomosis" and its reporting must be clearly specified in trials dealing with CRS. Other peroperative variables have been reported as significant prognostic factors for postoperative morbidity or for survival (total blood loss, duration of surgery, peritoneal fluid cytological examination before and after CRS and HIPEC procedure) and are listed in Table 8.2.

8.3 HIPEC Variables

Although no major differences in morbidity rates and survival results exist in the literature between series using closed or open abdomen techniques, precise description of variables during HIPEC procedures must be reported: technique of HIPEC used, number of inflow and outflow drains used, inflow and outflow temperatures, intraperitoneal temperatures, duration of HIPEC, flow rate, volume of peritoneal dialysis liquid, doses of drugs, timing of drug injection into the circuit, type of quality control during the whole procedure, etc. Up to now, only intraperitoneal temperature has been reported as a significant prognostic factor in one phase II study [21].

8.4 Postoperative Variables

As demonstrated for colorectal or gastric cancer without PC, the pathological type of tumor must be precisely reported in CRS trials: Appendiceal cancers must be reported apart from colorectal cancers, and mucinous-type colorectal cancers must be analyzed as a specific subgroup [8, 20, 22, 23].

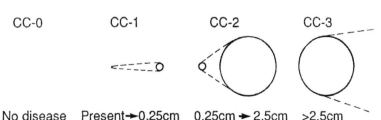

Fig. 8.2 Completeness of Cytoreduction Score

Table 8.2. Nonexhaustive proposed list for PC from colorectal cancer treated by CRS and HIPEC

	Variables	Subgroups	Other data	References[a]
Pre-operative variables	Age			
	Gender			
	WHO Performance Status			
	Location of primary tumor			22, 24
	pTNM of primary tumor			
	Type of PC	Synchronous	Neoadjuvant chemotherapy	
			Response to neoadjuvant chemotherapy	
			CRS + HIPEC at first or second look	
			Delay between first and second look	
		Metachronous	Type of initial treatment	
			Adjuvant chemotherapy	
			Disease-free interval	
			Number of surgical looks before CRS	
			Systemic chemotherapy before CRS	
			Response to systemic chemotherapy	
Per-operative variables	PCI	Before and after CRS		14, 22
	Gilly PC staging	Before and after CRS		8, 19
	Number of affected regions			8, 22
	Peritoneal fluid cytology	Before and after HIPEC		24
	Ascites			9, 24
	CCR score			8, 14, 20, 22
	R0, R1, R2 score			3, 24, 25
	Duration of surgery			19, 20, 21
	Number of resected organs			
	Number of anastomoses			19, 20
	Blood loss during surgery			20
	HIPEC variables	Inflow and IP temperatures		
		Drugs and dosage	Weight of the patient	
		Type of circuit		
		Temperature at drug introduction		
		Flow rate and duration		
		Volume of perfusate		
Post-operative variables	Pathological examination	Type and differentiation		8, 20, 22, 23
	Mortality	Within the 30 postoperative days		
	Morbidity	Grade 1		
		Grade 2		
		Grade 3		
		Grade 4		
	Parenteral nutrition			
	Duration hospital stay			
	Post-CRS treatment	Systemic chemotherapy		
		EPIC		
Survival	OS and DFS			
	Location of recurrence			
	Cause of death			

[a] References reporting variable as a significant prognostic factor
CRS, cytoreductive surgery; HIPEC, intraperitoneal chemohyperthermia; PCI, peritoneal cancer index; PC, peritoneal carcinomatosis; CCR, completeness of cytoreduction; OS, overall survival; DFS, disease-free survival; EPIC, immediate postoperative intraperitoneal chemotherapy

Two major postoperative variables must be clearly defined: mortality and morbidity. All trials evaluating CRS and HIPEC reported 0% to 10% mortality rates and 10% to 60% morbidity rates [2, 3, 12, 19]. A careful analysis of the literature reveals that mortality (restricted to the first 30 postoperative days) is easy to define while morbidity rates could be strongly different according to the selected criteria of morbidity. Some trials report an exhaustive list of postoperative complications (including urinary infections and superficial wound abscess), while other series only report severe postoperative complications.

An acceptable clinical research methodology could define the post-CRS and HIPEC morbidity according to the toxicity grading used by medical oncologists (Common Toxicity Criteria from NCI or WHO grades): The use of this grading system will allow us to compare morbidity rates between the different reported trials according to grade 1, 2, 3, and 4 toxicity.

Another important postoperative issue is the use of immediate postoperative intraperitoneal chemotherapy (EPIC) or the use of additional "adjuvant" systemic chemotherapy. In a recent multi-institutional study, a higher morbidity rate was observed for patients receiving EPIC compared with HIPEC alone [2].

8.5 Survival Results

Homogeneous presentation of survival results remains a key point in peritoneal surface oncology clinical research. Reporting both "overall survival" (OS) and "disease-free survival" (DFS) is obviously the minimum required. However, the exact "starting point" of the calculation has to be specified. Overall and DF survival could be calculated from the initial diagnosis of the disease, from the date of recurrence, or from the date of CRS and HIPEC. This point is of particular interest to be able to compare results of CRS and HIPEC to those obtained with systemic chemotherapy.

Of course, complete follow-up data of the trial must be added to the reported results, as well as the cutoff date for the analysis and the number of patients alive at the cutoff date.

8.6 Conclusion

Peritoneal surface malignancy represents a complex disease group since PC from colorectal cancer or from ovarian cancer, pseudomyxoma peritonei, or primary peritoneal neoplasms are obviously different disease processes. The experience we have accumulated in Lyon since 1989 reveals that a correct clinical research methodology is difficult to achieve for PC. Many research fields remain unexplored, such as the molecular biology of PC, which could represent a main prognostic factor for survival and therefore a main patient selection criterion. Many clinical research studies are ongoing, evaluating the respective impact of CRS and of HIPEC on outcomes, as well as patient quality of life after such aggressive treatments.

Taking into consideration the complexity of this field, we propose, as a challenge, a list of variables we need for clinical research in the field of PC arising from colorectal cancer treated with CRS and HIPEC. It is not an exhaustive list, and we hope that it can be improved by other experts.

References

1. Verwaal VJ, van Ruth S, de Bree E et al. (2003) Randomized trial of cytoreduction and hyperthermic intraperitoneal chemotherapy versus systemic chemotherapy and palliative surgery in patients with peritoneal carcinomatosis of colorectal cancer. J Clin Oncol 21:3737–3743
2. Glehen O, Kwiatkowski F, Sugarbaker PH, Elias D, Levine EA, De Simone M, Baronne R, Yonemura Y, Cavaliere F, Quenet F, Gutman M, Tentes AAK, Lorimier G, Bernard JL, Bereder JM, Porcheron J, Gomez Portilla A, Shen P, Deraco M, Rat P (2004). Cytoreductive surgery combined with perioperative intraperitoneal chemotherapy for the management of peritoneal carcinomatosis from colorectal cancer : a multi institutional study. J Clin Oncol 22:3284–3892
3. Glehen O, Mithieux F, Osinsky D et al. (2003) Sur-

gery combined with peritonectomy procedures and intraperitoneal chemohyperthermia in abdominal cancers with peritoneal carcinomatosis: a phase II study. J Clin Oncol 21:799–806
4. Glehen O, Cotte E, Schreiber V, Sayag Beaujard AC, Vignal J, Gilly FN (2004) Intraperitoneal chemohyperthermia and attempted cytoreductive surgery in patients with peritoneal carcinomatosis of colorectal origin. Br J Surg 91:747–754
5. Gilly FN, Carry PY, Sayag AC (1994) Regional chemotherapy (with mitomycin C) and intraoperative hyperthermia for digestive cancers with peritoneal carcinomatosis. Hepatogastroenterology 41:124–129
6. Sadeghi B, Arvieux C, Glehen O, et al. (2000) Peritoneal carcinomatosis from non gynecologic malignancies: results of the EVOCAPE 1 multicentric prospective study. Cancer 88:358–363
7. Rey Y, Porcheron J, Thalabard JN et al. (2000) Carcinoses péritonéales traitées par chirurgie de reduction tumorale et chimio-hyperthermie intrapéritonéale. Ann Chir 125:631–642
8. Glehen O, Cotte E, Schreiber V, Sayag Beaujard AC, Vignal J, Gilly FN (2004) Intraperitoneal chemohyperthermia and attempted cytoreductive surgery in patients with peritoneal carcinomatosis of colorectal origin. Br J Surg 91:747–754
9. Glehen O, Schreiber V, Cotte E, Sayag Beaujard AC, Osinsky D, Freyer G, François Y, Vignal J, Gilly FN (2004) Cytoreductive surgery and intraperitoneal chemohyperthermia for peritoneal carcinomatosis arising from gastric cancer. Arch Surg 139:20–26
10. Beaujard AC, Glehen O, Caillot JL, Francois Y, Bienvenu J, Panteix G et al. (2000) Intraperitoneal chemohyperthermia with mitomycin C for digestive tract cancer patients with peritoneal carcinomatosis. Cancer 88:2512–2519
11. Jacquet P, Sugarbaker PH (1996) Clinical research methodologies in diagnosis and staging of patients with peritoneal carcinomatosis. In: Sugarbaker PH (ed) Peritoneal carcinomatosis: principles of management. Kluwer Academic Publishers, Boston, pp 359–374
12. Elias D, Blot F, El Otmany A, Antoun S, Lasser P, Boige V et al. (2001) Curative treatment of peritoneal carcinomatosis arising from colorectal cancer by complete resection and intraperitoneal chemotherapy. Cancer 92:71–76
13. Sugarbaker PH (1999) Successful management of microscopic residual disease in large bowel cancer. Cancer Chemother Pharmacol 43:15–25
14. Gomez Portilla A, Sugarbaker PH, Chang D (1999) Second look surgery after cytoreductive and intraperitoneal chemotherapy for peritoneal carcinomatosis from colorectal cancer : analysis of prognostic features. World J Surg 23:23–29
15. Fujimoto S, Takahaschi M, Mutou T et al. (1997) Improved mortality rate of gastric cancer patients with peritoneal carcinomatosis treated with intraperitoneal hyperthermic chemoperfusion combined with surgery. Cancer 79:884–891
16. van der Vange N, van Goethem AR, Zoetmulder FAN et al. (2000) Extensive cytoreductive surgery combined with intraoperative intraperitoneal perfusion with cisplatin under hyperthermic conditions (OVHI-PEC) in patients with recurrent ovarian cancer. Eur J Surg Oncol 26:663–668
17. Yonemura Y, Fujimura T, Fuschida S et al. (1999) A new surgical approach (peritonectomy) for the treatment of peritoneal dissemination. Hepatogastroenterology 46:601–609
18. Sugarbaker PH, Chang D (1999) Results of treatment of 385 patients with peritoneal surface spread of appendiceal malignancy. Ann Surg Oncol 6:727–731
19. Glehen O, Osinsky D, Cotte E et al. (2003) Intraperitoneal chemohyperthermia using a closed abdominal procedure and cytoreductive surgery for the treatment of peritoneal carcinomatosis: morbidity and mortality analysis of 216 consecutive procedures. Ann Surg Oncol 10:863–869
20. Stephens AD, Alderman R, Chang D et al. (1999) Morbidity and mortality analysis of 200 treatments with cytoreductive surgery and hyperthermic intraoperative intraperitoneal chemotherapy using the Coliseum technique. Ann Surg Oncol 6:790–796
21. Jacquet P, Stephens AD, Averbach AM et al. (1996) Analysis of morbidity and mortality in 60 patients with peritoneal carcinomatosis treated by cytoreductive surgery and heated intraoperative intraperitoneal chemotherapy. Cancer 77:2622–2629
22. Verwaal VJ, van Tinteren H, van Ruth S et al. (2004) Predicting the survival of patients with peritoneal carcinomatosis of colorectal origin treated by aggressive cytoreduction and hyperthermic intraperitoneal chemotherapy. Br J Surg 91:739–746
23. Pilati P, Mocellin S, Rossi CR, Foletto M, Campana L, Nitti D et al. (2003) Cytoreductive surgery combined with hyperthermic intraperitoneal intraoperative chemotherapy for peritoneal carcinomatosis arising from colon adenocarcinoma. Ann Surg Oncol 10:508–513
24. Loggie BW, Fleming RA, McQuellon RP et al. (2000) Cytoreductive surgery with intraperitoneal hyperthermic chemotherapy for disseminated peritoneal cancer of gastrointestinal origin. Am Surgeon 66:561–568
25. Shen P, Levine EA, Hall J et al. (2003) Factors predicting survival after intraperitoneal hyperthermic chemotherapy with mitomycin C after cytoreductive surgery for patients with peritoneal carcinomatosis. Arch Surg 138:26–33

9 Lessons Learnt from Clinical Trials in Peritoneal Surface Oncology: Colorectal Carcinomatosis

Frans A. N. Zoetmulder and Vic J. Verwaal

Recent Results in Cancer Research, Vol. 169
© Springer-Verlag Berlin Heidelberg 2007

9.1 Introduction

Very few surgical cancer therapies have been tested in randomised studies. An obvious reason for this is the fact that most cancer operations were developed in the age when randomised studies were simply not heard of. By now many cancer operations have proved to be curative in a considerable percentage of patients, and neither patients nor surgeons would want to miss that chance of permanent cure. After Sugarbaker had shown in a small randomised study that post-operative intraperitoneal 5-flu-orouracil (5-FU) installations could prevent the development of peritoneal metastases in some high risk colon cancer patients [1] he developed this technique as treatment for patients with established peritoneal carcinomatosis (PC). As he could show some promising results, a group of enthusiasts grew who invested heavily in this new approach towards an, until then, incurable disease. The post-operative 5-FU installation technique evolved into the hyperthermic intraperitoneal chemotherapy (HIPEC) technique with either mitomycin C or oxaliplatin, which is at present used in many centres.

Notwithstanding promising results in phase II type studies from several centres [2–13], it proved impossible to convince the wider medical oncology community of the benefits of cytoreduction and HIPEC in these patients. Gradually it became clear that only convincing evidence from a randomised study could achieve this goal.

9.2 Randomised Study in PC of Colorectal Origin

There is only one randomised study comparing the HIPEC approach with conventional treatment of PC of colorectal origin [14]. In this study from the Netherlands Cancer Institute patients with proven PC were randomised either to undergo limited palliative surgery followed by systemic treatment with 5-FU/leucovorin or to undergo cytoreduction and HIPEC, followed by the same systemic chemotherapy. One hundred and five patients were randomised in a 3-year period, 51 in the standard arm and 54 in the experimental arm. Only 44 patients in the standard arm started their chemotherapy. Two patients refused the result of the randomisation and went abroad to undergo HIPEC treatment. The other patients did not start, mainly because of early progression.

In the experimental arm five patients did not get their HIPEC therapy. One patient died while on the waiting list, one patient refused at the last minute, and three patients developed distant metastases in the time between randomisation and the planned operation date.

HIPEC consisted of continuous peritoneal lavage with a solution containing mitomycin C at a dose of 35 mg/m2, with a maximum of 70 mg. Half of this dose was administered at the start of the lavage, 25% after 30 min and 25% after 60 min, with a total lavage time of 90 min. The temperature was kept between 40°C and 42°C, at three measuring points in the abdomen. Thirty-five patients started their systemic chemotherapy after recovery from the HIPEC treatment. The main reason for not starting was a complicated post-operative period. Detailed information on the extent of PC was only available for the patients undergoing HIPEC. Many patients had very extensive PC, with 54% having five or more of seven abdominal regions involved and over 30% having six or seven regions involved.

It was possible to resect all macroscopic PC in 38% of patients. In 43% small residues (<2.5 mm) were left behind, whereas in 19% larger residues remained. To achieve this level of cytoreduction a multitude of surgical resections had to be done, including omentectomy and multiple bowel resections in most patients. In accordance with this extensive surgery complications have been frequent. Most common complications were infectious, related to small bowel leakage. In 17 patients mild leucocytopenia occurred, with a nadir on day 10. Notwithstanding, the 30-day mortality was only 2% and the mean hospital stay 26 days. However, eight patients died within 3 months, commonly because of long-term post-operative complications and early cancer recurrence. All early deaths and the majority of complications occurred in patients with extensive PC (6 or 7 regions involved).

All patients were analysed according to the intention to treat principle. Survival data show that patients in the HIPEC arm lived significantly longer than patients undergoing conventional therapy (Fig. 9.1). The median survival almost doubled, from 12 to 22 months. Also in this study a survival plateau developed at 20%, with no additional death after 5 years.

A recent update from this study shows that the advantage of HIPEC therapy is still significant after a follow-up of 5 years.

Not all patients benefited equally. As in other series, the extent of disease at the start of cytoreduction and the completeness of cytoreduction are the dominant factors predicting long-term survival. None of the patients with truly diffuse disease, involving six or seven abdominal regions, survived long. Only patients without any macroscopic tumour residue survived longer than 5 years (Fig. 9.2).

Cost comparison between the two treatment arms showed that in the Netherlands setting, HIPEC treatment costs €17,284.00 per life year gained. Quality of life (QoL) comparison showed some reduction in the QoL score, 3 months after HIPEC treatment, but QoL scores were equal in both arms after 6 months.

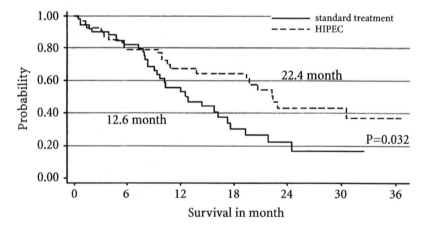

Fig. 9.1 Survival in 105 patients randomised to either undergo standard therapy or cytoreduction and HIPEC

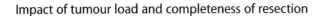

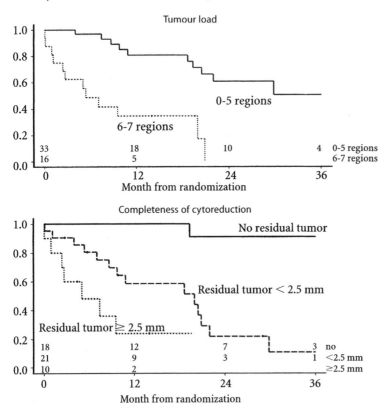

Fig. 9.2 Impact of extent of PC and completeness of cytoreduction on survival (Verwaal et al. [15])

9.3 Lessons from This Study

This randomised study convincingly proves that PC from colorectal cancer is a potentially curable disease, comparable to other limited colon cancer metastases, such as liver and lung. The combination of complete cytoreduction and HIPEC, followed by systemic chemotherapy, can cure some of these patients.

This has not been an easy study to perform. For many patients with PC of colorectal cancer HIPEC presents their last chance for cure, and few will willingly submit to randomisation that includes a treatment option without such a long-term perspective. The reason that this study succeeded was the fact that the investigators honestly doubted whether the advantages of the HIPEC approach could offset the early morbidity and mortality anticipated. Based on this honest uncertainly it proved possible to convince so many patients to take part. In this endeavor the down-to-earth attitude of many Dutchmen towards disease and death was of great help. It was also helpful that the Netherlands Cancer Institute, the institution which conducted this trial, was during this period the only HIPEC treatment centre in the country.

After this trial, however, it is clear that it will be impossible to conduct a new study without cytoreduction and HIPEC as standard treatment.

Patient selection has emerged as a key issue during this trial. When the trial was designed the understanding of the relationship between extent of disease before cytoreduction, the completeness of cytoreduction and the outcome was still not fully appreciated. Because of this many patients were included to whom we at present would not offer HIPEC therapy. A consequence of this has been a high rate of complications and toxicity. Since all early deaths occurred in patients with extensive disease, it seems obvious that exclusion of these patients will improve short-term outcome. Indeed, implementation of more strict selection criteria over the years has improved the percentage of completely resectable cases, reduced the complication rate and improved the median survival significantly (Fig. 9.3) [14].

Selection remains difficult, however. because of the difficulty of depicting PC on CT or MRI. The main source for reliable information on the extent of disease remains the observation during laparotomy. As in most cases PC is diagnosed during laparotomy, either for surgery of the primary, or during laparotomy for recurrence or obstruction, this information should be readily available. It is, however, disappointing how many surgeons still observe the presence of PC but do not take the effort to clearly describe the spread over the abdomen. However, the message gets through slowly, and it is clear that more and more surgeons in the Netherlands now understand the importance of proper registration of the extent of disease, especially of the involvement of the small bowel.

Small bowel involvement is the key factor deciding resectability of PC. Diffuse involvement, especially if the mesentery starts shrinking, turns a patient inoperable. If there is any suspicion in that direction, laparoscopy is probably indicated. If it is found during laparotomy, we do not proceed with the HIPEC procedure. At present this occurs in 10% of planned HIPEC procedures.

Many questions surrounding HIPEC treatment of PC of colorectal cancer are still open. For instance, is the addition of HIPEC to complete cytoreduction essential, or could the same result be reached by combining cytoreduction with modern multidrug systemic chemotherapy? Also, what is the best schedule of HIPEC, MMC as used in the randomized study, or can the same or better results be reached with the combination of preoperative systemic 5-FU and HIPEC with oxaliplatin?

Another interesting question is whether the sequence of first cytoreduction and HIPEC and afterwards systemic chemotherapy is really the best. Now that we have combination systemic chemotherapy which will reduce tumour burden in a majority of cases [15] it could be of benefit to reverse the sequence and give patients systemic chemotherapy first and do the cytoreduction and HIPEC at the point of maximum response.

All these questions are awaiting further well-designed multi-centre randomised stud-

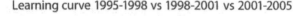
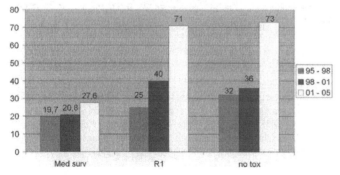

Fig. 9.3 Learning curve, influence on completeness of cytoreduction, complication rate and median survival. *R1*, complete cytoreduction; *No tox*, absence of complications; *Med surv*, median survival

ies, which hopefully will be conducted in the near future.

At this moment, however, cytoreduction and HIPEC with mitomycin C followed by systemic chemotherapy is the only curative treatment for patients with PC of colorectal cancer based on solid evidence.

References

1. Sugarbaker PH, Gianola FJ, Speyer JL et al. (1985) Prospective randomized trial of intravenous v intraperitoneal 5-FU in patients with advanced primary colon or rectal cancer. Semin Oncol 12:101–111
2. Sugarbaker PH, Jablonski KA (1995). Prognostic features of 51 colorectal and 130 appendiceal cancer patients with peritoneal carcinomatosis treated by cytoreductive surgery and intraperitoneal chemotherapy. Ann Surg 221:124–132
3. Sugarbaker PH, Schellinx ME, Chang D, Koslowe P, von Meyerfeldt M (1996). Peritoneal carcinomatosis from adenocarcinoma of the colon. World J Surg 20:585–591
4. Elias D, Blot F, El Otmany A et al. (2001) Curative treatment of peritoneal carcinomatosis arising from colorectal cancer by complete resection and intraperitoneal chemotherapy. Cancer 92:71–76
5. Loggie BW, Fleming RA, McQuellon RP, Russell GB, Geisinger KR (2000) Cytoreductive surgery with intraperitoneal hyperthermic chemotherapy for disseminated peritoneal cancer of gastrointestinal origin. Am Surg 66:561–568
6. Elias D, Marsaud M, Ede C et al. (2004) Efficacy of intraperitoneal chemohyperthermia with oxaliplatin in colorectal peritoneal carcinomatosis. Preliminary results in 24 patients. Ann Oncol 15:781–785
7. Glehen O, Kwiatkowski F, Sugarbaker PH et al. (2004) Cytoreductive surgery combined with perioperative intraperitoneal chemotherapy for the management of peritoneal carcinomatosis from colorectal cancer: a multi-institutional study. J Clin Oncol 22:3284–3292
8. Gilly FN, Beaujard A, Glehen O et al. (1999) Peritonectomy combined with intraperitoneal chemohyperthermia in abdominal cancer with peritoneal carcinomatosis: phase I–II study. Anticancer Res 19:2317–2321
9. Verwaal VJ, van Tinteren H, van Ruth S, Zoetmulder FA (2004) Predicting the survival of patients with peritoneal carcinomatosis of colorectal origin treated by aggressive cytoreduction and hyperthermic intraperitoneal chemotherapy. Br J Surg 91:739–746
10. Pilati P, Mocellin S, Rossi CR et al. (2003) Cytoreductive surgery combined with hyperthermic intraperitoneal intraoperative chemotherapy for peritoneal carcinomatosis arising from colon adenocarcinoma. Ann Surg Oncol 10:508–513
11. Cavaliere F, Perri P, Rossi CR et al. (2003) [Indications for integrated surgical treatment of peritoneal carcinomatosis of colorectal origin: experience of the Italian Society of Locoregional Integrated Therapy in Oncology]. Tumori 89:21–23
12. Shen P, Hawksworth J, Lovato J et al. (2004) Cytoreductive surgery and intraperitoneal hyperthermic chemotherapy with mitomycin C for peritoneal carcinomatosis from nonappendiceal colorectal carcinoma. Ann Surg Oncol 11:178–186
13. Kecmanovic DM, Pavlov MJ, Ceranic MS et al. (2005) Treatment of peritoneal carcinomatosis from colorectal cancer by cytoreductive surgery and hyperthermic perioperative intraperitoneal chemotherapy. Eur J Surg Oncol 31:147–152
14. Verwaal VJ, van Ruth S, Witkamp A et al. (2005) Long-term survival of peritoneal carcinomatosis of colorectal origin. Ann Surg Oncol 12:65–71
15. Verwaal VJ, van Ruth S, de Bree E et al. (2003) Randomized trial of cytoreduction and hyperthermic intraperitoneal chemotherapy versus systemic chemotherapy and palliative surgery in patients with peritoneal carcinomatosis of colorectal cancer. J Clin Oncol 21:3737–3743
16. Goldberg RM (2005) Advances in the treatment of metastatic colorectal cancer. Oncologist 10 [Suppl 3]:40–48, Review3

10 Experimental Models and Questions in Basic Science Research for Pseudomyxoma Peritonei

Laura A. Lambert, Donald H. Lambert, Paul Mansfield

10.1 Introduction

Pseudomyxoma peritonei (PMP) is a poorly understood disease characterized by mucinous ascites and disseminated peritoneal mucinous tumors, with a clinically protracted course. Although PMP has been ascribed to a variety of sources (Yasar et al. 1997; Lee and Scully 2000; Imaoka et al. 2006), clinical and molecular evidence is mounting that neoplastic mucin-producing goblet cells of the appendix are the primary cause of PMP. (Ronnett et al. 1995; Ronnett et al. 1997; Szych et al. 1999). Although PMP is not an intrinsically malignant process, it is not a benign process either. Not only does PMP replace the entire free space of the abdomen with mucin, it also causes fibrosis that often leads to complete bowel obstruction and ultimately death. Currently the only effective treatment for PMP is cytoreductive surgery (CRS) that removes all of the mucin and mucin-producing cells combined with hyperthermic intraperitoneal chemotherapy (HIPEC) (Sugarbaker 2006). Unfortunately, even with this aggressive treatment, patients with PMP may endure recurrent mucin accumulation and eventually die from the disease.

Clinical research has recently advanced our understanding of PMP in terms of its etiology and clinical significance. However, little is known of the subcellular, cellular, and extracellular mechanisms of PMP. Systematic scientific molecular- and cellular-level investigations have yet to be conducted. The current paucity of basic science knowledge of PMP is likely due to its rarity and the perception that it is an „orphan" disease. Additionally, there are no commercially available primary PMP cell lines or established animal models to facilitate PMP research. Consequently, basic science research in PMP is essentially unexplored. Owing to significant recent advances in technology and the understanding of cancer biology, the time to begin exploring the basic science of PMP has definitely arrived.

The recent advent of clinically effective, biological anticancer agents and targeted therapies has reinvigorated the fight against cancer, including peritoneum-based malignancies. The need and the rationale for developing treatments for patients with PMP are clear. The morbidity associated with CRS and HIPEC and the incidence of PMP-specific death following these treatments demand better and more benign treatment strategies. Because of the resistance of PMP to conventional, systemic chemotherapy, there are no treatment options for patients with inoperable disease. Investigation at the molecular and cellular levels may identify targets unique to the mucin-producing neoplastic cells that hopefully will lead to rational, targeted, and effective treatments. The purpose of this chapter is to review the basic science PMP literature, to outline some important goals of PMP basic science research, and to discuss potential avenues of future investigation.

10.2 The Challenge

Conventional DNA-damaging chemotherapy is largely effective because cancer cells replicate DNA and divide more frequently than normal cells. Theoretically, increased cell division renders cancerous cells more susceptible to DNA damage by chemotherapy agents than normal cells. Although this approach has some success in certain cancers, it is not effective in PMP for a number of reasons. (1) In most cases of PMP, the disease process is largely acellular. (2) The few cells that cause PMP are not exposed to therapeutic levels of systemically administered antineoplastic agents because of the peritoneum-blood barrier and the mucin they produce. (3) Based upon the indolent nature of the disease (Solkar et al. 2004), PMP-producing cells probably divide more slowly than the more rapidly dividing cells of chemosensitive malignancies. Nevertheless, the cells responsible for PMP, like those of any other type of neoplasm, are governed by the same requirements for neoplastic transformation: (1) genetic alteration, (2) deregulation of the cell cycle, (3) resistance to apoptosis, and (4) the ability to metastasize (although extraperitoneal metastases are an extremely rare event in this disease). Through research focused on the identification and exploitation of defects in these causes of neoplastic transformation, potential targets for curing PMP can be identified.

10.3 Neoplastic Mucin-Producing Goblet Cells of the Appendix

Most research efforts in PMP have been clinical and focused primarily on the origin, the pattern of spread, and the malignant transformation of the neoplasm. Although these studies have helped categorize and stratify various clinicopathological parameters, they have not significantly altered the management of the disease. Only a few studies have looked specifically at the genetic alterations of the PMP-producing cells. Szych et al. described the clonality of PMP-producing cells (Szych et al. 1999). They identified identical k-Ras proto-oncogene mutations in 16 of 16 (100%) PMP patients with synchronous appendiceal and ovarian tumors. They also observed a discordant pattern of allelic loss between the ovarian and appendiceal tumors at either one or two loci (on chromosomes 18q, 17p, 5q, or 6q) in six PMP patients. In all but one instance, heterozygosity was lost in the ovarian tumor, whereas both alleles were retained in the matched appendiceal lesion, suggesting a pattern of tumor progression in a secondary (metastatic) site (ovary). Based on these observations, the authors concluded that mucinous tumors involving the appendix and ovaries in women with PMP are clonal and derived from a single site, most likely the appendix. Cuatrecasas et al. and Kabbani et al. have reported similar findings (Cuatrecasas et al. 1996; Kabbani et al. 2002). Other studies have examined the presence of the mismatch repair genes and the loss of chromosome 18q in mucinous tumors of appendix (Maru et al. 2004; Misdraji et al. 2004). No obvious role in appendiceal malignant transformation has been identified.

Carr et al. characterized some aspects of cell cycle deregulation and apoptosis in epithelial neoplasms of the appendix and of the colorectum (Carr et al. 2002). They retrospectively reviewed 299 surgical immunohistochemistry (IHC) specimens of adenocarcinomas and adenomas of the appendix and colorectum. Their objectives were to determine differences in the numbers of proliferating and apoptotic cells and expression of p53. Outcome measures included expression of Ki-67 (proliferation), M30 (apoptosis), p53 (tumor suppressor), CD44s (cell adhesion molecule), and bcl-2 (anti-apoptosis). The authors examined 33 cases of well-differentiated mucinous adenocarcinoma of the appendix, of which 20 were associated with PMP and 48 patients with appendiceal adenomas (the associated number of patients with PMP was not described). Comparison of the colorectal versus appendiceal adenomas showed significant differences between the levels of Ki-67 ($P<0.001$), p53 ($P<0.01$), and bcl-2 ($P<0.01$), with the appendiceal neoplasms containing less of each marker. Comparison of the adenocarcinomas showed significant differences in Ki-67 (P<0.001), M30 (P<0.001), and CD44s (P<0.01), again with the appendiceal tumors containing less of each marker. However, only the M30 count was significantly different in the analysis of well-differentiated mucinous adenocarcinomas. The authors postulated that the lower rates of proliferation and apoptosis seen with appendiceal carcinomas are consistent with their more indolent behavior. They postulated also that the decreased expression of CD44s in the appendiceal neoplasms might be relevant to the relatively low rate of distant metastases. The most intriguing finding was that apoptosis (M30) and the apoptosis-to-proliferation ratio (M30: Ki-67) were not dependent on tumor morphology (mucinous vs. nonmucinous). Because the M30-to-Ki-67 ratio was lower in the appendix (vs. colorectal cancer), the lower appendiceal apoptotic rate could not be attributed to a reduction in cell proliferation. The authors suggested that the duration of apoptosis may be shorter in mucinous appendiceal tumors. In that case, the number of apoptotic cells in the tumor sample would be small. Alternatively, appendiceal neoplasms may have acquired a resistance to apoptosis.

The most striking feature of PMP is the overproduction of mucin. O'Connell et al. argue that it is the over production of mucin that causes PMP's morbidity and that this is where therapeutic efforts should be focused (O'Connell et al. 2002). Using a variety of experimental techniques, O'Connell et al. demonstrated that secretory MUC2 is the predominant mucin present in PMP. (MUC2 is the primary gastrointestinal mucin, and it is produced by highly differentiated goblet cells.) This finding supports the concept that the appendiceal goblet cell is the most likely origin of PMP, as the other likely candidates (the normal ovary or mucinous ovarian tumors) do not produce significant amounts of MUC2 . If MUC2 is the mucin of PMP, it could provide a molecular target that can differentiate the neoplastic cells (mucin-producing) from the normal cells (non-mucin producing) within the peritoneal cavity.

O'Connell et al. used IHC, in situ hybridization, and digital imaging techniques to compare the amount of mucin present in both normal and neoplastic appendiceal goblet cells. Because the expression of mucin was similar in both cell types, the authors concluded that the mucin overproduction in PMP was not due to abnormal mucin production per se. They next isolated and cultured epithelial cells found in PMP, performed DNA extractions, and digested the DNA with restriction enzymes. These experiments revealed no alterations in the MUC2 gene that might explain the excessive mucin production. In addition, there was no association between mucin production and the degree of malignant transformation. The authors concluded that the mucin overproduction was most likely due to an increased burden of mucin-producing cells. This is the only published study that has utilized primary PMP cell cultures. Although the authors were unable to generate an immortalized cell line, they successfully passaged in culture enough MUC2-expressing epithelial cells from PMP to perform their provocative experiments. This is remarkable considering the difficulties associated with primary cell culture and that one kilogram of PMP tissue yields only 10^7 cells!

The authors asked also whether the epigenetic phenomenon of DNA methylation plays a role in regulating MUC2 production. DNA methylation is an epigenetic process whereby DNA methyltransferase covalently attaches methyl groups to cytosine and guanine-rich areas of DNA. These regions, known as CpG islands, usually occur in gene promoters. Methylation of a gene promoter can result in decreased expression or complete silencing of the gene, including many tumor suppressor genes. After treatment of the PMP cells with 5'-azacytidine, and lipopolysaccharide (DNA demethylating agents), there was a significant increase in MUC2 mRNA production, presumably due to demethylation of the MUC2 promoter. The authors concluded that DNA methylation of the MUC2 promoter probably plays a role in the MUC2 production in PMP. Finally, the authors recommended that inhibition of MUC2 transcription be considered as an adjuvant therapy for PMP. Like many scientific endeavors, attempting to answer a question often creates many more.

10.4 Questions

Clearly these above-mentioned studies are the "tip of the molecular biology of PMP iceberg." An obvious and important question is which cancer-causing mutations are active in PMP? A cell cycle question unique to PMP is why is the rate of cell proliferation so slow compared to other neoplasms? Also, what is the role of cell cycle aberrations in the production of PMP? Are PMP cells more or less resistant to apoptosis than those of colorectal origin and if more resistant what survival pathways are involved? What determines the metastatic potential and the locoregional invasion profile of PMP? Finally, is there a relationship between the neoplastic transformation of appendiceal goblet cells and the mucin production in PMP?

During the past decade, major technological advances and their application to cancer research have increased our understanding of the genetic and biochemical mechanisms by which cancers arise. This knowledge has recently been translated into new therapies that target the genetic causes of cancer. Consequently, the direction of cancer research has shifted to a patient-centered model that is based on three important observations: (1) All neoplasms contain genetic alterations that drive their growth and/or mark their progression; (2) tumor behavior is influenced by the surrounding host tissue; and (3) individual differences in (1) and (2) affect the clinical course of the disease. As is taking place with most other cancers, these observations must be applied to PMP research as well.

10.5 Experimental Models

Before PMP researchers can take advantage of the technological advances occurring in molecular biology, a primary cell line must be developed. Five cell lines have been created from colon or rectum tumors, which are capable of forming mucin-producing tumors in nude mice (Park et al. 1987; Tibbetts et al. 1988; Yamachika et al. 2005). Only one of these is commercially available (Park et al. 1987), and there are no commercially available PMP cell lines. Immortalized cell lines are difficult to establish, even when starting with an aggressive primary tumor. Reports of mucin-producing cell lines capable of creating a PMP-like condition in nude mice, from primary colon cancers (Tibbetts et al. 1988) or from peritoneal implants (Park et al. 1987), illustrate the difficulties associated with this undertaking. Even transient primary PMP cultures, as detailed in the experience by O'Connell et al. is a formidable task (O'Connell et al. 2002). Some of the variables associated with this task include media, growth supplements, temperature, CO2 content, extracting fibroblasts, and whether to grow the cells in suspension or on a culture plate. Based upon recent experience in our laboratory, growing PMP cells in suspension is the most successful. Creation of xenografts may be another way of generating cells and a means of "jump-starting" a primary culture. In addition to establishing a primary culture, PMP research requires an animal model. While intraperitoneal and orthotopic xenographs of mucin-producing tumor cells are acceptable experimental systems, the creation of a transgenic PMP mouse would be ideal.

10.6 Genetics

The absence of a PMP cell line does not preclude PMP genetic analysis. It is possible to compare the gene sequences of healthy tissue with diseased tissue in order to understand genetic variations associated with a disease. Once genetic variations are identified, targeted sequencing studies of particular genes can then assess the presence of any cancer-causing mutations. Discovery of cancer-causing mutations by DNA sequencing has already led to the successful treatment of some cancers, such as c-kit positive gastrointestinal stromal tumors with c-kit inhibitor STI-571 (Sanborn and Blanke 2005). In general, cancer-causing mutations tend to occur in tumor suppressor genes that are inactivated by loss-of-function mutations or oncogenes, which are activated by gene amplification, gene translocation, or gain-of-function mutations. The list of cancer-causing mutations being considered for targeted anticancer strategies is long and getting longer (Table 10.1). As the potential genetic targets continue to grow, an understanding of PMP genetics will be essential for the treatment of PMP patients.

Table 10.1 Examples of potential targeted therapies

Biologic target	Target function	Potential therapeutic agent(s)	Mechanism of action
I. Signal transduction pathways			
Endothelial growth factor receptor (EGFR)	Tyrosine kinase; initiates intracellular signaling for cell proliferation	Cetuximab (Erbitux®, Bristol Meyers Squib, New York, NY)	Antagonistic monoclonal antibody
EGFR	Tyrosine kinase; initiates intracellular signaling for cell proliferation	Iressa (ZD1893)	Small molecule inhibitor
RAS	Mitogen-responsive proto-oncogene	Tipfarnib, Iofarnib	Farnesyl transferase inhibitors
RAF-1	Signal transduction kinase in RAS proto-oncogene pathway	BAY-43-9006	Kinase inhibition
II. Cell cycle			
Cyclin-dependent kinases	Cell cycle progression	Flavopiridol, roscovitine	Kinase inhibition
III. Apoptosis			
Tumor necrosis factor-apoptosis initiating ligand (TRAIL)	Induction of apoptosis	TRAIL	Agonistic antibody
IV. Angiogenesis			
Vascular endothelial growth factor (VEGF)	Promotion of angiogenesis	Avastin® (bevacizumab, BV, Genentech, San Francisco, CA)	Antagonistic monoclonal antibody
VEGF	Promotion of angiogenesis	PTK/ZK	Small molecule inhibitor
V. Other potential targets			
Matrix Metalloproteinases (MMPs)	Breakdown of extracellular matrix; promotion of metastases	Marimastat; prinostat; tanomastat;	MMP inhibition through direct binding
Cyclooxygenase 2 (COX2)	Conversion of arachidonic acid to prostaglandin; relation to cancer biology unclear	Sulindac, aspirin, rofecexib, celecoxib	Inhibits prostaglandin production
mTOR	Kinase; involved in protein translation of cell cycle genes	Rapamycin	Kinase inhibition
Proteasome	Degradation of negative cell cycle regulatory proteins	Bortezomib (PS-341, VelcadeTM, Millenium, Cambridge, MA)	Proteasome inhibitor
Heat shock protein-90 (HSP-90)	Stabilization of proteins involved in cell proliferation and survival	Geldamycin	HSP-90 inhibition

10.7 Cell Cycle

All neoplastic cells possess some form of cell cycle deregulation, and the cells that cause PMP are no exception. The cell cycle is the orderly sequence of events that ensures the appropriate and precise duplication and segregation of a cell's DNA during the process of cell division. The cycle is conventionally divided into four phases: (1) S phase, during which DNA replication occurs (S for synthesis); (2) M phase, during which the cell undergoes the process of mitosis; and two gap phases, (3) G1 and (4) G2, during which the remainder of the cell's contents are duplicated (Fig. 10.1).

Biochemical switches or checkpoints exist between each cell cycle phase to ensure that the proper sequence of events is followed. One of the most common and important sites of aberrant cell cycle regulation is known as the "restriction point." The restriction point is the biochemical switch created by the confluence of the pRb (tumor suppressor) and c-Myc (oncogene) pathways that governs the transition between the G1 and S phases (Blagosklonny and Pardee 2002) (Fig. 10.2) This checkpoint

Regulation of Restriction Point

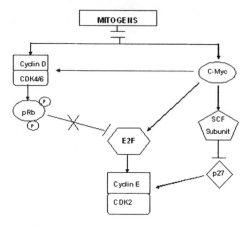

Fig. 10.2 The restriction point. The restriction point is the key checkpoint in late G_1 phase where the cell commits to replicating its DNA. This molecular switch revolves around the activity of Cdk2 and its G_1-associated cyclin, cyclin E, and the point of convergence of the RB (p16-Cdk4/6-cyclin D-pRb) tumor suppressor pathway and c-Myc proto-oncogene pathway

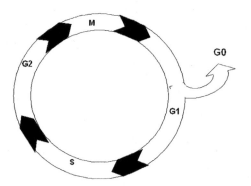

Fig. 10.1 The cell cycle. The cell cycle is divided into four major phases. Cells in G_1 can either progress through the cell cycle or exit to G_0 (quiescence). Passage of the cell from the G_1 phase to the S phase is controlled by the important biochemical switch known as the restriction point. Once through the restriction point, the cell is committed to DNA replication, which occurs in S phase. The G_2 phase ensures that the newly replicated DNA is ready for segregation into daughter cells. In M phase, the nucleus and then the cytoplasm divide

is particularly important because once a cell passes through it, the cell becomes committed to DNA replication. Loss of the restriction point results in inappropriate cell replication and the inability of the cell to stop cycling and enter a quiescence state known as G0. All aspects of the cell cycle have been associated with neoplastic transformation owing to mutation. Some of the more common mutations include the G1 cyclins (D, E), their negative regulators (p16, p53), and their downstream targets (pRb, cMyc). Because these types of mutations are directly associated with the neoplastic process, there is an interest in using small molecules that target the cell cycle. Identification of cell cycle defects in PMP will increase the number of potential PMP anticancer targets.

10.8 Apoptosis

It is well established that defects in apoptosis occur commonly in cancer. These defects contribute to all aspects of cancer including pathogenesis, progression, and therapeutic resistance. Consequently, targeting the apoptotic machinery is also appealing as an anticancer adjunct. It is reasonable to expect that some loss of regulation of apoptosis is also present in the neoplastic cells responsible for PMP.

The two most prominent pathways linked to apoptosis are the NF-kappaB family of transcription factors and the Akt protein kinase. NF-kappaB directly binds the promoters and induces expression of several antiapoptotic genes (Karin et al. 2002). Akt links growth factors and oncogenes to the apoptosis pathways (Testa and Bellacosa 2001). Defects in both of these pathways are associated with cancer. A better understanding of the cellular pathways controlling apoptosis-regulatory genes in normal, tumor, and PMP cells should aid in developing treatment strategies that can be optimized for individual patients based upon the genetic characteristics of their tumors (Reed and Tomaselli 2000; Reed 2001).

10.9 Metastasis

Although there are case reports of PMP metastasizing to distant organs (Mortman et al. 1997), PMP is ordinarily confined to the peritoneal cavity for the duration of the disease. A provocative study by Cho et al. suggests a definitive role for mucin-specific biological properties in the pattern of metastases from colorectal cancer. (Cho et al. 1997) This study examined two model human cell lines. One was derived from a mucinous colorectal carcinoma (Cla) and the other from a moderately differentiated, nonmucinous adenocarcinoma (HM3). The study aimed to determine the quantitative and qualitative differences in mucin synthesis, mucin gene expression, and biological properties in the two model cell lines. This study showed that MUC2 mRNA levels were significantly higher in the mucinous Cla cells compared with HM3 cells and the Cla mucins had mostly short carbohydrate side-chains, while HM3 cells had mostly longer side chains. Protein analysis of the cell homogenates showed higher expression of MUC2 apomucin and mucin-associated carbohydrate antigens (T, Tn and sialyl Tn), and decreased sialyl Lex expression in Cla cells compared with HM3. Sialyl Lex antigen is as a ligand to E-selectins, which are present on activated vascular endothelium (Bevilacqua and Nelson 1993). The sialyl Lex antigen is expressed on many colon cancer cells, which bind to endothelial cells (Kojima et al. 1992; Majuri et al. 1992). Therefore sialyl Lex is postulated to be involved in the adhesion of cancer cells to endothelial cells where subsequent extravasation possibly results in metastasis. A similar antigen expression profile was observed with IHC analysis of 35 colorectal adenocarcinoma and 25 mucinous colorectal carcinoma tissues. Further examination of these cell lines also showed that Cla cells had significantly higher in vitro invasive activity and significantly lower E-selectin binding and liver colonization activities in nude mice. The authors concluded that colorectal mucinous carcinoma cells differ qualitatively and quantitatively from nonmucinous colorectal adenocarcinoma cells, in the pattern of mucin gene expression and in the synthesis and secretion of mucin. Cho et al. suggest that the biological and mucin characteristics of mucinous carcinoma cells contribute to extensive local invasion by penetrating tissue stroma and that this is the predominant mechanism of tumor progression for these cells. On the other hand, the biological and mucin characteristics of well- to moderately differentiated colorectal adenocarcinoma progress via distant metastasis formation.

Although these findings are not specific to PMP, the concepts proposed by Cho for colorectal cells apply to research regarding metastases, patterns of spread, the role of adhesion molecules, and possibly progression of malignant transformation in PMP. In addition, characterization of the mucin epitopes suggests the possibility of a PMP vaccine providing a "double hit." For example, if mucin epitopes are adhesion molecules, using them as antigens could provide a specific target to recruit the immune system, and they could inhibit contact with other cells or the extracellular matrix. In normal cells, cell contact or "anchorage dependence" is essential for cell growth. Loss of anchorage triggers a subtype of apoptosis known as anoikis (Reddig and Juliano 2005). Although the role of anchorage dependence is unknown in PMP, strategies to disrupt cellular adhesion may be another therapeutic target.

10.10 MUC2

MUC2 expression is an obvious therapeutic target for PMP. However, although MUC2 inhibition could prevent the accumulation of intraperitoneal mucin, it could also have detrimental effects. For example, MUC2 is a potential tumor suppressor (Velcich et al. 2002). Currently, it is not known whether this is a protective effect of MUC2 against extrinsic carcinogenic effects on intestinal cells or whether it is an active function of MUC2 gene expression. However, if MUC2 is a tumor suppressor, it is possible that MUC2 expression is important to the indolent nature of PMP and the question regarding the relationship between MUC2 expression and the neoplastic transformation of the goblet cell of the appendix has an even greater significance. Inhibiting MUC2 may lessen intraperitoneal mucus but at the same time may also result in the loss of tumor suppression.

On the basis of staining normal and neoplastic appendiceal goblet cells, O'Connell et al. concluded that there was no relationship between MUC2 expression and neoplastic transformation (O'Connell et al. 2002). However, their findings could be technique related. Normal and neoplastic cells can contain only a limited volume of mucin. Unless the neoplastic mucin-producing cells are significantly larger than normal appendiceal goblet cells, antibody staining techniques are not likely to detect a difference in mucin volume. Furthermore, the staining antibodies require physical space, and this limits the amount of antibody binding in a given area. Because staining techniques provide only a "snapshot," a functional assay is necessary to determine the true mechanism of mucin production in PMP. Recent studies of mucin-producing colon cancer cell lines have begun to detail the complex regulation of MUC2 expression. These include the roles of various transcription factors like galectin-3, AP-1, RELP, and CDX2. (Yamamoto et al. 2003; Song et al. 2005; Heiskala et al. 2006) Although these results are not specific to PMP, the concepts apply to researching the mechanism of MUC2 production in PMP and its relationship to the neoplastic transformation of the goblet cell.

Unraveling the relationship between MUC2 and the transformation of PMP cells will require a model system in which MUC2 expression can be silenced. Currently, synthetic short-interfering RNA (siRNA) is commonly used to silence genes. If this method can be used to silence the MUC2 gene, then its effect on the cell cycle, resistance or susceptibility to apoptosis, and clonogenicity could be studied. In addition, phenotypic changes (epithelial-to-mesenchymal transition) associated with a cell's ability to metastasize could also be investigated. Unfortunately, a prerequisite to these experiments is the development of a PMP cell line.

10.11 Future Investigations

The concepts discussed above are speculative but offer a broad overview of potential basic science research efforts in PMP. Current investigations are looking at new potential areas of vulnerability such as the cyclooxygenase 2 enzyme (Gatalica and Loggie 2006), growth factor receptors (EGFR), and angiogenesis. Preclinical studies are optimizing intraperitoneal hyperthermia and the chemotherapy agents used with it, and novel intraperitoneal treatments are being investigated. (Verschraegen et al. 2003; Elias et al. 2006) Hopefully the information gleaned from the molecular and cellular research of mucinous neoplasms of the colon and rectum will apply to PMP. However, the many biological issues that are unique to PMP beg for efforts focused on PMP-producing cells. PMP's orphan disease status must not deter its investigation. The history of cancer research is replete with examples of advances owing to important discoveries made in orphan diseases (Mirchandani and D'Andrea 2006). Finally, because PMP relies so much on regional therapy, it is a unique model system for the surgeon-scientist to think "outside the box."

References

Bevilacqua MP, Nelson RM (1993) Selectins. J Clin Invest 91:379–387

Blagosklonny MV, Pardee AB (2002) The restriction point of the cell cycle. Cell Cycle 1:103–110

Carr NJ, Emory TS, Sobin LH (2002) Epithelial neoplasms of the appendix and colorectum: an analysis of cell proliferation, apoptosis, and expression of p53, CD44, bcl-2. Arch Pathol Lab Med 126:837–841

Cho M, Dahiya R, Choi SR et al. (1997) Mucins secreted by cell lines derived from colorectal mucinous carcinoma and adenocarcinoma. Eur J Cancer 33:931–941

Cuatrecasas M, Matias-Guiu X, Prat J (1996) Synchronous mucinous tumors of the appendix and the ovary associated with pseudomyxoma peritonei. A clinicopathological study of six cases with comparative analysis of c-Ki-ras mutations. Am J Surg Pathol 20:739–746

Elias D, Raynard B, Bonnay M et al. (2006) Heated intraoperative intraperitoneal oxaliplatin alone and in combination with intraperitoneal irinotecan: pharmacologic studies. Eur J Surg Oncol 32:607–613

Gatalica Z, Loggie B (2006) COX-2 expression in pseudomyxoma peritonei. Cancer Lett 244:86–90

Heiskala K, Giles-Komar J, Heiskala M et al. (2006) High expression of RELP (Reg IV) in neoplastic goblet cells of appendiceal mucinous cystadenoma and pseudomyxoma peritonei. Virchows Arch 448:295–300

Imaoka H, Yamao K, Salem AA et al. (2006) Pseudomyxoma peritonei caused by acute pancreatitis in intraductal papillary mucinous carcinoma of the pancreas. Pancreas 32:223–224

Kabbani W, Houlihan PS, Luthra R et al. (2002) Mucinous and nonmucinous appendiceal adenocarcinomas: different clinicopathological features but similar genetic alterations. Mod Pathol 15:599–605

Karin M, Cao Y, Greten FR et al. (2002) NF-kappaB in cancer: from innocent bystander to major culprit. Nat Rev Cancer 2:301–310

Kojima N, Handa K, Newman W et al. (1992) Inhibition of selectin-dependent tumor cell adhesion to endothelial cells and platelets by blocking O-glycosylation of these cells. Biochem Biophys Res Commun 182:1288–1295

Lee KR, Scully RE (2000) Mucinous tumors of the ovary: a clinicopathologic study of 196 borderline tumors (of intestinal type) and carcinomas, including an evaluation of 11 cases with "pseudomyxoma peritonei". Am J Surg Pathol 24:1447–1464

Majuri ML, Mattila P, Renkonen R (1992) Recombinant E-selectin-protein mediates tumor cell adhesion via sialyl-Le(a) and sialyl-Le(x). Biochem Biophys Res Commun 182:1376–1382

Maru D, Wu TT, Canada A et al. (2004) Loss of chromosome 18q and DPC4 (Smad4) mutations in appendiceal adenocarcinomas. Oncogene 23:859–864

Mirchandani KD, D'Andrea AD (2006) The Fanconi anemia/BRCA pathway: a coordinator of cross-link repair. Exp Cell Res 312:2647–2653

Misdraji J, Burgart LJ, Lauwers GY (2004) Defective mismatch repair in the pathogenesis of low-grade appendiceal mucinous neoplasms and adenocarcinomas. Mod Pathol 17:1447–1454

Mortman KD, Sugarbaker PA, Shmookler BM et al. (1997) Pulmonary metastases in pseudomyxoma peritonei syndrome. Ann Thorac Surg 64:1434–1436

O'Connell JT, Tomlinson JS, Roberts AA et al. (2002) Pseudomyxoma peritonei is a disease of MUC2-expressing goblet cells. Am J Pathol 161:551–564

Park JG, Oie HK, Sugarbaker PH et al. (1987) Characteristics of cell lines established from human colorectal carcinoma. Cancer Res 47:6710–6718

Reddig PJ, Juliano RL (2005) Clinging to life: cell to matrix adhesion and cell survival. Cancer Metastasis Rev 24:425–439

Reed JC (2001) Apoptosis-regulating proteins as targets for drug discovery. Trends Mol Med 7:314–319

Reed JC, Tomaselli KJ (2000) Drug discovery opportunities from apoptosis research. Curr Opin Biotechnol 11:586–592

Ronnett BM, Kurman RJ, Zahn CM et al. (1995) Pseudomyxoma peritonei in women: a clinicopathologic analysis of 30 cases with emphasis on site of origin, prognosis, and relationship to ovarian mucinous tumors of low malignant potential. Hum Pathol 26:509–524

Ronnett BM, Shmookler BM, Diener-West M et al. (1997) Immunohistochemical evidence supporting the appendiceal origin of pseudomyxoma peritonei in women. Int J Gynecol Pathol 16:1–9

Sanborn RE, Blanke CD (2005) Gastrointestinal stromal tumors and the evolution of targeted therapy. Clin Adv Hematol Oncol 3:647–657

Solkar MH, Akhtar NM, Khan Z et al. (2004) Pseudomyxoma extraperitonei occurring 35 years after appendicectomy: a case report and review of literature. World J Surg Oncol 2:19

Song S, Byrd JC, Mazurek N et al. (2005) Galectin-3 modulates MUC2 mucin expression in human colon cancer cells at the level of transcription via AP-1 activation. Gastroenterology 129:1581–1591

Sugarbaker PH (2006) New standard of care for appendiceal epithelial neoplasms and pseudomyxoma peritonei syndrome? Lancet Oncol 7:69–76

Szych C, Staebler A, Connolly DC et al. (1999) Molecular genetic evidence supporting the clonality and appendiceal origin of pseudomyxoma peritonei in women. Am J Pathol 154:1849–1855

Testa JR, Bellacosa A (2001) AKT plays a central role in tumorigenesis. Proc Natl Acad Sci USA 98:10983–10985

Tibbetts LM, Chu MY, Vezeridis MP et al. (1988) Cell culture of the mucinous variant of human colorectal carcinoma. Cancer Res 48:3751–3759

Velcich A, Yang W, Heyer J et al. (2002) Colorectal cancer in mice genetically deficient in the mucin Muc2. Science 295:1726–1729

Verschraegen CF, Kumagai S, Davidson R et al. (2003) Phase I clinical and pharmacological study of intraperitoneal cis-bis-neodecanoato(trans- R, R-1, 2-diaminocyclohexane)-platinum II entrapped in multilamellar liposome vesicles. J Cancer Res Clin Oncol 129:549–555

Yamachika T, Nakanishi H, Yasui K et al. (2005) Establishment and characterization of a human colonic mucinous carcinoma cell line with predominant goblet-cell differentiation from liver metastasis. Pathol Int 55:550–557

Yamamoto H, Bai YQ, Yuasa Y et al. (2003) Homeodomain protein CDX2 regulates goblet-specific MUC2 gene expression. Biochem Biophys Res Commun 300:813–818

Yasar A, De Keulenaer B, Opdenakker G et al. (1997) Pseudomyxoma peritonei in association with primary malignant tumor of the ovary and colon. J Belge Radiol 80:233–234

11 Peritoneal Carcinomatosis of Colorectal Origin: Recent Advances and Future Evolution Toward a Curative Treatment

Dominique Elias and Diane Goere

11.1 Introduction

Peritoneal carcinomatosis (PC) is generally considered a dramatic event in colorectal cancer. A recent prospective study of 349 patients with PC treated conventionally showed that median survival was 7 months (Jayne et al. 2002). A new therapeutic concept now allows selected patients with PC to achieve cure: It combines complete cytoreductive surgery (CCS), treating macroscopic disease, with immediate intraperitoneal chemohyperthermia (HIPEC), treating residual microscopic disease. This concept has become a reality for diffuse disease in the abdominal cavity but is also on the verge of becoming so for associated resectable visceral metastases located at different sites (Elias et al. 2005). In addition, it is noteworthy that the results currently obtained with CCS combined with HIPEC are similar to those obtained 10 years ago after hepatectomy for liver metastases from colorectal cancer (Elias et al. 2004). In this chapter, only treatments of colorectal PC performed with a curative intent (CCS being the first, indispensable step) are considered.

11.2 The Primordial Prognostic Impact of Complete Cytoreduction

That CCS is combined with HIPEC is critical, but the completeness of surgery is the key element in this new approach. This point was clearly demonstrated by a retrospective multicenter study of 506 patients with colorectal cancer and PC treated in 28 institutions (Glehen et al. 2004a). All patients had cytoreductive surgery and perioperative intraperitoneal chemotherapy (HIPEC and/or immediate postoperative intraperitoneal chemotherapy). Patients in whom cytoreductive surgery was complete (n=271) had a median survival of 32.4 months versus 8.4 months for patients whose lesions were not amenable to cytoreductive surgery (P<0.001). The 5-year survival rate was 31% for those patients with residual nodules measuring less than 5 mm versus 15% when residual nodules were greater than 5 mm, and none of the latter patients survived. In a randomized trial that was stopped prematurely (because patients refused to enter the trial), we treated 35 patients with CCS who were subsequently randomized to receive or not early postoperative intraperitoneal chemotherapy (Elias et al. 2004). Overall survival rates were similar but unexpectedly high in both groups (60% at 2 years), highlighting the impact of CCS. In conclusion, surgery combined with HIPEC is only efficient and logical if CCS is really complete. Performing HIPEC without CCS is unethical, dangerous, costly, and finally reprehensible.

11.3 Results of Phase II Studies with CCS

In the multicenter retrospective study of 506 patients treated with cytoreductive surgery and perioperative HIPEC in 28 different institutions, the morbidity and mortality rates were 23% and 4%, respectively (Glehen et al. 2004a). Until now, most teams have used mitomycin C as the cytotoxic drug and hyperthermia at 41°C over 90 min. Few teams prefer to use oxaliplatin (Elias et al. 2002) or oxaliplatin plus irinotecan (Elias et al. 2004a) at 43°C over 30 min associated with intravenous 5-fluorouracil (5-FU) and leucovorin.

In this chapter, only patients treated with CCS are considered because such treatment is illogical for macroscopic residual disease. Table 11.1 shows the survival rates obtained with this combined treatment.

Overall 5-year survival rates were generally between 30% and 45%, with median survival of between 24 and 60 months, which means that some patients can definitively be cured with this combined treatment. More than half of these patients never relapsed inside the peritoneum, underlining how the original concept has become a reality.

Between June 1998 and December 2002, 30 patients (mean age 49.8±9.8 years) with macroscopic colorectal PC underwent complete resection of PC followed by HIPEC with oxaliplatin in our Institute (Elias et al. 2006b). Eligibility criteria were as follows: a good general status and age below 65 years, no extraabdominal disease, no occlusive disorders, and no bulky clinical or radiological PC. Eleven patients had associated extraperitoneal lesions in the liver (n=5), the ovary (n=4), and the spleen (n=2). These additional lesions were resected during the same procedure. All patients had previously received intravenous chemotherapy containing oxaliplatin or irinotecan over a period of at least 3 months. Those who achieved an objective response received the same regimen postoperatively over 4 to 6 months. During the same period, eight other patients with PC and the same eligibility criteria were also operated on with a curative intent, but complete resection of PC was impossible so they did not receive HIPEC. The oxaliplatin solution (460 mg/m2 of oxaliplatin in 2 l/m2 of isosmotic 5% dextrose) was administered intraperitoneally, in an open abdominal cavity (coliseum technique), at a homogeneous temperature of 43°C (range:

Table 11.1. Survival of patients who underwent CCS in phase II studies

Reference	Year	No. of patients	Type of IP chemotherapy	Follow-up (months)	Median survival (months)	Survival (%) 2 years	Survival (%) 5 years
Pestiau and Sugarbaker	2000	44	HIPEC (MMC) + EPIC	40	24	–	30
Elias et al.	2001	64	HIPEC (MMC) or EPIC	52	36	60	27
Pilati et al.	2003	34	HIPEC (MMC + CDDP)	15	18	31	–
Shen et al.	2004	37	HIPEC (MMC)	15	28	55	34
Glehen et al.	2004	23	HIPEC (MMC)	60	33	54	21
Multicentric[a]	2004	271	HIPEC (MMC) or EPIC	53	32	–	31
Verwaal et al.	2005	59	HIPEC (MMC)	–	43	–	43
Elias et al.	2006b	30	HIPEC (Oxali)	55	60	73	48

[a] Multicentric study: Glehen et al. 2004a
CCS, complete cytoreductive surgery; HIPEC, intraperitoneal chemohyperthermia; MMC, mitomycin C; EPIC, early postoperative intraperitoneal chemotherapy; Oxali, oxaliplatin

44–42°C) over 30 min (strictly 30 min as soon as the minimal temperature of 42°C had been reached throughout the abdominal cavity, plus 5–8 min before to heat the infusate from 38°C to 42°C). Patients received an intravenous perfusion of 5-FU (400 mg/m2) with leucovorin (20 mg/m2) before starting HIPEC. 5-FU was administered intravenously because it potentiates the activity of oxaliplatin but cannot be mixed with the latter inside the peritoneal cavity (pH incompatibility). After resection, the size of residual tumor seeding was 0 mm in 19 patients and <2 mm in 11. No postoperative deaths occurred (0%), and grade 2–3 morbidity (requiring specific treatment) was 37%. Median follow-up was 55 months (range: 31–84). Twenty-two (73%) patients relapsed after a median interval of 14 months (range 2–46); 11 of them (37%) developed a peritoneal recurrence (3 times associated with an extraperitoneal recurrence). Seven of these 22 patients (32%) were amenable to repeat curative surgery (liver: 2, peritoneum: 2, lung: 2, and spleen: 1). Patients with unresectable recurrences were treated with intravenous (i.v.) chemotherapy. Contrary to all expectations, one of these patients achieved a complete response of multiple small lung metastases that had been present for 2 years. At 2, 3, and 5 years, overall survival rates (95% confidence interval) were 73% (59–88), 53% (9–72), and 48.5% (31–66), respectively. At 2, 3 and 5 years, disease-free survival rates were 48% (32–66), 41.5% (27–59), and 34% (19–52), respectively (Fig. 11.1). Median survival was 60.1 months.

It is important to remember that these good results are to a great extent due to patient selection: Subjects had a good general status and no extraperitoneal metastases, and their PC was completely resectable. For comparison purposes, it is interesting to recall the results of the prospective study of 349 patients with colorectal cancers in Singapore, conducted from 1989 to 1999 (Jayne et al. 2002): Patients with PC were treated with 5-FU and leucovorin and had a median survival of 7 months and a 2-year survival rate of 15%. This study also shows us that 60% of PC that were synchronous with the primary tumor were limited to the peritoneum (no associated visceral metastases), and two-thirds were localized and therefore resectable. Once again for comparison purposes, the study of the 50 patients randomized to the control arm in the Amsterdam study (Verwaal et al. 2003) who did not receive HIPEC showed better survival because they fulfilled inclusion criteria (no other metastases than PC, good general status). Among them, 7 underwent a radical resection of PC, 22 a palliative resection, 8 a bypass, and 13 only a laparotomy. They received monthly first-line

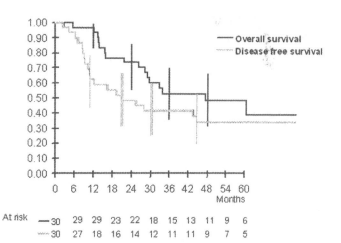

Fig. 11.1 Overall and disease-free survival rates of 30 patients with colorectal carcinomatosis treated with maximal cytoreductive surgery and intraperitoneal chemohyperthermia with oxaliplatin

systemic leucovorin and 5-FU chemotherapy and second-line irinotecan. Median survival of these patients was 12.8 months, and the 2-year survival rate was 25%. For the subgroup of patients who underwent a radical resection of PC, median survival was 17 months.

Very recently, we conducted a retrospective multicentric study of 50 patients (who fulfilled inclusion criteria for treatment with HIPEC) selected in five different Anticancer Centers in France (10 patients per center). These patients did not receive HIPEC and were treated conventionally by symptomatic surgery when necessary and mainly with the most recent chemotherapy regimens, all of them receiving oxaliplatin and irinotecan. Twenty of them received a third line of chemotherapy and 16 a fourth line. These optimal chemotherapeutic regimens yielded a median survival of 24.1 months. This median survival of 24.1 months is currently the real survival duration obtained with chemotherapy in these selected patients with colorectal PC. We can probably add 3 months (=27 months) when patients also receive the new antiangiogenic drugs. The 27 months obtained with this "conventional treatment" is what must be compared with the 60 months that have just been attained with CCS plus HIPEC.

11.4 Randomized Trial

The Netherlands Cancer Institute conducted a randomized trial comparing the CCS-HIPEC (attempted cytoreductive surgery plus HIPEC with mitomycin C) to conventional treatment of peritoneal carcinomatosis (see above) (Verwaal et al. 2003). Between February 1998 and August 2001, 105 patients were included in this intention-to-treat analysis. In the experimental arm (n=54), 37% underwent CCS, 43% had residual tumor deposits that were smaller than 2.5 mm, and 20% had residual deposits exceeding 2.5 mm. HIPEC was performed by the coliseum technique with mitomycin C at 40°C over 90 min. After a median follow-up of 22 months, median survival was 12.6 months in the standard therapy arm versus 22.3 months in the experimental therapy arm (P=0.03), corresponding to 2-year survival rates of 25% and 48%, respectively (Fig. 11.2). Only one death occurred among the 18 patients who underwent CCS. Patients with six or seven involved regions (among a total of 7) had very poor survival (median 5.4 months) compared with those with one to five involved regions (median >29 months) (P<0.001).

This randomized trial clearly demonstrates that cytoreductive surgery followed by HIPEC improves the survival of patients with PC. Patients were randomized before surgery, and because of this study design, only 37% of those in the experimental arm were amenable to CCS. Only this small group obtained considerable benefit from CCS-HIPEC. It is noteworthy that the temperature of HIPEC and the drug used were not optimal. If we consider that only patients with CCS should be selected to receive HIPEC, that the temperature can be increased up to 43°C, and that mitomycin C can be replaced by more potent drugs, then better survival results could potentially be observed. This notwithstanding, we owe a lot to the team in Amsterdam for conducting this difficult trial. A few attempts have been made to conduct similar trials in France and in the USA, but they have failed because patients refused to participate.

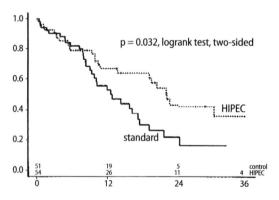

Fig. 11.2 Kaplan-Meier curves comparing overall survival after standard treatment to that after hyperthermic intraperitoneal chemotherapy (HIPEC). Netherlands randomized study. (Verwaal et al. 2003)

11.5 Validated and Unvalidated HIPEC Techniques for Colorectal PC

The strong prognostic impact of the completeness of the cytoreductive surgery has now clearly been demonstrated. The benefit of intraperitoneal chemotherapy, or better still, of chemohyperthermia has been proven by randomized studies in rat experimental models but not in humans. In addition, the great superiority of a high temperature (43°C) over a lower temperature (40° and 41°C) has only been demonstrated in vitro. A comparative study has never been conducted to test different peritoneal infusion durations. Finally, it is highly probable that multiagent regimens would be more efficient than single-agent regimens, as is the case with systemic chemotherapy, that new potent drugs such as oxaliplatin and irinotecan would be more active than the old drug (mitomycin C), and that it would be more logical to use high doses than low doses. Five parameters could be modified, temperature, duration, type of chemotherapy, different drug combinations, and their respective doses, giving rise to infinitely different combinations. Establishing the real superiority of one combination over another theoretically necessitates conducting a randomized study with at least 100 patients. It would be impossible to test all these possibilities, especially as new drugs are becoming available more and more rapidly. Our duty is to choose or define the most promising CCS-HIPEC combination and ensure its development in Phase II studies.

However, one important trial is about to be conducted in the near future to randomly compare HIPEC versus nothing after CCS in colorectal cancer patients with PC. Patients would be randomized during surgery, after CCS. The aim of this trial will be to prove that HIPEC after CCS yields better survival rates than the most recent systemic chemotherapy combined with targeted drugs or antibodies. Such a trial would be confronted with two challenges: (1) Design of the study: Adjuvant biochemotherapies (whatever the type) would have to be administered in the two arms. However, this biochemotherapy should be identical in both arms during the same period in a given center wherever it is administered. However, for obvious ethical reasons, they would have to be modified over time to ensure that patients receive the most powerful regimen. This study should be multicentric and not exceed 3 years, but agreement would have to be reached regarding the type of HIPEC (drug, doses, temperature, duration, coliseum technique or not). (2) Obtaining the consent of the patients who are frantically surfing the web to find more information about their disease: HIPEC has already been widely diffused by the media, and patients are reluctant to risk not having it. If we wanted to initiate a randomized study comparing hepatectomy to "no hepatectomy" in patients with resectable liver metastases, it would be unethical and refused by patients. To date, nowhere in the world has such a study been conducted and yet hepatectomy has become the gold standard treatment. HIPEC, whose efficacy is increasingly demonstrated outside randomized trials, which are difficult to conduct for all the reasons mentioned above, could experience a similar outcome.

11.6 Current Indications for CCS with HIPEC

There are no evidence-based medical data on this topic. However, there is a consensus among experts to approve the following points. Absolute contraindications to HIPEC are a poor general status, extra-abdominal disease, and the impossibility of performing CCS, which generally indicates that PC is massive and diffuse. Relative contraindications are (1) progression of PC during preoperative systemic chemotherapy, and/or the unsuccessful elimination of ascites with such treatment, because this generally signifies unresectability (Elias et al. 2005), and (2) the presence of resectable liver metastases (LM). We did in fact demonstrate in a group of 24 patients that the presence of one, two, or a maximum of three resectable LM does not automatically contraindicate HIPEC with a curative intent (Elias et al. 2006). Moderate PC was discovered in these patients at laparotomy performed to resect LM. They underwent complete resection of LM and PC plus HIPEC. Mortality was 4%, and morbidity was 58%. The 3-year overall survival rate was 42%, and the disease-free survival rate was 24%. Three patients relapsed in the peritoneum and 13 in the liver (3 underwent a repeat hepatectomy). The only significant prognostic factor was the number of LM [less than 3] (P<0.01). In a similar manner, the Washington Cancer Institute reported on 16 patients with synchronous PC and hematogenous metastasis in the liver or in the lung who underwent a complete resection at both sites (Carmignani et al. 2004). The median duration of survival was 21 months, confirming that extraperitoneal metastases are not an absolute contraindication to HIPEC, provided they are resectable.

Massive and diffuse PC is probably a contraindication for HIPEC. The analysis of 10 prognostic factors performed by Sugarbaker's team in 70 patients who underwent CCS (da Silva and Sugarbaker 2005) revealed that only a peritoneal carcinomatosis index >20 (P=0.001) and involved lymph nodes (P=0.03) had a significant negative impact; age, sex, histological differentiation or mucinous type, and the site (colon or rectum) had no impact. Unfortunately, none of the imaging techniques currently available is capable of depicting the real extent of PC. The CT scan (Dromain et al. 2003), MRI, and also the PET scan (recent prospective study performed in our Institute; data not shown) are unable to provide reliable information. Only naked eye inspection at laparotomy or coelioscopy is able to do so.

11.7 Probable and Potential Improvements of the HIPEC Technique

At this point in time, the best way to improve the results of this "combined modality" is to aim at complete cytoreduction, by using the coliseum technique, which is the only technique that allows bathing of all peritoneal surfaces and ensures thermal homogeneity (Elias et al. 2000). The temperature in the peritoneal cavity should be as close as possible to 43°C. In the medium term, drugs that are more active than mitomycin C and cisplatin could be used intraperitoneally against colorectal cancer cells. Recently, oxaliplatin and irinotecan demonstrated unequivocal efficiency against this type of cancer cell, which is why we subsequently conducted a phase I pharmacokinetics study with these agents during HIPEC in humans. The first study established tolerance and the recommended dose of oxaliplatin (Elias et al. 2002). Intraperitoneal oxaliplatin was associated with a preliminary i.v. infusion of 5-FU with leucovorin (because 5-FU potentiates oxaliplatin but cannot be mixed with it because of pH incompatibility). The recommended dose was 460 mg/m2 of oxaliplatin in 2 l/m2 of 5% dextrose with a dwell time of 30 min, as soon as the minimal intraperitoneal temperature of 42°C was obtained throughout the peritoneal cavity. The phase II study with this regimen included 30 patients with colorectal PC. A 5-year survival rate of 48.5% and a 5-year disease-free survival rate of 34% were obtained (Elias et al. 2006b). Because multiagent chemotherapy is more potent than single-agent chemotherapy, it was logical to add irinotecan to the peritoneal perfusate. We conducted the first phase II trial combining oxaliplatin and irinotecan in humans (Elias et al. 2004a). SN-38, the active metabolite of irinotecan, appears immediately in the peritoneum. We found that the recommended dose was 360 mg/m2 for the two drugs in 2 l/m2 of 5% dextrose with a dwell time of 30 min in the peritoneal cavity, once the temperature of the bath had reached 42°C. This study is ongoing.

Other chemotherapy agents can be used during HIPEC (Sugarbaker et al. 2005), and some new agents such as Dimate (Monneuse et al. 2005) or Albendazole (Pourgholami et al. 2205) are currently being tested. It also seems possible to use antitumor antibodies inside the peritoneal cavity (Stroehelein et al. 2005), but results are very preliminary.

11.8 Outlook for HIPEC in Colorectal PC

If we anticipate using new agents inside the peritoneal cavity (see above), three main directions need to be explored in future trials. However, it is very difficult to conduct prospective randomized trials for the following reasons: (1) in order to be rapid, they need to be multicentric, (2) there is no consensus about the gold standard HIPEC technique, and (3) patients frequently refuse to participate in trials in which there is "no treatment" (no HIPEC) in one arm.

We first need to conduct a randomized trial comparing HIPEC versus no HIPEC after CCS. In our opinion, any kind of systemic chemotherapy or new targeted treatment could be administered in the two arms, before or after surgery, because therapeutic advances are ever more rapid and standard treatment practices are too different from one country to another for an agreement to be reached on a unique adjuvant treatment.

Second, we need to test systematic second-look surgery in patients with a high risk of developing PC. Its aim should be the early detection and treatment of PC, which occurs in 80% of patients presenting simultaneously with the primary tumor: a perforation, minimal PC, involvement of neighboring organs, or ovarian metastasis. These patients would receive the standard adjuvant systemic chemotherapy for 6 months and would have systematic second-look surgery 6 months after the end of this chemotherapy.

Third, we need to test the efficacy of preventive HIPEC against the occurrence of PC in patients when the primary tumor is occlusive or perforated or invades the serosa or neighboring organs.

11.9 Conclusion

Recently, the curative treatment of colorectal PC has progressed rapidly and has already attained the same survival rates as those obtained with hepatectomy for the treatment of resectable liver metastases. Future progress in imaging of PC, in the HIPEC technique, and in new agents should allow us to improve our current results. Multicentric prospective trials concerning the role and the modalities of HIPEC are advisable.

References

Carmignani CP, Ortega-Perez G, Sugarbaker PH (2004) The management of synchroneous peritoneal carcinomatosis and hematogeneous metastasis from colorectal cancer. EJSO 30:391–398

Da Silva RG, Sugarbaker PH (2005) Analysis of 10 prognostic factors in patients having a complete cytoreduction plus intraoperative intraperitoneal chemotherapy for carcinomatosis from colorectal cancer (abstract). Eur J Cancer 3:175

Dromain C, Bisdorff A, Elias D, Antoun S, Boige V, Lasser P et al. (2003) Computed tomographic features of peritoneal carcinomatosis treated with intraperitoneal chemohyperthermia. J Comut Assist Tomogr 27:327–332

Elias D, Antoun, S, Goharin A, El Othmany A, Puizillout JM, Lasser PH (2000) Research on the best chemohyperthermia technique for treatment of peritoneal carcinomatosis after complete resection. Int J Surg Invest 1:431–439

Elias D, Blot F, El Otmany A, Antoun S, Lasser P, Boige V et al. (2001) Curative treatment of peritoneal carcinomatosis from colorectal cancer by complete resection and intraperitoneal chemotherapy. Cancer 92:71–76

Elias D, Bonnay M, Puizillou JM, Antoun S, Demirdjian S, El Otmany A et al. (2002) Heated intra-operative intraperitoneal oxaliplatin after complete resection of peritoneal carcinomatosis: pharmacokinetics and tissue distribution. Ann Oncol 13:267–272

Elias D, Matsuhisa T, Sideris L, Liberale G, Drouard-Troalen L, Raynard B et al. (2004a) Heated intra-operative intraperitoneal oxaliplatin plus irinotecan after complete resection of peritoneal carcinomatosis: pharmacokinetics, tissue distribution and tolerance. Ann Oncol 15:1558–1565

Elias D (2004) Peritoneal carcinomatosis or liver metastases from colorectal cancer: similar standards for a curative surgery? Ann Surg Oncol 11:122–123

Elias D, Delperro JR, Sideris L, Benhammou E, Pocard M, Baton O et al. (2004b) Treatment of peritoneal carcinomatosis from colorectal cancer: impact of the complete cytoreductive surgery and difficulties in conducting randomized trials. Ann Surg Oncol 11:518–521

Elias D, Liberale G, Vernerey D, Pocard M, Ducreux M, Boige V, Malka D, Pignon JP, Lasser P (2005a). Hepatic and extrahepatic colorectal metastases: when resectable, their localization does not matter, but their total number has a prognostic effect. Ann Surg Oncol 12:1–10

Elias D, Benizri E, Vernerey D, Eldweny H, Dipietroantonio D, Pocard M (2005b). Preoperative criteria of incomplete resectability of peritoneal carcinomatosis from non-appendiceal colorectal carcinoma. Gastroenterol Clin Biol 29:1010–1013

Elias D, Benizri E, Pocard M, Ducreux M, Boige V, Lasser P (2006a). Peritoneal carcinomatosis with liver metastases from colorectal origin treated with complete resection and intraperitoneal chemotherapy: feasibility and results. EJSO (in press)

Elias D, Raynard B, Farhondeh F, Goere D, Rouquie D, Ciuchendea R, Ducreux M. (2006b) Peritoneal carcinomatosis of colorectal origin: long term results of intraperitoneal chemohyperthermia with oxaliplatin following complete cytoreductive surgery. Gastroentrol Clin Biol 30:1200–1208

Glehen O, Kwiatowsky F, Sugarbaker P, Elias D, Levine E, De Simone M et al. (2004a) Cytoreductive surgery combined with intraperitoneal chemotherapy for management of peritoneal carcinomatosis from colorectal cancer: a multi-institutional study. J Clin Oncol 22:3284–3292

Glehen O, Cotte E, Schreiber V, Sayag-Beaujard A, Vignal J, Gilly FN (2004b). Intraperitoneal chemohyperthermia and attempted cytoreductive surgery in patients with peritoneal carcinomatosis of colorectal origin. Br J Surg 91:747–754

Jayne DG, Fook S, Loi C, Seow-Choen F (2002) Peritoneal carcinomatosis from colorectal cancer. Br J Surg 89:1545–1550

Monneuse O, Mestrallet JP, Quash G, Gilly JF, Glehen O (2005) Intraperitoneal treatment with Dimate combined with surgical debulking is effective for experimental peritoneal carcinomatosis in a rat model. J Gastrointest Surg 9:769–774

Pestiau SR, Sugarbaker PH (2000) Treatment of primary colon cancer with peritoneal carcinomatosis: comparison of concomitant versus delayed management. Dis Colon Rectum 43:1341–1346

Pilati P, Mocellin M, Rossi CR, Foletto M, Campana L, NittiD et al. (2003) Cytoreductive surgery combined with intraperitoneal intraoperative chemotherapy for peritoneal carcinomatosis arising from colon adenocarcinoma. Ann Surg Oncol 10:508–513

Pourgholami MH, Akhter J, Wang L, Lu Y, Morris D (2005) Antitumor activity of albendazole against the human colorectal cancer-line HT-29: in vitro and in a xenograft model of peritoneal carcinomatosis. Cancer Chemother Pharmacol 55:425–432

Shen P, Hawksworth J, Lovato J, Loggie B, Geisinger K, Fleming R et al. (2004) Cytoreductive surgery and intraperitoneal hyperthermic chemotherapy with mitomycin C for peritoneal carcinomatosis from nonappendiceal colorectal carcinoma. Ann Surg Oncol 11:178–786

Strohelein M, Lordick F, Ruettinger D, Gruetzner U, Menzel H, Bartheileim K et al. (2005) Intraperitoneal application of the trifunctional antibody catumaxomab for the treatment of peritoneal carcinomatosis due to GI cancer. A phase I trial (abstract). Eur J Cancer 3:186

Sugarbaker PH, Torres Mora J, Carmignani P, Anthony Stuart O, Yoo D. (2005) Update on chemotherapeutic agents utilized for perioperative intraperitoneal chemotherapy. Oncologist 10:112–122

Verwaal V, van Ruth S, de Bree E, van Slooten G, van Titeren G, Boot H et al. (2003) Randomized trial of cytoreduction and hyperthermic intraperitoneal chemotherapy versus systemic chemotherapy and palliative surgery in patients with peritoneal carcinomatosis of colorectal cancer. J Clin Oncol 21:3737–3743

Verwaal V, van Ruth S, Whitkamp A, Boot H, van Slooten G, Zoetmulder FA. (2005) Long-term survival of peritoneal carcinomatosis of colorectal origin. Ann Surg Oncol 12:65–71

12 Pathologic Characterization and Differential Diagnosis of Malignant Peritoneal Mesothelioma

Nelson G. Ordóñez

Recent Results in Cancer Research, Vol. 169
© Springer-Verlag Berlin Heidelberg 2007

12.1 Introduction

Mesotheliomas are characterized by their ability to exhibit a broad range of cytomorphological features and to grow in a wide variety of histological patterns. Based on their appearance, three major histological types of mesotheliomas are recognized: epithelioid, mixed epithelioid and sarcomatoid (biphasic), and sarcomatoid. Although the distribution of these histological types varies from series to series, epithelioid mesothelioma is the most common. Of the 157 cases included in the two largest series of peritoneal malignant mesotheliomas, 132 (84%) were epithelioid, 22 (14%) biphasic, and 3 (2%) sarcomatoid (Baker et al. 2005; Kannerstein and Churg. 1977). The purpose of this chapter is to discuss the morphological variants of mesothelioma and to review the roles of immunohistochemistry and electron microscopy in the diagnosis of peritoneal mesothelioma. Particular emphasis is placed on the uncommon morphological variants of mesothelioma, some of which have only recently been described, as well as on the immunohistochemical markers that have most recently become available and for which there is evidence that they could be useful in the diagnosis of mesothelioma.

12.2 Epithelioid Mesothelioma

Since the histological features of epithelioid mesotheliomas are highly variable, these tumors can be confused with a variety of carcinomas that can metastasize to the peritoneum. Epithelioid mesotheliomas most frequently exhibit either a tubulopapillary, acinar (glandular), or solid pattern that can occur alone or in combination. On occasion, however, they may present other histological patterns, including signet ring, deciduoid, clear cell, or rhabdoid. Given that there is a general lack of awareness of the latter patterns, diagnostic difficulties may be encountered, especially in biopsy specimens.

12.2.1 Tubulopapillary Pattern

The tubulopapillary pattern is one of the most common histological patterns of epithelioid mesothelioma. It is also the pattern that most frequently needs to be distinguished from adenocarcinoma metastatic to the peritoneum. The tubulopapillary pattern consists of a mixture of small tubules and papillary structures with fibrovascular cores lined by a layer of relatively uniform cuboidal cells. In women, peritoneal mesotheliomas exhibiting tubulopapillary morphology should be distinguished from serous carcinoma of the ovary and peritoneum (Fig. 12.1).

12.2.2 Acinar (Glandular) Pattern

In the acinar pattern, most of the neoplastic cells appear to form glandular-like structures of varying size and shape. The differential

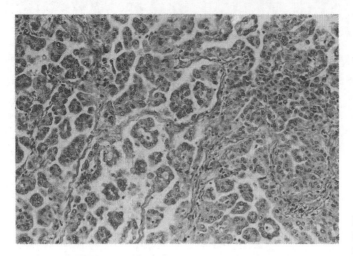

Fig. 12.1 Peritoneal mesothelioma showing prominent papillary features

diagnosis of mesotheliomas exhibiting this pattern is with metastatic adenocarcinomas of different origins that can metastasize to the peritoneum.

12.2.3 Solid Pattern

The solid pattern is one of the most common histological patterns of epithelioid peritoneal mesothelioma. In this pattern, the neoplastic cells are arranged in nests, cords, or sheets. Individually, the cells are round or cuboidal, relatively uniform, and often discohesive. The differential diagnosis of these cases depends on the degree of differentiation. If the tumor is well differentiated, it can be confused with reactive mesothelial hyperplasia. The differential diagnosis in less differentiated mesotheliomas includes a variety of metastatic carcinomas exhibiting a solid morphology.

12.2.4 Signet Ring Pattern

Mesotheliomas with signet ring-like morphology are relatively uncommon. This pattern is characterized by the presence of vacuolated cells with eccentric nuclei. Electron microscopy studies demonstrate that the main cause of the signet ring feature seen on light microscopy is the presence of an intracytoplasmic lumen that often displaces the nucleus to the periphery of the cell. The differential diagnosis of mesotheliomas with signet ring features is primarily with metastatic signet ring adenocarcinomas to the peritoneum.

12.2.5 Deciduoid Pattern

In 1985, Talerman et al. reported a primary epithelioid peritoneal mesothelioma in a 13-year-old girl that was initially diagnosed as diffuse pseudotumoral deciduosis (Talerman et al. 1985). Two additional cases exhibiting the same morphological features and occurring in young women, ages 23 and 24 years, respectively, were reported by Nascimento et al. in 1994. These authors coined the term deciduoid mesothelioma (Nascimento et al. 1994). In 1999, Orosz et al reported another example of this morphological variant of peritoneal mesothelioma in a 15-year-old girl (Orosz et al. 1999). Because all four of these cases occurred in young females, were confined to the peritoneum, and presented an unusually aggressive clinical behavior, it was initially considered that deciduoid mesothelioma was a distinct entity. Subsequent investigations by Shank et al. and by this author demonstrated that deciduoid features can also be seen in mesotheliomas arising in the pleura in elderly men with a history of asbestos exposure (Ordóñez 2000a; Shanks et al. 2000).

Mesotheliomas with deciduoid features are uncommon, and at present only about 30 cases, the majority of which occurred in the peritoneum, have been documented in the literature (Ordóñez 2000a; Shanks et al. 2000; Serio et al. 2002; Shia et al. 2002; Chung et al. 2003; Asioli et al. 2004; Maeda et al. 2004; Kimura et al. 2005; Mourra et al. 2005). Histologically, mesotheliomas with deciduoid features are characterized by a diffuse proliferation of large, round, ovoid, and polygonal epithelioid cells with sharp cellular outlines, abundant densely eosinophilic cytoplasm, and round, vesicular nuclei (Fig. 12.2). In a given tumor, the deciduoid morphology may be generalized or predominant, or it may be a component of a mesothelioma exhibiting a conventional tubular or papillary pattern. The differential diagnosis of deciduoid mesothelioma includes a variety of tumors composed of large epithelioid cells with abundant, dense, eosinophilic cytoplasm.

12.2.6 Clear Cell Pattern

Mesotheliomas entirely or predominantly composed of clear cells are uncommon, and only a few examples of epithelioid mesotheliomas exhibiting clear cell morphology have been documented in the literature (Ordóñez et al. 1996; Cavazza 2002; Dessy 2001; Ordóñez 2005b).

In a recent published series of 20 clear cell mesotheliomas, 17 originated in the pleura and 3 in the peritoneum. The most frequent cause of the cytoplasmic clearing was the accumulation of large amounts of intracytoplasmic glycogen (Fig. 12.3). Other less common factors included the accumulation of large amounts of lipid, mitochondrial swelling, the presence of numerous intracytoplasmic vesicles, or a large number of intracytoplasmic lumens. Peritoneal mesotheliomas with clear cell morphology can be confused with a variety of carcinomas that can metastasize to the peritoneum and can also present clear cell features. These include renal cell carcinomas, clear cell carcinomas of the ovary, and squamous carcinomas and adenocarcinomas of the lung. Both immunohistochemical and ultrastructural studies can be very useful in assisting in the differential diagnosis between these malignancies (Ordóñez 2005b).

12.2.7 Rhabdoid Pattern

Mesotheliomas with rhabdoid features are rare and have been reported to originate not only in the pleura (Puttagunta et al. 2000) but also in the peritoneum (Matsukuma et al. 1996; Ordóñez 2006b). Histologically, they are characterized by a proliferation of noncohesive or loosely cohesive cells having abundant cytoplasm, a large eccentric nucleus with a prominent nucleolus, and a hyaline intracytoplasmic inclusion displacing the nucleus. Electron microscopy studies have shown that these inclusions consist of aggregates of intermediate filaments

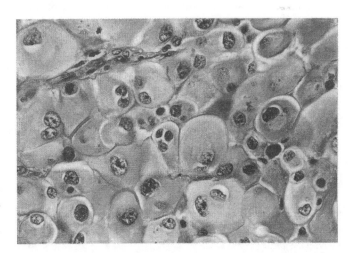

Fig. 12.2 Peritoneal mesothelioma exhibiting a deciduoid pattern. The tumor is composed of confluent sheets of large polygonal cells with dense cytoplasm

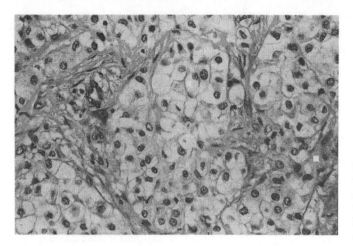

Fig. 12.3 Peritoneal mesothelioma with clear cell morphology. In this case, the cytoplasmic clearing was the result of the accumulation of large amounts of glycogen in the cytoplasm

arranged in interlacing bundles or whorllike arrays. Mesotheliomas with rhabdoid features can be confused with a variety of tumors with similar morphology that can involve the serosal membranes. The four tumors with the greatest potential of being confused with rhabdoid mesotheliomas are carcinomas with rhabdoid features, proximal-type epithelioid sarcomas, synovial sarcomas, and rhabdomyosarcomas. Immunohistochemical and electron microscopy studies can assist in establishing the differential diagnosis (Ordóñez 2006b).

12.3 Sarcomatoid Mesothelioma

Sarcomatoid mesotheliomas originating in the peritoneum are rare. Histologically, they are characterized by being composed of spindle cells arranged in fascicles or in a storiform pattern (Fig. 12.4). Depending on histological features, the differential diagnosis includes a variety of sarcomas with spindle or pleomorphic morphology, sarcomatoid carcinomas, and spindle cell melanomas. On occasion, sarcomatoid mesotheliomas can present lymphohistiocytic features and be associated with lymphoplasmocytic infiltrate (lymphohistiocytic pattern) (Khalidi et al. 2000). Mesotheliomas exhibiting this pattern can potentially be confused with either a reactive inflammatory process or lymphoma.

12.4 Mixed (Biphasic) Mesothelioma

About 15% to 20% of the peritoneal mesotheliomas can exhibit a mixture of epithelioid and sarcomatoid components (Kannerstein and Churg 1977; Baker et al. 2005). Peritoneal mesotheliomas presenting this pattern should be distinguished from other malignancies exhibiting biphasic morphology, such as synovial sarcomas and carcinosarcomas.

12.5 Immunohistochemistry

Of the various ancillary techniques that have been recognized as being useful in the diagnosis of mesothelioma, immunohistochemistry is, at present, regarded as having the most practical utility, especially in distinguishing epithelioid mesotheliomas from metastatic carcinomas involving the peritoneum. Since an absolutely specific and sensitive marker for mesothelioma has not yet been identified, the immunohistochemical diagnosis of this tumor depends largely on the use of panels that combine markers that are commonly expressed in mesotheliomas, but not in carcinomas (positive mesothelioma markers), with those that are frequently expressed in carcinomas, but not in mesotheliomas (positive carcinoma markers). These panels, however, are continuously changing as a result of the identification

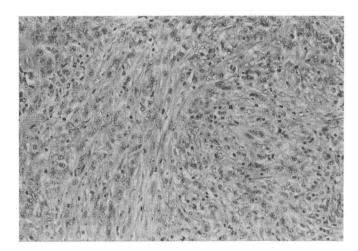

Fig. 12.4 Sarcomatoid mesothelioma composed of spindle cells

of new markers that could be useful in distinguishing epithelioid mesotheliomas from the different types of carcinomas with which they may be confused.

12.5.1 Positive Mesothelioma Markers

12.5.1.1 Podoplanin and the D2-40 Monoclonal Antibody

Podoplanin, a 38-kDa transmembrane mucoprotein, is the most recently recognized positive mesothelioma marker (Fig. 12.5). Although podoplanin and the recently commercially available D2-40 monoclonal antibody were initially regarded as two different mesothelioma markers (Ordóñez 2005a), recent investigations have shown that podoplanin and the so-called M2A oncofetal antigen expressed in germ cell tumors and recognized by the D2-40 antibody are identical proteins (Schacht et al. 2005). Recently, several studies have been published on the value of podoplanin in the diagnosis of mesothelioma (Chu et al. 2005; Kimura and Kimura 2005; Ordóñez 2005a, 2006a). The results of these investigations showed that podoplanin is frequently expressed in epithelioid mesotheliomas but is absent in sarcomatoid mesotheliomas (Ordóñez 2005a; Sienko et al. 2005). The percentages of positivity reported in epithelioid mesotheliomas have ranged from 86% to 100% of the cases (Chu et al. 2005; Kimura and Kimura 2005; Ordóñez 2005a; Sienko et al. 2005). Additionally, several groups of investigators have shown that lung adenocarcinomas are almost invariably negative for podoplanin, and therefore it could serve as a marker for discriminating between these malignancies and epithelioid mesotheliomas (Chu et al. 2005; Ordóñez 2005a; Sienko et al. 2005). However, the value of podoplanin in assisting in the differential diagnosis between epithelioid mesotheliomas and serous carcinomas of the ovary is less clear. In a recent investigation by this author, podoplanin expression was demonstrated in 37 (93%) of 40 peritoneal mesotheliomas and in 6 (13%) of 45 serous carcinomas (Ordóñez 2006a). While the reaction in the mesotheliomas was often strong and diffuse, the staining in the serous carcinomas was invariably focal. These results indicate that, although podoplanin is a useful marker for assisting in the differential diagnosis between lung adenocarcinomas and pleural mesotheliomas, its value in discriminating between peritoneal mesotheliomas and serous carcinomas is more limited.

12.5.1.2 Calretinin

Calretinin is a 29-kDa protein that was first described in the neurons of the central and peripheral neural systems and, subsequently, in certain nonneural cells, including steroid-producing cells of the testis and ovary, adipocytes, eccrine glands, keratinizing thymic

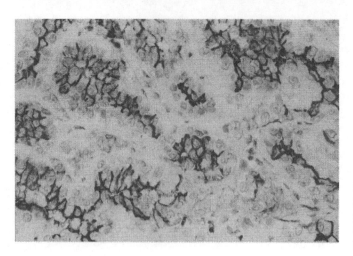

Fig. 12.5 Peritoneal mesothelioma stained with the D2-40 anti-podoplanin antibody. Typically, the reaction occurs primarily along the apical cell membrane

epithelial cells, and mesothelial cells (Doglioni et al. 1996; Dei Tos and Doglioni 1998). In 1996, Doglioni et al reported strong calretinin expression in all 36 epithelioid mesotheliomas, but only focal positivity was obtained in 28 (10%) of 294 adenocarcinomas of various origins (Doglioni et al. 1996). Based on these results, these investigators concluded that calretinin was a useful immunohistochemical marker for the diagnosis of mesothelioma. Subsequent investigations have confirmed the observation by Doglioni et al., and calretinin is, at present, regarded as being the most sensitive and one of the most specific of the positive mesothelioma markers (Ordóñez 1998c, 2003a). Because of this, it has been recommended as one of the primary markers in the various panels that are currently used in the diagnosis of mesothelioma. The reported percentages of calretinin expression reported in recent investigations have ranged from 31% to 38% in serous carcinomas (Cathro and Stoler 2005; Chu et al. 2005; Ordóñez 2006a), 6% to 10% in lung adenocarcinomas (Carella et al. 2001; Comin et al. 2001; Abutaily et al. 2002; Ordóñez 2003a), and 0% to 10% in renal cell carcinomas (Martignoni et al. 2001; Osborn et al. 2002; Lugli et al. 2003; Ordóñez 2004). The staining in the positive cases was often focal. This is in contrast to epithelioid mesotheliomas, which almost invariably exhibit strong calretinin positivity (Fig. 12.6). Because of the frequent and strong expression of calretinin in epithelioid mesotheliomas, a negative staining for this marker should be regarded as an indication against such a diagnosis. It should be mentioned that calretinin expression has been reported in up to two-thirds of the sarcomatoid mesotheliomas (Oates and Edwards 2000; Lucas et al. 2003), and therefore it is one of the few markers that have proved to be useful in distinguishing sarcomatoid mesotheliomas from other malignancies exhibiting similar morphologic features.

12.5.1.3 Keratin 5/6

Keratin 5/6 is another positive mesothelioma marker that has been found to be useful in the diagnosis of mesothelioma (Clover et al. 1997; Ordóñez 1998d, 2003a). Although this marker is useful for discriminating between pleural mesotheliomas and lung adenocarcinomas, its utility for distinguishing between peritoneal mesotheliomas and serous carcinomas is less defined. In a recent investigation, 93% of the epithelioid peritoneal mesotheliomas and 31% of the serous carcinomas were reported to express keratin 5/6 (Ordóñez 2006a). These results indicate that immunostaining for this marker has little practical utility for discriminating between these malignancies. Nor does keratin 5/6 have any value in the differential diagnosis between peritoneal mesotheliomas and squamous carcinomas, as it is almost invariably expressed in the latter tumors (Ordóñez 1998d). In contrast, because keratin

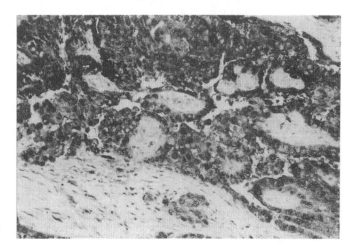

Fig. 12.6 Peritoneal mesothelioma showing diffuse, strong nuclear and cytoplasmic positivity for calretinin

5/6 is not expressed in renal cell carcinomas, it can be useful for distinguishing these tumors from mesotheliomas (Ordóñez 2004).

12.5.1.4 Mesothelin

Mesothelin is a 40-kDa cell surface glycoprotein of unknown function that was first described as the antigenic target of the K1 monoclonal antibody that was generated using the OVCAR-2 ovarian cell line as immunogen (Chang et al. 1992). Early immunohistochemical studies reported strong expression in epithelioid mesotheliomas, but negative staining in lung adenocarcinomas, and suggested that this marker could assist in discriminating between these malignancies. Since serous carcinomas usually express mesothelin, it was also indicated that immunostaining for this marker had no utility for discriminating between these malignancies. More recent studies using the 5B2 antibody have shown that about one-third of the adenocarcinomas and squamous carcinomas of the lung exhibit mesothelin expression (Ordóñez 2003b). Despite its low specificity, a negative staining for mesothelin is a strong indication against the diagnosis of epithelioid mesothelioma because of the common strong membranous reactivity seen in these tumors. Because of this common, strong expression of mesothelin in mesotheliomas, recent studies have even indicated that this marker could serve as a serum marker for monitoring disease progression in patients with mesothelioma, as well as for screening individuals with a history of asbestos exposure for early evidence of the disease (Robinson et al. 2003).

12.5.1.5 Wilms Tumor 1 Protein

Wilms tumor 1 (WT1) protein is one of the most recently recognized positive mesothelioma markers. Depending on the type of antibody used, WT1 expression has been demonstrated in 43% to 93% of the epithelioid mesotheliomas (Amin et al. 1995; Oates and Edwards 2000; Ordóñez 2000c, 2003a; Foster et al. 2001; Miettinen et al. 2001). Since WT1 is not expressed in either squamous carcinomas or adenocarcinomas of the lung, it has been proven to be a useful immunohistochemical marker for distinguishing between these malignancies and epithelioid mesotheliomas (Ordóñez 2003a, 2006c). However, WT1 expression has been demonstrated in the large majority of serous carcinomas (Ordóñez 2000c; Goldstein et al. 2001; Goldstein and Uzieblo 2002; Hashi et al. 2003); therefore, immunostaining for this marker has no utility in distinguishing these tumors from peritoneal mesotheliomas.

12.5.1.6 Thrombomodulin

Thrombomodulin (CD141) was the first of the positive mesothelioma markers to be recognized as useful in the diagnosis of mesothelioma (Collins et al. 1992). However, the importance of this marker has declined in recent years as a result of the identification of more specific and sensitive mesothelioma markers. According to recent investigations, thrombomodulin expression can be demonstrated in about 77% of the epithelioid mesotheliomas (Ordóñez 2003a), 7% of the lung adenocarcinomas (Ordóñez 2003a), and 4% of the serous carcinomas (Ordóñez 2006a), but it is absent in renal cell carcinomas (Ordóñez 2004). These findings indicate that thrombomodulin can be useful, particularly in distinguishing between the latter tumors and mesotheliomas. Since thrombomodulin is often expressed in squamous carcinomas (Ordóñez 1997), immunostaining for this marker has no utility in distinguishing these tumors from mesotheliomas.

12.5.2 Positive Carcinoma Markers

12.5.2.1 Monoclonal Antibody MOC-31

MOC-31 is a monoclonal antibody that recognizes an epithelial cell adhesion molecule (Ep-CAM) that is strongly expressed in carcinomas, but not in mesotheliomas. According to most recent investigations, 98% of the serous carcinomas of the ovary and peritoneum (Ordóñez 2006a), 90% to 100% of the lung adenocarcinomas (Edwards and Oates 1995; Sosolik et al. 1997; Ordóñez 2003a), and 97% of the squamous carcinomas strongly react with MOC-31 (Ordóñez 2006c). This is in contrast to epithelioid mesotheliomas, in which only 2% to 10% have been reported to be positive in small focal areas of the tumor or in scattered neoplastic cells (Ordóñez 2003a). Because of its high sensitivity and specificity, MOC-31 is regarded as one of the best positive carcinoma markers for discriminating between the previously mentioned carcinomas and epithelioid peritoneal mesotheliomas. Since only 50% of the renal cell carcinomas have been reported to react with MOC-31 (Ordóñez 2004), immunostaining for this marker has only limited utility for distinguishing between these tumors and mesotheliomas.

12.5.2.2 Monoclonal Antibody Ber-EP4

Ber-EP4 is another anti-Ep-CAM antibody that, like MOC-31, is often used to distinguish epithelioid peritoneal mesotheliomas from carcinomas involving the peritoneum (Barnetson et al. 2006; Ordóñez 2006a). Ber-EP4 positivity has been reported in 100% of the lung adenocarcinomas and serous carcinomas of the ovary and peritoneum (Ordóñez 2003a, 2006a), 87% of the squamous carcinomas of the lung (Ordóñez 2006c), and 42% of the renal cell carcinomas (Ordóñez 2004) in most recent studies. Only 10% to 18% of the epithelioid mesotheliomas included in those recent investigations showed Ber-EP4 positivity in small areas of the tumor or in a few cells (Barnetson et al. 2006; Ordóñez 2003a, 2006a, 2006c). This is in contrast to the usually strong and diffuse reactivity seen in carcinomas, particularly those originating in the lung, ovary, and peritoneum (Fig. 12.7). The results of these investigations indicate that Ber-EP4 is a useful marker for discriminating between epithelioid mesotheliomas and lung adenocarcinomas (Ordóñez 1998b, 2003a), serous carcinomas (Ordóñez 1998a, 2006a; Barnetson et al. 2006), and squamous carcinomas of the lung (Ordóñez 2006c), but it has no utility for assisting in distinguishing epithelioid mesotheliomas from renal cell carcinomas (Ordóñez 2004).

12.5.2.3 Monoclonal Antibody BG-8

BG-8 is a monoclonal antibody that reacts with the blood group Lewisy (Jordon et al. 1989). In 1997, Riera et al., using this antibody, were able to demonstrate strong Lewis^Y expression in 187 (89%) of 211 adenocarcinomas of various origins, but weak positivity was seen in only 5 (9%) of 57 epithelioid mesotheliomas (Riera et al. 1997). The conclusion of that investigation was that BG-8 immunostaining could be useful for assisting in the diagnosis of mesotheliomas. The reported percentages of BG-8 positivity have ranged from 89% to 100% for adenocarcinomas of the lung (Ordóñez 2000c, 2003a), 80% to 83% for squamous carcinomas (Lyda and Weiss 2000; Ordóñez 2006c), and 73% for serous carcinomas of the ovary and peritoneum (Ordóñez 2006a). These results indicate that BG-8 immunostaining could be useful for distinguishing mesotheliomas from those types of carcinomas previously men-

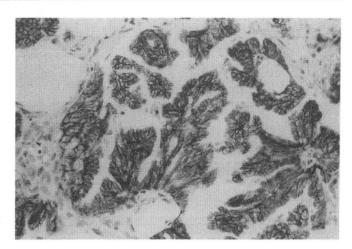

Fig. 12.7 Metastatic serous carcinoma to the peritoneum showing strong reactivity with the Ber-EP4 antibody

tioned. However, because the large majority of the renal cell carcinomas have been reported to be BG-8 negative (Ordóñez 2004), immunostaining for this marker has no utility for discriminating these tumors from mesotheliomas.

12.5.2.4 Carcinoembryonic Antigen

Carcinoembryonic antigen (CEA) was the first marker that was recognized as being useful in distinguishing between epithelioid mesotheliomas and adenocarcinomas of the lung (Wang et al. 1979). Current information indicates that approximately 80% of the lung adenocarcinomas express this marker, while epithelioid mesotheliomas are almost always negative (Ordóñez 2003a). Because of its high sensitivity and specificity, CEA is still regarded as being a good marker for distinguishing between these two malignancies. Since CEA is expressed in only a minority of serous carcinomas (Ordóñez 1998a; Barnetson et al. 2006) and is absent in renal cell carcinomas (Ordóñez 2004), immunostaining for this marker has no value in assisting in the differential diagnosis between these malignancies and epithelioid peritoneal mesotheliomas.

12.5.2.5 B72.3 Monoclonal Antibody

B72.3 is one of the earliest immunohistochemical markers that was recognized as being useful in the diagnosis of mesotheliomas. The percentages of B72.3 positivity reported for lung adenocarcinomas have ranged from 75% to 85% (Ordóñez 2003a) and from 70% to 75% for serous carcinomas (Ordóñez 1998a, 2006a), whereas mesotheliomas have been almost invariably negative for this marker (Ordóñez 2003a, 2006a). Since renal cell carcinomas do not react with this antibody (Ordóñez 2004), immunostaining for B72.3 has no utility in discriminating these tumors from mesotheliomas.

12.5.2.6 Leu-M1 (CD15)

Leu-M1 (CD15) is another of the early positive carcinoma markers that was recognized as being useful in the diagnosis of mesothelioma. According to recent investigations, 50% to 70% of the lung adenocarcinomas (Roberts et al. 2001; Ordóñez 2003a) and 30% to 60% of the serous carcinomas of the ovary and peritoneum (Attanoos et al. 2002; Ordóñez 2006a) are leu-M1 positive, whereas mesotheliomas are negative for this marker. These results indicate that even though leu-M1 is highly specific for discriminating between these tumors and mesotheliomas, its sensitivity is relatively low, especially compared with other currently available positive carcinoma markers. It should be mentioned, however, that because the large majority of conventional and papillary renal cell carcinomas react with leu-M1 (Ordóñez 2004), immunostaining with this antibody can be very useful in distinguishing these tumors from mesotheliomas.

12.5.3 Miscellaneous Markers

12.5.3.1 Estrogen and Progesterone Receptors

Because estrogen receptors are often expressed in serous carcinomas of the ovary and peritoneum, but not in mesotheliomas, it has recently been suggested that they could serve as an immunohistochemical marker for distinguishing between these malignancies (Ordóñez 2005c; Barnetson et al. 2006). In two recently published studies, estrogen receptors were reported in approximately 90% of the serous carcinomas, but in none of the peritoneal mesotheliomas investigated (Ordóñez 2005c; Barnetson et al. 2006). The conclusion of both investigations was that immunostaining for estrogen receptors could be very useful for discriminating between these malignancies. Since, in these same studies, progesterone receptors were demonstrated in 30% to 60% of the serous carcinomas and the staining in these cases was often focal and weak, it was concluded that immunostaining for progesterone receptors had no practical utility in the diagnosis of peritoneal mesotheliomas.

12.5.3.2 Renal Cell Carcinoma Marker

Renal cell carcinoma marker (RCC Ma) is the designation given to a monoclonal antibody that recognizes a 200-kDa glycoprotein present in the normal proximal tubule of the kidney (Yoshida and Imam 1989). The percentages of RCC Ma positivity reported in conventional renal cell carcinomas have ranged from 75% to 85% of the cases and for papillary renal cell carcinomas from 75% to 95% (Avery et al. 2000; McGregor et al. 2001; Ordóñez 2004). Only one study has investigated the expression of RCC Ma in mesotheliomas (Ordóñez 2004). In that study, only 3 (8%) of 45 epithelioid mesotheliomas exhibited focal positivity in small areas of the tumor or in a few scattered tumor cells. The conclusion of that investigation was that RCC Ma immunostaining was useful for assisting in the differential diagnosis between epithelioid peritoneal mesotheliomas and renal cell carcinomas by establishing the renal origin of the tumor.

12.5.3.3 Thyroid Transcription Factor 1

Thyroid transcription factor 1 (TTF-1) is a tissue-specific transcription factor that is expressed in normal lung and thyroid, as well as in carcinomas derived from these organs (Ordóñez 2000b). TTF-1 is expressed in approximately 75% of the lung adenocarcinomas (Ordóñez 2000c, 2003a), but it is absent in squamous carcinomas of the lung (Ordóñez 2006c). Since TTF-1 expression is absent in mesotheliomas, immunostaining for this marker can assist not only in distinguishing these tumors from lung adenocarcinomas, but also in determining the lung origin of metastatic adenocarcinomas to the peritoneum.

12.5.3.4 P63

P63 is a recently characterized transcription factor that is strongly expressed in squamous carcinomas, but not in epithelioid mesotheliomas (Ordóñez 2006c). Since epithelioid mesotheliomas are, on occasion, confused with squamous carcinomas metastatic to the serosal membranes, immunostaining for p63 can assist in discriminating between these malignancies.

12.6 Electron Microscopy

Although malignant mesotheliomas have no specific ultrastructural features, electron microscopy is a very useful technique for assisting in the diagnosis of these tumors, especially when distinguishing epithelioid mesotheliomas from carcinomas (Ordóñez 2006a). Epithelioid mesotheliomas are characterized by a profusion of long, slender, wavy microvilli along any of the cell surfaces (Fig. 12.8). In contrast, the microvilli in adenocarcinomas are less abundant, short, straight, and usually limited to the apical surface of the cells. In addition, the cell membranes in adenocarcinomas are often intimately apposed, while in epithelioid mesotheliomas intercellular gaps, often exhibiting microvilli, are a common finding (Fig. 12.9). Large collections of intermediate filaments, often arranged in tonofibrillary bundles, are common in mesotheliomas, while they are usually absent in adenocarcinomas. Electron

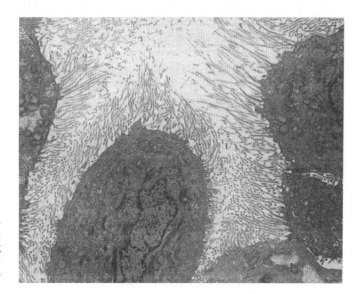

Fig. 12.8 Electron micrograph showing a group of mesothelioma cells with a profusion of long microvilli on the apical and lateral surfaces of the cell membrane (×7,000)

microscopy can also provide a better understanding of the morphological features of mesotheliomas that are seen by light microscopy. For example, as previously mentioned, the clearing of the cytoplasm seen in some mesotheliomas can be caused by a variety of factors, including the intracytoplasmic accumulation of large amounts of glycogen and/or lipid, marked swelling of mitochondria, massive dilatation of the endoplasmic reticulum, or the presence of large numbers of intracytoplasmic vesicles or intracytoplasmic lumens. Although the presence of glycogen can be demonstrated by the use of special stains, such as periodic acid Schiff (PAS), all of the other factors can only be demonstrated by electron microscopy.

The diagnostic value of electron microscopy in sarcomatoid mesotheliomas is somewhat more limited than in epithelioid mesotheliomas, but tonofibrillary bundles, intercellular junctions, an incomplete basal lamina, and rare surface microvilli are features that, when present, will support this diagnosis (Oury et al. 1998). Additionally, there are a variety of ultrastructural features that are useful in the diagnosis of some soft tissue tumors that can be confused with sarcomatoid mesotheliomas. In these instances, their presence or absence in a given tumor could assist in establishing the differential diagnosis.

12.7 Conclusions

Because peritoneal mesotheliomas can present a wide spectrum of histological patterns, they can be confused with a variety of other neoplastic conditions that can involve the peritoneum. At present, a large number of immunohistochemical markers that can assist in the diagnosis of mesotheliomas are available. However, as previously stated, an absolutely specific and sensitive mesothelioma marker has yet to be identified. From this review, it is evident that since the diverse markers that can assist in the diagnosis of mesothelioma are expressed differently among the various types of carcinomas, the selection of the markers to be used in a particular case depends on the differential diagnosis. For example, if the tumor has papillary features and occurs in a woman, the differential diagnosis is between peritoneal mesothelioma and metastatic serous carcinoma of the ovary or primary peritoneal serous carcinoma, but if the tumor is primarily composed of clear cells or exhibits solid or squamoid features, the differential diagnosis should include metastases from a renal cell carcinoma or a squamous carcinoma, respectively. In my experience, an immunohistochemical panel consisting of two positive mesothelioma markers and two positive carcinoma markers, the selection of which is based on the differential diagnosis of a specific tumor, usually allows a diagnosis to be established. Finally, in those instances in which the results obtained by the different panels of markers are equivocal, electron microscopy can be very helpful in assisting in establishing the differential diagnosis between mesothelioma and the various types of malignancies that can occur in the peritoneum.

References

Abutaily AS, Addis BJ, Roche WR (2002) Immunohistochemistry in the distinction between malignant mesothelioma and pulmonary adenocarcinoma: a critical evaluation of new antibodies. J Clin Pathol 55:662–668

Amin KM, Litzky LA, Smythe WR, Mooney AM, Morris JM, Mews DJY, Pass HI, Kari C, Rodeck U, Rauscher FJ III, Kaiser LR, Albelda SM (1995) Wilms' tumor 1 susceptibility (WT1) gene products are selectively expressed in malignant mesothelioma. Am J Pathol 146:344–356

Asioli S, Dal Piaz G, Damiani S (2004) Localised pleural malignant mesothelioma. Report of two cases simulating pulmonary carcinoma and review of the literature. Virchows Arch 445:206–209

Attanoos RL, Webb R, Dojcinov SD, Gibbs AR (2002) Value of mesothelial and epithelial antibodies in distinguishing diffuse peritoneal mesothelioma in females from serous papillary carcinoma of the ovary and peritoneum. Histopathology 40:237–244

Avery AK, Beckstead J, Renshaw AA, Corless CL (2000) Use of antibodies to RCC and CD10 in the differential diagnosis of renal neoplasms. Am J Surg Pathol 24:203–210

Baker PM, Clement PB, Young RH (2005) Malignant peritoneal mesothelioma in women. A study of 75 cases with emphasis on their morphologic spectrum and differential diagnosis. Am J Clin Pathol 123:724–737

Carella R, Deleonardi G, D'Errico A, Salerno A, Egarter-Vigl E, Seebacher C, Donazzan G, Grigioni WF (2001) Immunohistochemical panels for differentiating epithelial malignant mesothelioma from lung adenocarcinoma: a study with logistic regression analysis. Am J Surg Pathol 25:43–50

Cathro HP, Stoler MH (2005) The utility of calretinin, inhibin, and WT1 immunohistochemical staining in the differential diagnosis of ovarian tumors. Hum Pathol 36:195–201

Cavazza A, Pasquinelli G, Agostini L, Leslie KO, Colby TV (2002) Foamy cell mesothelioma. Histopathology 41:369–371

Chang K, Pai LH, Batra JK, Pastan I, Willingham MC (1992) Characterization of the antigen (CAK1) recognized by monoclonal antibody K1 present on ovarian cancers and normal mesothelium. Cancer Res 52:181–186

Chu AY, Litzky LA, Pasha TL, Acs G, Zhang PJ (2005) Utility of D2-40, a novel mesothelial marker, in the diagnosis of malignant mesothelioma. Mod Pathol 18:105–110

Chung DJ, Kang YW, Kim BK, Park JY, An YS, Yang JM, Kim JH (2003) Deciduoid peritoneal mesothelioma: CT findings with pathologic correlation. Abdom Imaging 28:614–616

Clover J, Oates J, Edwards C (1997) Anti-cytokeratin 5/6: a positive marker for epithelioid mesothelioma. Histopathology 31:140–143

Collins CL, Ordóñez NG, Schaefer R, Cook CD, Xie SS, Granger J, Hsu PL, Fink L, Hsu SM (1992) Thrombomodulin expression in malignant pleural mesothelioma and pulmonary adenocarcinoma. Am J Pathol 141:827–833

Comin CE, Novelli L, Boddi V, Paglierani M, Dini S (2001) Calretinin, thrombomodulin, CEA, and CD15: a useful combination of immunohistochemical markers for differentiating pleural epithelial mesothelioma from peripheral pulmonary adenocarcinoma. Hum Pathol 32:529–536

Dei Tos AP, Doglioni C (1998) Calretinin: a novel tool for diagnostic immunohistochemistry. Adv Anat Pathol 5:61–66

Dessy E, Falleni M, Braidotti PI, Curto B, Panigalli T, Pietra GG (2001) Unusual clear cell variant of epithelioid mesothelioma. Arch Pathol Lab Med 125:1588–1590

Edwards C, Oates J (1995) OV 632 and MOC 31 in the diagnosis of mesothelioma and adenocarcinoma: an assessment of their use in formalin-fixed and paraffin wax embedded material. J Clin Pathol 48:626–630

Foster MR, Johnson JE, Olson SJ, Allred DC (2001) Immunohistochemical analysis of nuclear versus cytoplasmic staining of WT1 in malignant mesotheliomas and primary pulmonary adenocarcinomas. Arch Pathol Lab Med 125:1316–1320

Goldstein NS, Bassi D, Uzieblo A (2001) WT1 is an integral component of an antibody panel to distinguish pancreaticobiliary and some ovarian epithelial neoplasms. Am J Clin Pathol 116:246–252

Goldstein NS, Uzieblo A (2002) WT1 immunoreactivity in uterine papillary serous carcinomas is different from ovarian serous carcinomas. Am J Clin Pathol 117:541–545

Hashi A, Yuminamochi T, Murate S-I, Iwamoto H, Honda T, Hoshi K (2003) Wilms tumor gene immunoreactivity in primary serous carcinomas of the fallopian tube, ovary, endometrium, and peritoneum. Int J Gynecol Pathol 22:374–377

Jordon D, Jagirdar J, Kaneko M (1989) Blood group antigens, Lewisx and Lewisy, in the diagnostic discrimination of malignant mesothelioma versus adenocarcinoma. Am J Pathol 135:931–937

Kannerstein M, Churg J (1977) Peritoneal mesothelioma. Hum Pathol 8:83–94

Khalidi HS, Medeiros LJ, Battifora H (2000) Lymphohistiocytoid mesothelioma: an often misdiagnosed variant of sarcomatoid malignant mesothelioma. Am J Clin Pathol 113:649–654

Kimura N, Kimura I (2005) Podoplanin as a marker for mesothelioma. Pathol Int 55:83–86

Kimura N, Ogasawara T, Asonuma S, Hama H, Sawai T, Toyota T (2005) Granulocyte-colony stimulating factor and interleukin 6-producing diffuse deciduoid peritoneal mesothelioma. Mod Pathol 18:446–450

Lucas DR, Pass HI, Madan SK, Adsay NV, Wali A, Tabaczka P, Lonardo F (2003) Sarcomatoid mesothelioma and its histological mimics: a comparative immunohistochemical study. Histopathology 42:270–279

Lugli A, Forster Y, Haas P, Nocito A, Bucher C, Bissig H, Mirlacher M, Storz M, Mihatsch MJ, Sauter G (2003) Calretinin expression in human normal and neoplastic tissues: a tissue microarray analysis on 5233 tissue samples. Hum Pathol 34:994–1000

Lyda MH, Weiss LM (2000) Immunoreactivity for epithelial and neuroendocrine antibodies are useful in the differential diagnosis of lung carcinomas. Hum Pathol 31:980–987

Maeda S, Hosone M, Katayama H, Azuma K, Yokota A, Nakai A, Liu A, Naito Z (2004) Deciduoid mesothelioma in the pelvic cavity. Pathol Int 54:67–72

Martignoni G, Pea M, Chilosi M, Brunelli M, Scarpa A, Colato C, Tardanico R, Zamboni G, Bonetti F (2001) Parvalbumin is constantly expressed in chromophobe renal carcinoma. Mod Pathol 14:760–767

Matsukuma S, Aida S, Hata Y, Sugiura Y, Tamai S (1996) Localized malignant peritoneal mesothelioma containing rhabdoid cells. Pathol Int 46:389–391

McGregor DK, Khurana KK, Cao C, Tsao CC, Ayala G, Krishnan B, Ro JY, Lechago J, Truong LD (2001) Diagnosing primary and metastatic renal cell carcinoma: The use of the monoclonal antibody 'renal cell carcinoma marker'. Am J Surg Pathol 25:1485–1492

Miettinen M, Limon J, Niezabitowski A, Lasota J (2001) Calretinin and other mesothelioma markers in synovial sarcoma: analysis of antigenic similarities and differences with malignant mesothelioma. Am J Surg Pathol 25:610–617

Mourra N, de Chaisenmartin C, Goubin-Versini I, Parc R, Flejou JF (2005) Malignant deciduoid mesothelioma: a diagnostic challenge. Arch Pathol Lab Med 129:403–406

Nascimento AG, Keeney GL, Fletcher CD (1994) Deciduoid peritoneal mesothelioma. An unusual phenotype affecting young females. Am J Surg Pathol 18:439–445

Oates J, Edwards C (2000) HBME-1, MOC-31, WT1 and calretinin: as assessment of recently described markers for mesothelioma and adenocarcinoma. Histopathology 36:341–347

Ordóñez NG (1997) Value of thrombomodulin immunostaining in the diagnosis of mesothelioma. Histopathology 31:25–30

Ordóñez NG (1998a) Role of immunohistochemistry in distinguishing epithelial peritoneal mesotheliomas from peritoneal and ovarian serous carcinomas. Am J Surg Pathol 22:1203–1214

Ordóñez NG (1998b) Value of the Ber-EP4 antibody in differentiating epithelial pleural mesothelioma from adenocarcinoma. The M.D. Anderson experience and a critical review of the literature. Am J Clin Pathol 109:85–89

Ordóñez NG (1998c) Value of calretinin immunostaining in differentiating epithelial mesothelioma from lung adenocarcinoma. Mod Pathol 11:929–33

Ordóñez NG (1998d) Value of cytokeratin 5/6 immunostaining in distinguishing epithelial mesothelioma of the pleura from lung adenocarcinoma. Am J Surg Pathol 22:1215–1221

Ordóñez NG (1998e) Value of the MOC-31 monoclonal antibody in differentiating epithelial pleural mesothelioma from lung adenocarcinoma. Hum Pathol 29:166–169

Ordóñez NG (2000a) Epithelial mesothelioma with deciduoid features: report of four cases. Am J Surg Pathol 24:816–823

Ordóñez NG (2000b) Thyroid transcription factor-1 is a marker of lung and thyroid carcinomas. Adv Anat Pathol 7:123–127

Ordóñez NG (2000c) Value of thyroid transcription factor-1, E-cadherin, BG8, WT1, and CD44S immunostaining in distinguishing epithelial pleural mesothelioma from pulmonary and nonpulmonary adenocarcinoma. Am J Surg Pathol 24:598–606

Ordóñez NG (2003a) The immunohistochemical diagnosis of mesothelioma: a comparative study of epithelioid mesothelioma and lung adenocarcinoma. Am J Surg Pathol 27:1031–1051

Ordóñez NG (2003b) Value of mesothelin immunostaining in the diagnosis of mesothelioma. Mod Pathol 16:192–197

Ordóñez NG (2004) The diagnostic utility of immunohistochemistry in distinguishing between mesothelioma and renal cell carcinoma: a comparative study. Hum Pathol 35:697–710

Ordóñez NG (2005a) D2-40 and podoplanin are highly specific and sensitive immunohistochemical markers of epithelioid malignant mesothelioma. Hum Pathol 36:372–380

Ordóñez NG (2005b) Mesothelioma with clear cell features: an ultrastructural and immunohistochemical study of 20 cases. Hum Pathol 36:465–473

Ordóñez NG (2005c) Value of estrogen and progesterone receptor immunostaining in distinguishing between peritoneal mesotheliomas and serous carcinomas. Hum Pathol 36:1163–1167

Ordóñez NG (2006a) The diagnostic utility of immunohistochemistry and electron microscopy in distinguishing between peritoneal mesotheliomas and serous carcinomas: a comparative study. Mod Pathol 19:34–48

Ordonez NG (2006b) Mesothelioma with rhabdoid features: an ultrastructural and immunohistochemical study of 10 cases. Mod Pathol (in press)

Ordóñez NG (2006c) The diagnostic utility of immunohistochemistry in distinguishing between epithelioid mesotheliomas and squamous carcinomas of the lung: a comparative study. Mod Pathol (in press)

Ordonez NG, Myhre M, Mackay B (1996) Clear cell mesothelioma. Ultrastruct Pathol 20:331–336

Orosz Z, Nagy P, Szentirmay Z, Zalatnai A, Hauser P (1999) Epithelial mesothelioma with deciduoid features. Virchows Arch 434:263–266

Osborn M, Pelling N, Walker MM, Fisher C, Nicholson AG (2002) The value of mesothelium-associated antibodies in distinguishing between metastatic renal cell carcinoma and mesotheliomas. Histopathology 41:301–307

Oury TD, Hammar SP, Roggli VL (1998) Ultrastructural features of diffuse malignant mesotheliomas. Hum Pathol 29:1382–1392

Puttagunta L, Vriend RA, Nguyen GK (2000) Deciduoid epithelial mesothelioma of the pleura with focal rhabdoid change. Am J Surg Pathol 24:1440–1443

Riera JR, Astengo-Osuna C, Longmate JA, Battifora H (1997) The immunohistochemical diagnostic panel for epithelial mesothelioma. A reevaluation after heat-induced epitope retrieval. Am J Surg Pathol 21:1409–1419

Roberts F, Harper CM, Downie I, Burnett RA (2001) Immunohistochemical analysis still has a limited role in the diagnosis of malignant mesothelioma: a study of thirteen antibodies. Am J Clin Pathol 116:253–262

Robinson BW, Creaney J, Lake R, Nowak A, Musk AW, de Klerk N, Winzell P, Hellstrom KE, Hellstrom I (2003) Mesothelin-family proteins and diagnosis of mesothelioma. Lancet 362:1612–1616

Schacht V, Dadras SS, Johnson LA, Jackson DG, Hong Y-K, Detmar M (2005) Up-regulation of the lymphatic marker podoplanin, a mucin-type transmembrane glycoprotein, in human squamous cell carcinomas and germ cell tumors. Am J Pathol 166:913–921

Serio G, Scattone A, Pennella A, Giardina C, Musti M, Valente T, Pollice L (2002) Malignant deciduoid mesothelioma of the pleura: report of two cases with long survival. Histopathology 40:348–352

Shanks JH, Harris M, Banerjee SS, Eyden BP, Joglekar VM, Nicol A, Hasleton PS, Nicholson AG (2000) Mesotheliomas with deciduoid morphology: a morphologic spectrum and a variant not confined to young females. Am J Surg Pathol 24:285–294

Shia J, Erlandson RA, Klimstra DS (2002) Deciduoid mesothelioma: a report of 5 cases and literature review. Ultrastruct Pathol 26:355–363

Sienko A, Zander DS, Killen D, Singhal N, Barrios R, Haque A, Cagle PT (2005) D2-40 is a novel new marker of malignant mesothelioma (MM): Tissue microarray study of 45 MM versus 409 lung carcinomas and primary non-mesothelial neoplasms of the pleura and chest wall [abstract]. Mod Pathol 18 [Suppl 1]:318A

Sosolik RC, McGaughy VR, De Young BR (1997) Anti-MOC-31: A potential addition to the pulmonary adenocarcinoma versus mesothelioma immunohistochemistry panel. Mod Pathol 10:716–719

Talerman A, Montero JR, Chilcote RR, Okagaki T (1985) Diffuse malignant peritoneal mesothelioma in a 13-year-old girl. Report of a case and review of the literature. Am J Surg Pathol 9:73–80

Yoshida SO, Imam A (1989) Monoclonal antibody to a proximal nephrogenic renal antigen: immunohistochemical analysis of formalin-fixed, paraffin-embedded human renal cell carcinomas. Cancer Res 49:1802–1809

Wang NS, Huang SN, Gold P (1979) Absence of carcinoembryonic antigen-like material in mesothelioma. An immunohistochemical differentiation from other lung cancers. Cancer 44:937–943

13 Advances in Clinical Research and Management of Diffuse Peritoneal Mesothelioma

Marcello Deraco, Dario Baratti, Nadia Zaffaroni, Antonello Domenico Cabras, Shigeki Kusamura

Diffuse malignant mesothelioma is a tumor arising from the serosal surfaces of the pleura, peritoneum, pericardium, or tunica vaginalis testis. Although the tumor is exceedingly uncommon, there is a substantial interest in this disease, as either biological or occupational and medical-legal issues are concerned: asbestos is the principal carcinogen associated with malignant mesothelioma, and up to 8 million living persons in the USA have been occupationally exposed to asbestos over the last five decades (Robinson and Lake 2005).

Diffuse malignant peritoneal mesothelioma (DMPM) is a rapidly fatal disease for which conventional therapy, such as palliative surgery, radiotherapy, and systemic or intraperitoneal (IP) chemotherapy is unsatisfactory. Only in recent years, prospective trials of multimodality treatment consisting of cytoreductive surgery (CRS) and hyperthermic intraperitoneal chemotherapy (HIPEC) have reportedly resulted in a survival advantage for selected patients.

13.1 Epidemiology

About 2,500 new cases of mesothelioma are registered each year in the United States (Price 1997). The incidence of malignant mesothelioma has been rising worldwide since 1970, and it has been estimated that a 5%–10% increase in annual mortality rate will be observed worldwide at least until 2020 (Peto et al. 1995). The disease has likely already reached the incidence peak in the USA (Archer and Rom 1983). In contrast, in Europe (Peto et al. 1999) and Australia (Leigh and Robinson 2002) the peaks are not expected to occur for another 10–15 years. In Japan, as well as in other countries where wide use of asbestos was observed later then in the western world, peak incidence of mesothelioma is delaying (Murajama 2004). Moreover, the increased use of asbestos in developing countries is expected to result in an increase of mesothelioma incidence unless stringent occupational controls are put in place (Takayhashi 2004).

Mesothelioma is approximately threefold more common in males than in females. Incidence rises with age and is about 10-fold higher in individuals 60 to 64 year-old than in those 30 to 34 year-old (Price 1997).

Peritoneal mesothelioma accounts for 10% to 20% of all forms of malignant mesothelioma. A recent analysis of the Surveillance Epidemiology and End Results (SEER) database estimated a yearly incidence of 250 cases in the USA (Price 2003).

13.2 Etiology

The link between malignant mesothelioma and asbestos exposure was first reported by Wagner in 1960 in South Africa's Cape Province (Wagner et al 1960). In the 1960s and 1970s many case-controlled studies confirmed the association between both occupational and occasional asbestos exposure and this neoplasm (Spirtas et al. 2004). McDonald summarized data from 43 cohort studies and observed an overall proportional cancer-specific mortality rate of 2.5 to 102.3 in individuals exposed to asbestos (McDonald 2000). Subjects at risk for developing asbestos-related mesothelioma can be categorized as follows: workers directly exposed to asbestos during its mining or milling; workers exposed during use or manufacture of asbestos products, such as plumbers, carpenters, defense personnel, and insulation installers; people exposed incidentally to environmental asbestos contamination (Leigh and Robinson 2002).

No asbestos exposure can be documented in approximately 20% to 40% of patients with mesothelioma. Furthermore, the neoplasm is characterized by a long latency (up to 40 years) from asbestos exposure (McDonald 1985). These data suggest that other etiological factors may be determinant and that multiple somatic genetic events are required for mesothelioma oncogenesis.

13.2.1 Asbestos-Induced Oncogenesis

Asbestos induces mesothelioma by means of the following mechanisms: (1) asbestos fibers penetrate into the lung and hence enter the pleura, originating scarring (plaques) and malignant disease; (2) asbestos fibers may sever or pierce the mitotic spindle and disrupt mitosis, resulting in aneuploidy or other chromosomal damage; (3) asbestos induces the generation of iron-related reactive oxygen species that cause DNA alterations; (4) asbestos induces phosphorylation of the mitogen-activated protein kinases and the extracellular signal-regulated kinases. Such alterations increase the expression of early-response proto-oncogenes (Robinson et al. 2005). Crocidolite fiber is the most oncogenic form of asbestos; other fibers have less convincing evidence for causing mesothelioma (Pisick and Salgia 2005).

The role of asbestos exposure in the origin of DMPM has not been as well established as in pleural mesothelioma, especially in women. Spirtas et al. recorded in a case-control study 88% of pleural mesothelioma and 58% of peritoneal mesothelioma directly related to past asbestos exposure among men. By contrast, only 20% of women with peritoneal mesothelioma had past asbestos exposure (Spirtas et al. 1994). Several epidemiological studies have reported increased incidence of DMPM in men working in crocidolite mines and in male insulation workers. Risk of developing DMPM was significantly related to intensity of exposure to asbestos (Hassan and Alexander 2005). A case-control study was conducted at the Washington Cancer Institute on 40 patients with confirmed diagnosis of DMPM; 16 of them were females. A strong association between occupational asbestos exposure and DMPM was observed in men but not in women. Therefore, it has been suggested that the epidemiology and progress of DMPM may differ between men and women (Sugarbaker et al. 2003). Other possible etiologies of DMPM are abdominal external beam radiation for testicular carcinoma or cervical cancer (Antman et al. 1983), chronic peritonitis, and administration of thorotrast (Maurer and Egloff 1975).

13.2.2 Oncogenesis Not Related to Asbestos

Simian virus 40 (SV40) is a DNA virus that has been implicated as a possible cofactor in mesothelioma oncogenesis, although its role remains controversial. SV40 has demonstrated to be an oncogenic virus in rodent and human cells by a mechanism of tumor-suppressor gene blocking; SV40 DNA sequences have been found in malignant mesothelioma as well as in atypical mesothelial proliferation and noninvasive mesothelial lesions (Gazdar and Carbone 2004).

The hypothesis of a genetic susceptibility with an autosomal dominant pattern is based on the observations gathered in Cappadocia. Among inhabitants of two villages built from stone that contains a large amount of asbestos fibers, it has been documented that approximately 50% of deaths can be attributed to malignant mesothelioma (Baris et al. 1978).

Interestingly, in a nearby town that was built with stone from the same cave, no cases of mesothelioma were recorded. The researcher found that about 50% of descendants of affected parents develop the disease; when a person from an unaffected family marries a member of an affected family, their descendants develop mesothelioma (Roushdy-Hammady et al. 2001).

13.2.3 Molecular Biology

The biology of peritoneal mesothelioma is largely unknown, and the cellular and molecular bases for its proliferative potential and relative resistance to therapy have not yet been elucidated. One of the hallmarks of cancer cells is their limitless replicative potential. In a high percentage of human tumors the attainment of immortality is due to the reactivation of telomerase, an RNA-dependent DNA polymerase that stabilizes telomeres and allows cells to avoid the senescence checkpoint (Blackburn 2001), and may therefore contribute to tumorigenesis and neoplastic progression (Hahn et al. 1999). The core enzyme consists of an RNA component (hTR) that provides the template for the de novo synthesis of telomeric DNA and a catalytic subunit (hTERT, human telomerase reverse transcriptase) with reverse transcriptase activity (Cong et al. 2002). Some tumors, however, maintain their telomeres by one or more mechanisms referred to as alternative lengthening of telomeres (ALT) (Bryan et al. 1997). Telomere dynamics in ALT cells are consistent with a recombination-based mechanism, and characteristics of ALT cells include unusually long and heterogeneous telomeres and subnuclear structures termed ALT-associated promyelocytic leukemia (PML) bodies (APBs) that contain telomeric DNA, telomere-specific binding proteins. and proteins involved in DNA recombination and replication (Dunham et al. 2000). Based on the limited information available thus far, it appears that ALT is more frequently present in tumors of mesenchymal origin than in those of epithelial origin, possibly because of a tighter repression of telomerase in normal mesenchymal than in epithelial cells (Henson et al. 2002). Although it is well known that telomerase is largely expressed in pleural mesotheliomas (Kumaki et al. 2002), no information is available thus far concerning the presence of telomere maintenance mechanisms in DMPM. In this context, we analyzed the expression of telomere maintenance mechanisms in 28 DMPM specimens obtained from patients who underwent cytoreductive surgery at our Institute. Telomerase activity, as detected by the Telomeric Repeat Amplification Protocol (TRAP) assay, was present in 19 of 28 cases (67.9%). Moreover, in all telomerase-positive specimens a full-length hTERT transcript was detected. All telomerase-negative cases were characterized by the presence of APBs, as assessed by a combined PML immunofluorescence/telomere FISH approach, in sufficient percentage of cells (>0.5%) to be defined as ALT-positive according to Henson (Henson et al. 2005). Moreover, when we measured telomere length in individual cases by gel electrophoresis and Southern blot hybridization we found that telomeres were significantly longer in ALT-positive than in telomerase-positive specimens (unpublished observations). Overall, these preliminary results indicate the presence of multiple telomere maintenance mechanisms in peritoneal mesothelioma and suggest the requirement for telomere maintenance during the development of this malignancy.

Since apoptotic cell death is the major mode by which chemical and physical anticancer agents kill tumor cells, it is likely that dysregulation of the apoptotic pathways plays a role in sustaining peritoneal mesothelioma cell chemoresistance as already demonstrated for pleural mesothelioma. In fact, previous investigations have shown overexpression of antiapoptotic proteins belonging to the Bcl-2 family (Bcl-2 and Bcl-XL) and inhibitors of apoptosis protein (IAP) family (IAP-1 and survivin) in pleural mesothelioma cell lines and surgical specimens (Gordon et al. 2002). Moreover, through the use of antisense-mediated inhibition approaches, these studies also demonstrated a cytoprotective role of such proteins toward spontaneous and anticancer drug-induced apoptosis (Xia et al. 2002). The identification of points in the apoptotic pathways at which dysregulation occurs in DMPM could open new opportunities for the design of novel therapeutic strategies targeting the molecular determinants of treatment resistance of this malignancy. For this purpose, we examined the expression of antiapoptotic proteins belonging to the IAP family (survivin, c-IAP1, c-IAP2 and X-IAP), as well as proapoptotic proteins such as SMAC/Diablo, by immunohistochemistry in 32 peritoneal mesothelioma specimens. Overexpression of survivin and other IAP proteins was observed in a high percentage of tumors, ranging from 69% to 100%, and in an elevated fraction of tumor cells within individual specimens. Conversely, SMAC/Diablo immunostaining was detectable in only 34% of tumors. Accordingly, a low apoptotic index (median percentage of apoptotic cells, 0.45%; range, 0.01%–5.8%) was consistently observed (unpublished observations). To investigate whether antiapoptotic proteins represent potential targets for new therapeutic interventions in this disease, we tested the effects of survivin knockdown accomplished through RNA interference in a peritoneal mesothelioma cell line. Survivin is a structurally unique member of the IAP family whose expression is associated with clinical progression in some tumor types. Accumulating evidence supports the existence of a multifunctional survivin pathway positioned at the interface between mitotic progression and apoptosis inhibition and required to preserve the viability of proliferating tumor cells (Altieri 2003). Survivin also appears to be involved in tumor cell resistance to some anticancer agents as well as ionizing radiation. On the basis of these findings, survivin has been proposed as a promising target for new anticancer interventions (Altieri 2003). In this context, we transfected peritoneal mesothelioma cells with a 21-mer double-stranded small interfering RNA (siRNA) targeting survivin mRNA and observed a strong inhibition of survivin expression at mRNA and protein levels, which was followed by a time-dependent reduction of cell growth and a significant increase of caspase-9-mediated apoptotic rate. Moreover, sequential exposure of siRNA-transfected mesothelioma cells to anticancer drugs (cisplatin and doxorubicin) induced additive antiproliferative effects and markedly increased the apoptotic response to individual drug treatment (unpublished observations). Overall, our results indicate that peritoneal mesothelioma is characterized by dysregulation of apoptosis pathways, in terms of increased expression of antiapoptotic proteins, and suggest that strategies aimed at interfering with such proteins may provide a novel approach for the treatment of this malignancy.

13.3 Pathology

The histological features of malignant peritoneal mesothelioma are usually the same as their pleural counterparts and may be subdivided into epithelial, sarcomatoid, and biphasic tumors. Epithelial tumors predominate in both pleural and peritoneal locations. In a series of 82 peritoneal tumors, 75.6% were epithelial, 22% biphasic, and 2.4% sarcomatoid (Kannerstein and Churg 1977). The data are similar in our experience. Immunohistochemistry is an important ancillary technique in the diagnosis of mesothelioma. Mesotheliomas demonstrate a similar immunohistochemical profile, regardless of the site of origin (pleura or peritoneum). The more common antigens expressed in mesotheliomas are calretinin, cytokeratin 5/6, HMBME, N-cadherin, and thrombomodulin (Ordonez 1998).

The diagnostic microscopy and immunohistochemistry features of peritoneal mesothelioma along with a detailed pathological description of its different morphological types and subtypes is comprehensively described in Chap. 12 of this book.

13.4 Natural History

Patients are usually diagnosed with peritoneal mesothelioma when presenting signs and symptoms of advanced disease (see Fig. 13.1). DMPM growth is characterized by peritoneal seeding, eventually leading to the patient's death due to tumor encasement, bowel obstruction, and intractable malignant ascites (Moertel 1972). This pattern of spread supports the potential usefulness of selectively increasing cytotoxic drug concentrations by direct IP chemotherapy administration (Antman et al. 1980).

13.4.1 Clinical Presentation

The clinical presentation of DMPM can be varied. Signs and symptoms may last for months before the disease is diagnosed. Patients typically present with abdominal pain, increasing abdominal girth, bloating, weight loss, alteration in bowel habits, abdominal masses, ascites, or fever (Chan et al. 1975). The initial symptoms of DMPM were outlined in a series of 68 patients (Sugarbaker et al. 2003). Increased abdominal girth was the most common sign, reported in 56% of cases. The second most common initial symptom was pain, reported in 44% of patients. A new-onset hernia was seen in 13% of patients and was statistically more common in men. Occasionally DMPM may be discovered in asymptomatic individuals undergoing abdominal exploration or laparoscopy for other causes. In the above-mentioned series, incidental diagnosis was reported in 38% of the women and in 19% of the men; this difference was statistically significant (P=0.016). Clinical presentation was related to survival after surgical cytoreduction and HIPEC, since patients with DMPM diagnosed by incidental findings had significantly longer survival than those with symptomatic mesothelioma.

13.4.2 Pattern of Spread

Intraperitoneal malignancies spread according to three different patterns: direct extension, cell dissemination via peritoneal fluid, and surgical manipulation (Carmignani et al. 2003). As a consequence of the latter modality, viable exfoliated tumor cells become entrapped in avascular scar tissue, thus becoming relatively resistant to intravenous chemotherapy (CT). The dissemination within the peritoneal cavity was defined by Sugarbaker as a redistribution phenomenon, indicating a complete

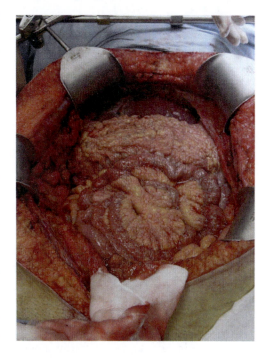

Fig. 13.1 Peritoneal carcinomatosis due to diffuse malignant peritoneal mesothelioma

and sequential invasion of the peritoneal cavity with large tumor volume localization at predetermined anatomical sites and minimal invasion at other sites (Sugarbaker 1994). Large pores are present on the peritoneal surface of the omentum, and lymphatic lacunae are open at the diaphragm undersurface. Consequently, a large volume of tumor rapidly localizes at these anatomical sites. Cells then settle by gravity within the abdomen, with accumulation in the pelvis, in the right retrohepatic space, in the left abdominal gutter, and at the Treitz ligament, while the ileum usually remains tumor free. Progression will eventually compromise gastrointestinal function because of bowel compression (Deraco et al. 1999).

The disease is generally confined to the peritoneal cavity and rarely metastasizes to the liver. Only in advanced stages may direct extension to the pleural cavity and distant spread be noted. An autopsy study demonstrated that two-thirds of the examined patients had tumor only in the abdominal cavity and that 78% of patients had died because of complications directly related to intra-abdominal disease, such as bowel obstruction (Antman et al. 1980).

13.5 Diagnosis

Definitive diagnosis of peritoneal mesothelioma is usually a difficult clinical problem (Whitaker 2000). Cytological diagnosis in ascitic fluid is often inconclusive, since cells frequently resemble elements with mesothelial hyperplasia. Only in recent years have cytological and ultrastructural methods enhanced the diagnostic accuracy of cytological assessment (Robinson et al. 2005). In the series of the Washington Cancer Institute, diagnosis was made by fluid sampling in none of 68 patients. Laparotomy was required in 44% of patients, laparoscopy in 52%, and US/CT-scan guided biopsy in 4% (Sugarbaker et al. 2003). Mesothelioma has a high propensity to implant in laparoscopic trocar tracts or abdominal incisions. Therefore, biopsies should be performed in the midline along the linea alba, as dissemination within the abdominal wall may result from placement of lateral ports (Brigand et al. 2006).

As discussed in Chap. 12, the differential diagnosis from carcinoma of ovarian or digestive origin may be problematic. Appropriate immunocytochemical stains are required. A positive calretinin, cytokeratin 7, EMA, WT1, and mesothelin stain has significant diagnostic sensitivity. In contrast, negative immunostaining for epithelial antigens such as CEA or B72.3 is highly suggestive of peritoneal mesothelioma (Ordonez 1998).

A clinicopathological study on 35 patients treated with cytoreductive surgery and locoregional hyperthermic CT has been carried out in our institution (Nonaka et al. 2005). Calretinin and WT-1 were expressed in all cases to a variable degree, while expression of polyclonal CEA and Ber-EP4 also were negative in all cases. MMP-2 was expressed in all cases, generally in a diffuse and strong fashion, whereas MMP-9 was expressed in 30 cases but was found to be of variable intensity and distribution. EGFR was expressed in a membranous pattern in all but two cases. Conversely, p16 was found to be only focally positive, with a nuclear staining pattern noted in 21 cases (60%) (see Table 13.1).

13.5.1 Radiological Imaging

The radiological features of peritoneal mesothelioma at CT scan have been reviewed recently. Diffuse disease distribution throughout the peritoneal cavity was observed, with large tumor volume in the midabdomen and in the pelvis in a majority of patients. These findings may raise the suspicion that a patient with malignant ascites could be affected by DMPM. A classification of mesothelioma involvement of small bowel and its mesentery has been proposed (see Table 13.2). Such classification provides important information on the extent of the disease and on the functional bowel impairment that may be expected (Yan et al. 2005).

Table 13.1. Immunohistochemical staining in 35 patients with malignant peritoneal mesothelioma

Score	Calretinin	WT-1	pCEA	Ber-Ep4	EGFR	p16	MMP-2	MMP-9
0	0	0	35	35	2	14	0	5
+1	0	5	0	0	1	11	2	9
+2	1	6	0	0	3	6	3	8
+3	6	5	0	0	7	2	7	8
+4	28	19	0	0	22	2	23	5

pCEA, polyclonal carcinoembryonic antigen; EGFR, epidermal growth factor receptor; MMP, matrix metalloproteinase

Table 13.2. Classification of small bowel and mesentery CT scan features

Class	Presence of ascites	Small bowel and mesentery involvement	Loss of mesenteric vessel clarity	CT scan interpretation
0	No	No	No	Normal appearance
I	Yes	No	No	Ascites only
II	Yes	Thickening, enhancing	No	Solid tumor present
III	Yes	Nodular thickening, segmental obstruction	Yes	Loss of normal architecture

CT, computed tomography

The role of preoperative abdominal and pelvic CT scan in the identification of patients most likely to benefit from a comprehensive treatment of CRS and HIPEC has been assessed. Tumor mass >5 cm in the epigastric region and loss of normal architecture of the small bowel and its mesentery were the radiological features related to failure in adequately removing all the macroscopic tumor. In a composite analysis, none of the patients with both of these radiological features had an adequate cytoreduction. Conversely, patients who lacked these two preoperative CT scan findings had a 94% probability of adequate cytoreduction (Yan et al 2005).

13.5.2 Serum Markers

Serum mesothelin-related proteins are a soluble form of mesothelin that has reported to be elevated in 84% of patients with pleural mesothelioma and in only 2% with other pulmonary diseases (Pass et al. 2005). Serum osteopontin levels were shown to be significantly higher in patients with pleural mesothelioma than in those with asbestos exposure (Robinson et al. 2003). No data are presently available about the clinical utility of these antigens in DMPM management. We conducted a study on the clinical role of serum markers in patients with DMPM. (Baratti et al. 2006). Baseline diagnostic sensitivity was 58% for CA125, 50% for CA15.3, 2.3% for Ca19.9, and 0 for CEA. These data may be of some help in the initial assessment of peritoneal dissemination of unknown origin, since they demonstrate that an elevated CA125 should not exclude a diagnosis of DMPM, although the tumor is less common than ovarian cancer, with which it is easily confused. Serial postoperative CA125 and CA15.3 measurements were effective in assessing response to treatment and disease progression after surgery and HIPEC.

13.6 Staging

In contrast to pleural mesothelioma, no staging system is universally accepted for peritoneal mesothelioma. A standard assessment of tumor burden would be of help in selecting patients for aggressive multimodality treatment, planning cytoreductive surgery, and predicting patient outcome. Furthermore, as addressed in Chap. 8, standard disease staging might assist in comparing results from different investigators.

Currently, four intraoperative staging systems are used in peritoneal malignancies. The Japanese Research Society for Gastric Cancer system was originally proposed to classify carcinomatosis from gastric primary cancer. Such classification is very simple and quantifies peritoneal involvement according to location and number of tumor nodules (Iwamoto et al. 1989). It is described in detail in Chap. 8. Correlation between survival and this classification was found in several studies investigating the impact of cytoreductive surgery followed by HIPEC for gastric cancer (Fujimoto et al. 1997), but it has never been applied to peritoneal mesothelioma.

A major drawback of this staging system is its inaccurate anatomic definition and the lack of size assessment of the cancer implants.

The Gilly peritoneal carcinomatosis staging system was first described in 1994 (Gilly et al. 1994). It is detailed in Chap. 8 (Table 8.1). In a recent paper, Gilly score was related to survival also among patients with peritoneal mesothelioma (Brigand et al. 2006). Simplicity and reproducibility are the main advantages of this system. However, the distribution of peritoneal surface implants, which is a prognostic determinant, is difficult to assess in stages 3 and 4. Large-size peritoneal implants confined to one portion of the abdomen may imply a favorable outcome; conversely, if tumor nodules <5 mm are diffuse all over the abdominal cavity, prognosis may be certainly worse (Harmon and Sugarbaker 2005).

The Peritoneal Cancer Index (PCI) was introduced by Sugarbaker and presently is the most widely used system for staging peritoneal malignancies. The PCI quantitatively combines tumor distribution in 13 abdominal anatomical regions with lesion size (Jacquet et al. 1996). It is described in detail in Chap. 8 (Fig. 8.1). In patients with carcinomatosis from invasive cancer, PCI correlates to the probability of performing a complete cytoreduction and prognosis after CRS with HIPEC (Harmon and Sugarbaker 2005). Sugarbaker and Elias independently established the correlation between PCI and survival in a large number of patients with carcinomatosis from colorectal cancer (Elias et al. 2001; Sugarbaker et al. 1999). Tentes and colleagues validated the PCI for ovarian cancer (Tentes et al. 2003). Sugarbaker reported that PCI>28 correlated to significantly lower survival rates in patients affected by peritoneal mesothelioma undergoing CRS and HIPEC (Sugarbaker et al. 2003). PCI score is presently adopted in our center to stage peritoneal malignancies, but we have not observed correlation to prognosis in patients with DMPM (Deraco et al. 2005). The main drawback of PCI is its complexity. Moreover, complete tumor removal could be difficult to achieve in cases with low PCI, if invasive large tumor is present at crucial anatomic sites, such as the hepatic hilum (Fig. 13.2)

The Simplified Peritoneal Cancer Index (SPCI) was introduced at the Netherlands Cancer Institute and has been used for colorectal and appendiceal cancer staging. There are marked similarities between the SPCI and the PCI. However, in the SPCI, there are seven anatomic regions (see Table 13.3) (Witkamp et al. 2001). Verwaal established that SPCI is able to predict not only patient outcome but also morbidity and mortality rates (Verwaal et al. 2004).

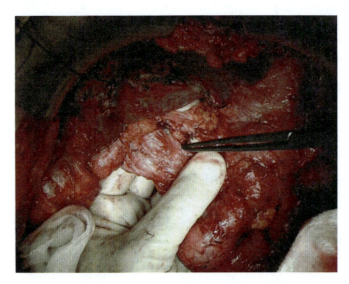

Fig. 13.2 Hepatic hilum dissection

Table 13.3. Simplified peritoneal cancer index (SPCI)

Abdominopelvic regions	Tumor diameter
1. Small pelvis	0=none
2. Ileocecal region	1=≤1 cm
3. Omentum/transverse colon	2=>1 cm, ≤5 cm
4. Small bowel/mesentery	3=>5 cm
5. Subhepatic area/stomach	
6. Left subdiaphragmatic area	
7. Right subdiaphragmatic area	

13.7 Conventional Treatment

13.7.1 Systemic Chemotherapy and Biological Therapies

The optimal chemotherapeutic regimen for DMPM is unclear. Treatment schedules that have been used in this disease include many drugs that have shown activity in pleural mesothelioma, but most of them showed a response rate of 10% to 15% (Krug 2005). Combination schedules have improved the response rate to about 25% (Hassan et al. 2006). Cisplatin has shown a good activity rate as a single agent or in combination; in a systematic meta-analysis including 83 different phase II trials it had the best single-agent activity. Other platinum analogs (i.e., carboplatin or oxaliplatin) have shown comparable results (Berghmans et al. 2002). The combination of cisplatin and gemcitabine has yielded response rates of 48% and 33%, respectively, in two different phase II trials, but these results have not been confirmed in other studies (Krug 2005). Antifolates (pemetrexed and raltitrexed) have shown more favorable results, particularly in combination with platinum compounds. A phase III clinical trial of pemetrexed plus cisplatin versus cisplatin alone showed an increased response rate and overall survival (OS). Median survival in the pemetrexed/cisplatin arm was 12.1 months versus 9.3 months in the control arm ($P=0.020$, two-sided log-rank test). Median time to progression was significantly longer in the pemetrexed/cisplatin arm: 5.7 months versus 3.9 months. Pemetrexed/cisplatin is currently considered the regimen of choice in the pleural form of the disease by many oncologists (Vogelzang et al. 2003). There is little information on the effectiveness of this combination for DMPM. The preliminary results of a nonrandomized trial started in June 2002 account for an overall objective response rate of 26% among 73 evaluable patients with DMPM. Median survival was 13.1 months for previously treated patients and has not been reached for chemotherapy-naive patients (Janne et al. 2006).

13.7.2 Intraperitoneal Chemotherapy

Since DMPM remains confined to the peritoneal cavity for most of its clinical course, several authors have investigated intraperitoneal chemotherapy (IP CT). Such procedure has the theoretical advantage of increased locoregional concentration along with reduced systemic toxicity. The disadvantages are the poor drug penetration in tumor tissue, the need for indwelling catheters, and intra-abdominal visceral adherences resulting in obstacle to free fluid circulation (Hassan and Alexander 2005). Cisplatin, mitomycin C, 5-fluoruracil, doxorubicin, and paclitaxel have been used in this setting (Vlasveld et al. 1991). In one of the largest series, IP CT with cisplatin and mitomycin was administered to 19 patients; 5-year OS was 10% (Markman and Kelsen 1992). IP CT has never been tested in a randomized fashion; this makes results difficult to evaluate.

13.7.3 Combined Treatment

Although the median survival of patients with DMPM reported in most series is short, long-term survival has been reported. In a series of 10 patients treated with sequential debulking surgery, CT (5IP and 1 intravenous) and whole abdominal irradiation, six patients achieved complete remission at 19–78 months. Conversely, those who did not receive this combined approach died after 2–15 months (Lederman et al. 1987). In Langer's study, 10 patients were treated with surgical debulking and IP cisplatin, sodium thiosulfate, and etoposide. Median survival was 22 months for patients with residual tumors <2 cm before IP treatment and 5 months for those with residual disease >2 cm; this difference was statistically significant. (Langer et al. 1993). Eltabbakh published a study of 15 women with DMPM treated with various combinations of surgery followed by systemic CT. Patients who underwent CRS survived longer than those who underwent biopsy only (Eltabbakh et al. 1999). Taken together, these data suggest the relevance of extensive debulking surgery on outcome. However, it is impossible to draw conclusions, as these studies were conducted on small series of patients, with a short follow-up, ill-defined eligibility criteria, and an absence of control groups.

13.8 Cytoreductive Surgery and Intraperitoneal Hyperthermic Perfusion

Most therapeutic options have failed to demonstrate significant results in the treatment or palliation of peritoneal mesothelioma. In the 1980s, a new integrated approach to peritoneal surface malignancies renewed the interest of the scientific community in this challenging field (Sugarbaker 2001). It consisted of aggressive cytoreductive surgery by means of peritonectomy procedures and other visceral resections along with HIPEC. Recent phase I and II prospective trials have reported promising results in selected patients undergoing this multimodality treatment protocol (Stewart et al. 2005).

13.8.1 Rationale

In patients with peritoneal mesothelioma the tumor remains confined within the abdominal cavity until advanced stages of the disease occur. This makes a combined locoregional approach attractive. Theoretically, CRS is aimed at removing all the visible tumor deposits and HIPEC is performed to treat microscopic residual disease.

13.8.1.1 Cytoreductive Surgery

The idea of reducing tumor volume for peritoneal surface malignancies was first reported for ovarian cancer as an important factor in achieving tumor response to CT (Eisenkop et al. 1998). The rationale is based on the enhancement of neoplastic chemosensitivity due to the recruitment of tumor cells to the growth phase and the possibility of surgically remove chemoresistant cellular clones. It is well known that the penetration of IP chemotherapy into tumor nodules is limited to 2–5 mm, even when combined with heat. Thus the goal of cytoreductive surgery for curative intent is to achieve maximum reduction of tumor volume (Ruth et al. 2003).

It is important to underline the difference between simple debulking and the surgical cytoreduction included in the combined protocol adopted in our center. We believe that more extensive surgery is required to minimize postoperative residual disease, including parietal peritonectomy and/or multiple organ resection. Such an aggressive surgical approach is an attempt to remove not only all the intracavitary tumor load but also the anatomic structure (i.e., the peritoneum) where the tumor originates and which represents a potential site of disease progression (see Fig. 13.3). In our experience, surgical procedures, such as colectomy, splenectomy, greater and lesser omentectomy, small bowel resection, and cholecystectomy, are frequently performed.

13.8.1.2 Intraperitoneal Chemotherapy

Systemic CT for peritoneal surface malignancies is largely ineffective because of its limited entry into the peritoneum. As with any locoregional antiblastic therapy, the objective of IP drug administration is to expose the tumor to a high drug concentration and to reduce systemic toxicity (Stewart et al. 2005). The presence of a peritoneal-plasma partition has been hypothesized (Dedrick and Flessner 1997). Pharmacokinetic studies have demonstrated that drugs delivered into the peritoneal cavity have a clearance inversely proportional to the square root of their molecular weight. Therefore, hydrophilic properties and

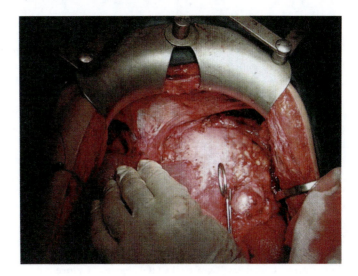

Fig. 13.3 Right diaphragmatic peritonectomy

high molecular weight result in an optimal pharmacokinetic profile for IP use, with low peritoneal absorption rate and rapid systemic clearance (Kuzuya et al. 1994). An optimal ratio between the areas under the curve of mitomycin C, doxorubicin, and cisplatin administered intraperitoneally and those obtained by systemic administration has been demonstrated (Deraco et al. 2003).

Not only the route but also the timing of administration is of relevance. HIPEC is performed before the development of intraabdominal adhesions, allowing a uniform drug distribution. Moreover, the procedure is carried out before exfoliated tumor cells are entrapped in avascular scar tissue, becoming relatively resistant to CT (Sugarbaker et al. 1990).

13.8.1.3 Antitumor Effect of Hyperthermia

Heat is a fundamental component of this new treatment, because of its own cancericidal property and chemosensitivity-modulating capacity. The direct cytotoxic activity of heat has been demonstrated in vitro at 42°C. The biophysical effects of hyperthermia are not completely understood but probably include membrane protein denaturalization (Arancia et al. 1989), increased vascular permeability (DuBose et al. 1998), alterations in the cytoskeleton and in complexes such as insulin receptors (Calderwood and Hahn 1983), and changes in enzyme complexes for DNA synthesis and repair (Xu et al. 2002). Moreover, the vasculature in solid tumors is chaotic, resulting in regions with low pH, hypoxia, and glucose level. This susceptible microenvironment makes solid tumors more sensitive to hyperthermia (Vaupel 1997). In addition, at 40°C to 42°C, the neoplastic cell becomes more chemosensitive because of an increase of intracellular drug concentration, the drug activation process (especially for alkylating agents), and an alteration in DNA repairing (Ozols and Young 1987). Heating cells to 43°C during platinum (CDDP) exposure has been found to increase drug accumulation in CDDP-resistant cell lines, with little effect on CDDP-sensitive cell lines. Ongoing platinum-DNA adduct formation after the end of CDDP exposure is also enhanced and/or adduct removal is decreased in heated cells, resulting in considerably more DNA damage (Hettinga et al. 1997). Mild hyperthermia increases the antitumor activity also of oxaliplatin, doxorubicin, and mitomycin C (Engelhardt 1987). It has been observed that the synergy between heat and mitomycin C occurs independently of the cell cycle; hence, a relevant tumoricidal effect is obtained even with brief drug exposure (Barlogie et al. 1980).

13.8.2 Patient Selection

The integrated procedure described herein is expensive in terms of financial resources, operative time, and technological facilities. A considerable rate of major morbidity has been reported by some groups (Kusamura et al. 2006). Patient selection is important to maximize the results of treatment, excluding patients who will not benefit from a high-morbidity and potentially life-threatening therapy. Preoperative clinical conditions have been shown to be a relevant prognostic factor for pleural mesothelioma (Robinson et al. 2005). Data from our institution demonstrate that performance status according to the Eastern Cooperative Oncology Group (ECOG) score (Oken et al. 1982) was related to progression-free (PFS) survival in patients with DMPM undergoing CRS and HIPEC (Deraco et al. 2006).

In the management of peritoneal malignancies the extent of previous surgery before definitive cytoreduction with HIPEC may have a negative impact on prognosis (Harmon et al. 2003). According to the cancer cell entrapment hypothesis, the raw surfaces of surgically dissected tissue planes are favorable sites for cancer cell adherence. Cancer progression deep to peritoneal surfaces, especially if imbedded in scar, is difficult or impossible to eradicate (Eggermont et al. 1987). The prior surgical score (PSS) has been introduced by Sugarbaker to rate the extent of surgery prior to definitive combined treatment. The assessment uses a diagram similar to that for PCI but excludes regions 9–12: PSS 0=no prior surgery or only a biopsy was performed; PSS 1=one region with prior surgery; PSS 2=2/5 regions previously dissected; PSS 3=more than 5 regions previously dissected. Five-year OS was 70% in appendiceal cancer patients with PSS=0–2 and 51% in those with PSS=3 (P=0.001) (Sugarbaker et al. 1999). Among patients with DMPM treated with CRS and HIPEC at the Centre Hospitalier Lyon Sud median OS was not statistically different between patients with PSS=0/1 and those with PSS=2/3 (Brigand et al. 2006).

At the National Cancer Institute of Milan inclusion criteria are the following:

- Confirmed pathological diagnosis of DMPM
- Age 75 years
- ECOG performance status 2
- No significant impairment of cardiorespiratory, renal, hepatic, and bone marrow function
- No parenchymal hepatic and/or extra-abdominal metastases
- No massive retroperitoneal disease
- Completely resectable (or at least potentially significantly reducible) peritoneal disease
- Written informed consent statement signed by the patient

13.8.3 Operative Technique

Cytoreductive surgery by means of peritonectomy procedures combined with HIPEC was described by Sugarbaker (Sugarbaker 2003). We present here the procedure adopted in our institution (Deraco et al. 2003, 2004).

13.8.3.1 Cytoreductive Surgery

Patients are placed in a supine position, with gluteal folds advanced to the break in the operating table to allow full access to the perineum. A three-way bladder catheter is inserted for cold lavage during hyperthermia in order to avoid mucosal damage.

The surgical procedure starts with a xyphopubic midline cutaneous incision. The deeper layers of the abdominal wall are dissected until the parietal peritoneum is visualized. The parietal peritoneum is then stripped from the abdominal wall. During this time the peritoneum remains closed to facilitate the procedure. Ureters, iliac arteries and veins, deferent ducts, and gonadal vessels are bilaterally visualized and spared. A 2-mm ball-tip electrosurgical handpiece is used on pure cut at high voltage as the standard tool to dissect peritoneal surfaces. At this point, the peritoneum is opened and lysis of adhesions is performed to allow full exploration of the peritoneal cavity. The Thompson self-retaining retractor is used to achieve generous abdominal exposure.

CRS is carried out on the basis of disease extension by the following steps: (1) greater omentectomy, right parietal peritonectomy, right colon resection; (2) pelvic peritonectomy with sigmoid colon resection ± hystero-annexectomy; (3) antrectomy, cholecystectomy, lesser omentectomy, and dissection of the duodenal-hepatic ligament; (4) right-upper-quadrant peritonectomy and Glissonian capsule resection; (5) left-upper-quadrant peritonectomy-splenectomy and left parietal peritonectomy; and (6) other intestinal resection and/or abdominal mass resection. In our institution the main goal of cytoreductive surgery is to remove all macroscopic tumor deposits, leaving no residual nodules >2.5 mm. However, not all six peritonectomy procedures are required in all patients. The surgical procedures and visceral resections are planned after careful assessment of disease extent and distribution (see Fig. 8.1). In those locations where only minimal tumor deposits involve parietal or visceral peritoneal surfaces, such as the stomach or bowel, local resection is attempted. Peritonectomies are performed in case of major serosal involvement, and segmental resections are carried out only when massive visceral involvement is observed. Anastomoses are completed before HIPEC; ostomies are constructed at the end of the entire procedure.

13.8.3.2 Hyperthermic Intraperitoneal Chemotherapy

In our institution HIPEC is performed according to the closed abdomen technique. After CRS, two inflow catheters (one in the right subdiaphragmatic cavity and one at deep pelvic level) and two outflow catheters (one in the left subdiaphragmatic cavity and one at superficial pelvic level) are inserted. Six temperature probes are placed in the abdominal cavity. After abdominal skin closure, the catheters are connected to the extracorporeal perfusion circuit [Performer LRT; RAND, Medolla (MO) Italy]. The device consists of a roller pump, a heat exchanger, a reservoir, an integrated control of temperature, flow, and pressure, and software for real time data monitoring, analysis and registration (see Fig. 13.4). The polysaline perfusate consists of a solution of 2/3 of Normosol R and 1/3 of Emagel (4–6 l) containing cisplatin (43 mg/l) plus doxorubicin (15.25 mg/l). The perfusion is carried out at a mean flow of 600 ml/min for 90 min, starting from the true hyperthermic phase (42.5°C).

A major technical variant is represented by the open-abdomen or "coliseum" technique,

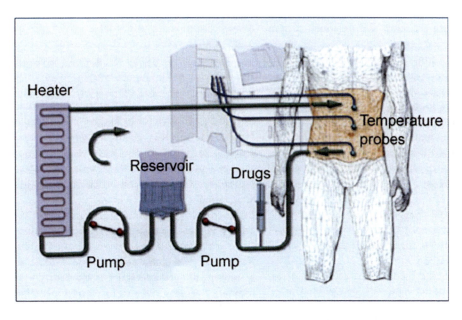

Fig. 13.4 The device and the extracorporeal circuit of hyperthermic intraperitoneal chemotherapy (HIPEC)

which involves covering the abdomen with a plastic sheet during the perfusion (Sugarbaker et al. 1999). Proponents of the open technique report that it provides optimal thermal homogeneity and spatial diffusion. In contrast, proponents of the closed technique suggest that the increased intra-abdominal pressure implies deeper drug penetration (Leunig et al. 1992). To date, no prospective trials have compared the two techniques.

13.8.4 Assessment of the Completeness of the Cytoreduction

Presently, two classification systems are used to rate the completeness of cytoreduction. We use the completeness of cytoreduction (CC) score devised by Sugarbaker and colleagues. The extent of the residual disease is scored after the completion of the surgical cytoreduction, as follows: cc-0=no residual disease; CC-1=residual disease ≤2.5 mm; CC-2=residual disease >2.5 mm ≤2.5 cm; CC-3=residual disease >2.5 cm (Jacquet and Sugarbaker 1996). Other authors have used the following classification system: R0=no gross disease with negative microscopic margins; R1=no gross disease with positive microscopic margins; R2a=residual tumor ≤5 mm; R2b=residual tumor >6 mm ≤2 mm; R2c=residual tumor >20 mm (Stewart et al. 2005). The CC-1 nodule size (2.5 mm) is thought to reflect the maximum tissue penetration of locoregionally delivered drugs. Nevertheless, no data in the literature are found to determine the superiority of one system over the other. Complete cytoreduction has been confirmed in all trials of CRS and HIPEC as one of the most relevant determinants of survival and can be defined in both systems as CC-0/1 or R0/1/2a, respectively.

13.9 Results

Few centers have reported prospective non-randomized trials evaluating surgical cytoreduction and HIPEC in patients affected by peritoneal mesothelioma. The National Cancer Institute in Bethesda, Maryland reported 18 patients included in three consecutive phase I trials (Park et al. 1999) and more recently a larger series of 49 patients with longer follow-up (Feldman et al. 2003). Results on 68 patients treated at the Washington Hospital Center were reported by Sugarbaker (Sugarbaker et al. 2003), updating a previous paper on 33 patients from the same institution (Sebbag et al. 2000). The National Cancer Institute of Milan has published a preliminary report on 19 patients (Deraco et al. 2003), a clinicopathological study on 33 patients (Nonaka et al. 2005), and a recent update on 49 patients with multivariate statistical analysis of prognostic factors (Deraco et al. 2006). Prospective trials on 12 and 15 patients, respectively, were conducted at the Centre Hospitalier Lyon Sud (Brigand et al. 2006) and at Wake Forest University (Loggie et al. 2001). In general, criteria for patient selection and treatment parameters are not consistent from one center to another as far as type, dose, temperature, and duration of hyperthermic chemotherapy are concerned. Furthermore, no standard definition of adequate cytoreduction seems to be universally accepted, as the surgical procedure in the different centers was aimed at obtaining residual disease nodules ranging from 2.5 to 25 mm in diameter. However, these studies demonstrate median survival times of 34 to 67 months, which is a significant improvement over the previously reported median survival time.

Malignant ascites is a common presentation and a major factor in disease-related morbidity and mortality. In the above-mentioned studies, palliation in the form of relief from ascites occurred in 86% to 99% of cases after HIPEC for malignant mesothelioma (Stewart et al. 2005).

13.9.1 Morbidity and Mortality

Because of the complexity of this combined treatment of CRS and HIPEC, morbidity and mortality rates may be significant. Operative mortality ranges from 0 to 11% and major morbidity ranges from 8% to 26% of peritoneal mesothelioma patients (Stewart et al. 2005).

13.9.2 Prognostic Factors

In the study of Sugarbaker the following factors were related to reduced OS: male sex, age>53 years, weight loss, nonincidental diagnosis, PCI>28, sarcomatous/biphasic histology, CC score=3, and presence of metastases (Sugarbaker et al. 2003). Prognostic factors were tested by multivariate analysis in Feldman's paper (Feldman et al. 2003). A history of previous debulking surgery and absence of deep tissue invasion were independent determinant of both improved OS and PFS; residual disease <1 cm and age <60 years were recognized as independent prognostic factors only for improved OS. Immunohistochemical stains for p53, p27, and Ki-67, as well as desmoplasia, were not related to prognosis. In the small series of the centre Hospitalier Lyon Sud, Gilly score 1–2 and CC score 1–2 were related to prolonged OS by univariate analysis (Brigand et al. 2006).

We observed that the CC score and the mitotic count (MC) presented the strongest association with OS at multivariate analysis. The estimated hazard rate was eight times higher for patients with residual disease >2.5 mm than for those with residual disease <2.5 mm, after adjustment for other variables. Whether this survival benefit resulted from lower tumor aggressivity or from the surgical effort itself is difficult to ascertain. However, this series included only the most malignant subtypes of DMPM, an aspect that could support the validity of aggressive surgical approach.

The second variable that remained in the Cox model as a factor influencing the OS was MC. Patients with an MC >5 per 50 HPFs presented a hazard rate 10 times higher compared with those with a lower MC. Data about this issue in the literature are conflicting. In two case series patients with high MC survived for a significantly shorter time than those with low MC (Ramael et al. 1994; Beer et al. 2000), whereas Kerrigan did not reach the same conclusion (Kerrigan et al 2002). However, the prognostic relevance of both variables (CC and MC) should be taken cautiously because the 95% confidence intervals for their respective hazard rates are fairly wide (2.05–36.24 for CC and 1.98–55.23 for MC).

Multivariate analysis of factors influencing PFS showed that performance status and MC remained in the model after the backward-elimination method. Preoperative clinical condition has been largely shown to be a prognostic factor for pleural mesothelioma, but the same finding has not been demonstrated for the peritoneal counterpart. In this series, it is noteworthy that the performance status was not related to OS. This could be attributed to the fact that the great majority of patients (89%) had an ECOG performance status of 0 and the number of deaths due to disease progression was not high enough. The independent association between MC and PFS emerged after the multivariate analysis even in the absence of a significant correlation at univariate analysis. This could have resulted from the presence of a confounding factor among the clinicopathological variables. Other factors possibly related to prognosis according to the literature, such as age at diagnosis, sex, and previous debulking, were not predictive of outcome in our series.

13.9.3 Biological Markers

P16, also known as INK4a, is a tumor-suppressor gene located on chromosome 9 in the region 9p21. Two alternatively spliced gene products are encoded by p16: the proteins P16 and p14ARF. The p16(INK4a) protein, by inhibiting cyclin-dependent kinase, downregulates Rb-E2F and leads to cell cycle arrest in the G1 phase. The p14(ARF) protein interacts with the MDM2 protein and neutralizes MDM2-mediated degradation of p53. Because p53/Rb genes are not altered in malignant mesothelioma, additional components of these pathways, such as p16 (INK4a) and p14(ARF), are candidates for inactivation. The recent molecular genetic study on 45 malignant mesothelioma specimens revealed alterations of p16 in 31% of cases, promoter methylation in 9%, deletion in 22%, and point mutation in 2% (Hirao et al. 2002). In our series, the immunoreaction of p16 was absent or reduced in 25 cases (71%), in agreement with previous reports (Kratzke et al. 1995).

EGFR is a cell surface receptor involved in the regulation of cell growth and differentiation. The binding of the ligand to the receptor causes activation of its intrinsic tyrosine kinase activity and rapid internalization of the receptor-ligand complex into the cell; this leads to an increase in cellular proliferation, an increase in angiogenesis, inhibition of apoptosis, and expression of extracellular matrix proteins. The overexpression of EGFR is associated with a poor prognosis in some cancers. An earlier study showed EGFR immunoexpression in 69% of the epithelial type of diffuse malignant pleural mesothelioma, 44% of the sarcomatoid type, and 22% of the mixed type. No correlation between EGFR overexpression and prognosis was identified. Twenty-two (63%) of 35 cases showed diffuse and strong immunoreactivity for EGFR, a finding consistent with a previous study (Trupiano et al. 2004).

The pattern of DMPM progression within the abdominal cavity suggests an important role of proteases, including the MMPs, in the evolution of the disease. Our study demonstrated the constant expression of MMP-2 and, to a lesser degree, of MMP-9. All the cases expressed MMP-2 to some extent, and 23 patients showed a 4+ staining intensity in DMPM cells. Overexpression of MMPs, particularly MMP-2 (gelatinase A), MMP-9 (gelatinase B), and MMP-11 (stromelysin 3), is related to tumor progression and metastasis in various carcinomas, including gastric, colonic, and pulmonary carcinomas (Cox et al. 2000). In a study of pleural mesotheliomas using semiquantitative gelatin zymography, increasing MMP-2 and pro-MMP-2 activity were independently associated with a poor prognosis, but MMP-9 activity had no prognostic significance (Edwards et al. 2003). Only a few small studies have investigated MMP immunohistochemically on surgical specimens of DMPM. The results were variable and not always consistent with those found by reverse transcriptase-polymerase chain reaction, Western blot, and gelatin zymography on mesothelioma cell lines, as well as fresh tissue (Liu et al. 2002).

13.10 Future Perspectives

Future directions in DMPM research should involve biological studies on tumor pathogenesis to elucidate the molecular mechanisms and the possible etiological role of asbestos in peritoneal mesothelioma oncogenesis. The comprehensive therapeutic approach to DMPM represented by CRS and HIPEC has attracted an increasing consensus as the treatment of choice for this disease in selected patients, but several technical issues need to be rationalized by means of larger prospective, possibly multicentric, trials (Sugarbaker et al. 2006). Since not all the patients with DMPM are candidates for surgery and HIPEC and many of them ultimately relapse, development of novel cytotoxic agents is needed. Promising approaches may be represented by new monoclonal antibodies directed against mesothelium, inhibitors blocking cellular signaling pathways, antiangiogenetic agents, and gene therapy (Hassan et al. 2006).

References

Altieri DC (2003a) Validating survivin as a cancer therapeutic target. Nat Rev Cancer 3:46–54

Altieri DC (2003b) Survivin, versatile modulation of cell division and apoptosis in cancer. Oncogene 22:8581–8589

Antman KH, Blum RH, Greenberger JS et al. (1980) Multimodality therapy for malignant mesothelioma based on a study of natural history. Am J Med 68:356–362

Antman KH, Corson JM, Li FP et al. (1983) Malignant mesothelioma following radiation exposure. J Clin Oncol 1:695–700

Arancia G, Crateri Trovalusci P, Mariutti G et al. (1989) Ultrastructural changes induced by hyperthermia in Chinese hamster V79 fibroblasts. Int J Hyperthermia 5:341–350

Archer VE, Rom WN (1983) Trends in mortality of diffuse malignant mesothelioma of pleura. Lancet 2:112–113

Baratti D et al. (2007) Circulating CA125 in patients with peritoneal mesothelioma treated by cytoreductive surgery and intraperitoneal hyperthermic perfusion. Ann Surg Oncol 14:500–508

Baris YI, Sahin AA, Ozesmi M et al. (1978) An outbreak of pleural mesothelioma and chronic fibrosing pleurisy in the village of Karain/Urgup in Anatolia. Thorax 33:181–192

Barlogie B, Corry PM, Drewinko B (1980) In vitro thermochemotherapy of human colon cancer cells with cis-dichlorodiammineplatinum(II) and mitomycin C. Cancer Res 40:1165–1168

Berghmans T et al. (2002) Activity of chemotherapy and immunotherapy on malignant mesothelioma: a systematic review of the literature with metaanalysis. Lung Cancer 38:112–121

Blackburn EH (2001) Structure and function of telomeres. Nature 350:569–573

Brigand C, Monneuse O, Mohamed F et al. (2006) Peritoneal mesothelioma treated by cytoreductive surgery and intraperitoneal hyperthermic chemotherapy: results of a prospective study. Ann Surg Oncol 13:405–412

Bryan TM, Englezou A, Dalla-Pozza L et al. (1997) Evidence for an alternative mechanism for maintaining telomere length in human tumors and tumor-derived cell lines. Nat Med 3:1271–1274

Cain J, Nori D, Huvos A et al. (1983) The role of radioactive colloids in malignant peritoneal mesotheliomas. Gynecol Oncol 16:263–274

Calderwood SK, Hahn GM (1983) Thermal sensitivity and resistance of insulin-receptor binding. Biochim Biophys Acta 756:1–8

Carmignani CP, Sugarbaker TA, Bromley CM et al. (2003) Intraperitoneal cancer dissemination: mechanisms of the patterns of spread. Cancer Metastasis Rev 22:465–472

Chan PS, Balfour TW, Bourke JB et al. (1975) Peritoneal nesothelioma. Br J Surg 62:576–580

Churg A, Cagle PT, Roggli VL (2006) Tumors of the serosal membranes. In: Atlas of tumor pathology, IV series. AFIP, Washington DC

Cong YS et al. (2002) Human telomerase and its regulation. Microbiol Mol Biol Rev 66:407–425

Dedrick RL, Flessner MF (1997) Pharmacokinetic problems in peritoneal drug administration: tissue penetration and surface exposure. J Natl Cancer Inst 89:480–487

Deraco M, Santoro N, Carraro O et al. (1999) Peritoneal carcinomatosis: feature of dissemination. A review. Tumori 85:1–5

Deraco M, Rossi CR, Pennacchioli E et al. (2001) Cytoreductive surgery followed by intraperitoneal hyperthermic perfusion in the treatment of recurrent epithelial ovarian cancer: a phase II clinical study. Tumori 87:120–126

Deraco M, Raspagliesi F, Kusamura S et al. (2003a) Management of peritoneal surface component of ovarian cancer. Surg Oncol Clin N Am 12:561–583

Deraco M, Casali P, Inglese MG et al. (2003b) Peritoneal mesothelioma treated by induction chemotherapy, cytoreductive surgery, and intraperitoneal hyperthermic perfusion. J Surg Oncol 83:147–153

Deraco M, Baratti D, Inglese MG et al. (2004) Peritonectomy and intraperitoneal hyperthermic perfusion (IPHP): a strategy that has confirmed its efficacy in patients with pseudomyxoma peritonei. Ann Surg Oncol 11:393–398

DuBose DA, Hinkle JR, Morehouse DH et al. (1998) Model for environmental heat damage of the blood vessel barrier. Wilderness Environ Med 9:130–136

Dunham MA, Neumann AA, Fasching CL et al. (2000) Telomere maintenance by recombination in human cells. Nat Genet 26:447–450

Eggermont AM et al. (1987) Laparotomy enhances intraperitoneal tumor growth and abrogates the antitumor effects of interleukin-2 and lymphokine-activated killer cells. Surgery 102:71–78

Eisenkop SM, Friedman RL, Wang HJ (1998) Complete cytoreductive surgery is feasible and maximizes survival in patients with advanced epithelial ovarian cancer: a prospective study. Gynecol Oncol 69:103–108

Elias D, Blot F, El Otmany A et al. (2001) Curative treatment of peritoneal carcinomatosis arising from colorectal cancer by complete resection and intraperitoneal chemotherapy. Cancer 92:71–76

Eltabbakh GH, Piver MS, Hempling RE et al. (1999) Clinical picture, response to therapy, and survival of women with diffuse malignant peritoneal mesothelioma. J Surg Oncol 70:6–12

Engelhardt R (1987) Hyperthermia and drugs. Rec Res Cancer Res 104:136–203

Feldman AL, Libutti SK, Pingpank JF et al. (2003) Analysis of factors associated with outcome in patients with malignant peritoneal mesothelioma undergoing surgical debulking and intraperitoneal chemotherapy. J Clin Oncol 21:4560–4567

Fujimoto S, Takahashi M, Mutou T et al. (1997) Improved mortality rate of gastric carcinoma patients with peritoneal carcinomatosis treated with intraperitoneal hyperthermic chemoperfusion combined with surgery. Cancer 79:884–891

Gazdar AF, Carbone M (2003) Molecular pathogenesis of mesothelioma and its relationship to Simian virus 40. Clin Lung Cancer 5:177–181

Gilly FN, Carry PY Sayag AC et al. (1994) Regional chemotherapy (with mitomycin C) and intra-operative hyperthermia for digestive cancers with peritoneal carcinomatosis. Hepatogastroenterology 41:124–129

Glehen O, Mithieux F, Osinsky D et al. (2003) Surgery combined with peritonectomy procedures and intraperitoneal chemohyperthermia in abdominal cancers with peritoneal carcinomatosis: a phase II study. J Clin Oncol 21:799–806

Gordon GJ, Appasani K, Parcells JP et al. (2002) Inhibition of apoptosis protein-1 promotes tumor cell survival in mesothelioma. Carcinogenesis 23:1017–1024

Hahn WC, Counter CM, Lundberg AS et al. (1999) Creation of human tumour cells with defined genetic elements. Nature 400:464–468

Harmon RL, Sugarbaker PH (2005) Prognostic indicators in peritoneal carcinomatosis from gastrointestinal cancer. Int Semin Surg Oncol 2:3–13

Hassan R, Alexander R (2005) Nonpleural mesotheliomas: mesothelioma of the peritoneum, tunica vaginalis ad pericardium. Hemat Oncol Clin N Am 19:1067–1087

Hassan R, Alexander R, Antman K et al. (2006) Current treatment options and biology of peritoneal mesothelioma: meeting summary of the first NIH peritoneal mesothelioma conference. Ann Oncol (in press)

Henson JD, Neumann AA, Yeager TR et al. (2002) Alternative lengthening of telomeres in mammalian cells. Oncogene 21:598–610

Henson JD, Hannay JA, McCarthy SW et al. (2005) A robust assay for alternative lengthening of telomeres in tumours shows the significance of alternative lengthening of telomeres in sarcomas and astrocytomas. Clin Cancer Res 11:217–225

Hettinga JV, Lemstra W, Meijer C et al. (1997) Mechanism of hyperthermic potentiation of cisplatin action in cisplatin-sensitive and -resistant tumor cells. Br J Cancer 75:1735–1743

Iwamoto A (1989) [Intraoperative chemotherapy with intraperitoneal activated carbon particles adsorbing mitomycin C against peritoneal dissemination of gastric cancer]. Gan To Kagaku Ryoho 16:2748–2751

Janne PA, Wozniak AJ, Belani CP et al. (2006) Open-label study of pemetrexed alone or in combination with cisplatin for the treatment of patients with peritoneal mesothelioma: outcomes of an expanded access program. Clin Lung Cancer 7:40–46

Jacquet P, Sugarbaker PH (1996) Current methodologies for clinical assessment of patients with peritoneal carcinomatosis. J Exp Clin Cancer Res 15:49–58

Kannerstein M, Churg J (1977) Peritoneal mesothelioma. Hum Pathol 8:83–94

Krug LM (2005) An overview of chemotherapy for mesothelioma. Hemat Oncol Clin N Am 19:117–136

Kumaki F, Kawai T, Churg A et al. (2002) Expression of telomerase reverse transcriptase in malignant mesotheliomas. Am J Surg Pathol 26:365–370

Kusamura S, Younan R, Baratti D et al. (2006) Cytoreductive surgery followed by intraperitoneal hyperthermic perfusion in the treatment of peritoneal surface malignancies: analysis of morbidity and mortality in 209 cases treated with closed abdomen technique. Cancer 106:1144–1153

Kuzuya T, Yamauchi M, Ito A et al. (1994) Pharmacokinetic characteristics of 5-fluorouracil and mitomycin C in intraperitoneal chemotherapy. J Pharm Pharmacol 46:685–689

Langer JC et al. (1993) Intraperitoneal cisplatin and etoposide in peritoneal mesothelioma: favorable outcome with multimodality approach. Cancer Chemother Pharmacol 32:204–208

Lederman GS, Recht A, Herman T et al. (1987) Long-term survival in peritoneal mesothelioma: the role of radiotherapy and combined modality treatment. Cancer 59:1882–1886

Leigh J, Robinson BWS (2002) The history of mesothelioma in Australia. In: Robinson BWS, Chahinian PA (eds) Mesothelioma. Martin Dunitz, London, pp 55–210

Leunig M, Goetz AE, Dellian M et al. (1992) Interstitial fluid pressure in solid tumors following hyperthermia: possible correlation with therapeutic response. Cancer Res 52:487–490

Loggie BW, Fleming RA, Mc Quellon RP et al. (2001) Prospective trial for the treatment of malignant peritoneal mesothelioma. Am Surg 67:999–1003

Markman M, Kelsen D (1992) Efficacy of cisplatin-based intra-peritoneal chemotherapy as treatment of malignant peritoneal mesothelioma. J Cancer Res Clin Oncol 118:547–550

Maurer F, Egloff B (1975) Malignant peritoneal mesothelioma after cholangiography with thorotrast. Cancer 36:1381–1385

McDonald JC (1985) Health implications of environmental exposure to asbestos. Environ Health Perspect 62:318–329

McDonald JC (2000) Asbestos. In: McDonald JC (ed) Epidemiology of work related disease. BMJ Books, London, pp 85–108

Moertel CG (1972) Peritoneal mesothelioma. Gastroenterology 63:346–350

Murajama T (2004) Emerging health effects of asbestos in Asia. In: Proceedings of the global asbestos congress, Tokyo, November 19–21, 2004: 17, abstract

Nonaka D, Kusamura S, Baratti D et al. (2005) Diffuse malignant mesothelioma of the peritoneum. Cancer 104:2181–2188

Oken MM, Creech RH, Tormey DC et al. (1982) Toxicity and response criteria of the Eastern Cooperative Oncology Group. Am J Clin Oncol 5:649–655

Ordonez NG (1998) Value of cytokeratin 5/6 immunostaining in distinguish epithelial mesothelioma of the pleura from lung adenocarcinoma. Am J Surg Pathol 22:1215–1221

Ozols RF, Young RC (1987) Ovarian cancer. Curr Probl Cancer 11:57–122

Park BJ, Alexander HR, Libutti SK et al. (1999) Treatment of primary peritoneal mesothelioma by continuous hyperthermic peritoneal perfusion (CHPP). Ann Surg Oncol 6:582–590

Pass HI, Lott D, Lonardo F et al. (2005) Asbestos exposure, pleural mesothelioma, and serum osteopontin levels. N Engl J Med 353:1564–1573

Peto J, Hodgson JT, Matthews FE et al. (1995) Continuing increase in mesothelioma mortality in Britain. Lancet 345:535–539

Peto J, Decarli A, La Vecchia C et al. (1999) The European mesothelioma epidemic. Br J Cancer 79:666–672

Pisick E, Salgia R (2005) Molecular biology of malignant mesothelioma: a review. Hemat Oncol Clin N Am 19

Price B (1997) Analysis of current trends in the United States mesothelioma incidence. Am J Epidemiol 45:211–218

Robinson BWS, Creaney J, Lake R et al. (2003) Mesothelin-family proteins and diagnosis of mesothelioma. Lancet 362:1612–1616

Robinson BWS, Lake RA (2005) Advanced in malignant mesothelioma. N Engl J Med 353:1591–603

Robinson BWS, Musk AW, Lake RA et al. (2005) Malignant mesothelioma. Lancet 366:397–408

Roushdy-Hammady I, Siegel J, Emri S et al. (2001) Genetic-susceptibility factor and malignant mesothelioma in the Cappadocian region of Turkey. Lancet 357:444–445

van Ruth S, Verwaal VJ, Hart AA et al. (2003) Heat penetration in locally applied hyperthermia in the abdomen during intra-operative hyperthermic intraperitoneal chemotherapy. Anticancer Res 23:1501–1508

Sadeghi B, Arvieux C, Glehen O et al. (2000) Peritoneal carcinomatosis from non-gynaecologic malignancies. Results of the EVOCAPE1 multicentric prospective study. Cancer 88:358–363

Sebbag G, Yan H, Shmookler BM et al. (2000) Results of treatment of 33 patients with peritoneal mesothelioma. Br J Surg 87:1587–1593

Shen P, Levine EA, Hall J et al. (2003) Factors predicting survival after intraperitoneal hyperthermic chemotherapy with mitomycin C after cytoreductive surgery for patients with peritoneal carcinomatosis. Arch Surg 138:26–33

Spirtas R, Heineman EF, Bernstein L et al. (1994) Malignant mesothelioma: attributable risk of asbestos exposure. Occup Environ Med 51:804–811

Stewart JH, Shen P, Levine EA (2005) Intraperitoneal hyperthermic chemotherapy for peritoneal surface malignancy: current status and future directions. Ann Surg Oncol 12:765–777

Sugarbaker PH (1994) Pseudomyxoma peritonei: a cancer whose biology is characterized by a redistribution phenomenon. Ann Surg 219:109–111

Sugarbaker PH (1999a) Results of treatment of 385 patients with peritoneal surface spread of appendiceal malignancy. Ann Surg Oncol 6:727–731

Sugarbaker PH (1999b) Successful management of microscopic residual disease in large bowel cancer. Cancer Chemother Pharmacol 43 [Suppl]:S15–S25

Sugarbaker PH (2003) Peritonectomy procedures. Surg Oncol Clin North Am 12:703–727

Sugarbaker PH, Graves T, DeBruijn EA et al. (1990) Early postoperative intraperitoneal chemotherapy as an adjuvant therapy to surgery for peritoneal carcinomatosis from gastrointestinal cancer: pharmacological studies. Cancer Res 50:5790–5794

Sugarbaker PH, Welch LS, Mohamed F et al. (2003) A review of peritoneal mesothelioma at the Washington Cancer Institute. Surg Oncol Clin North Am 12:605–621

Sugarbaker PH et al. (2006) Comprehensive management of diffuse malignant peritoneal mesothelioma. EJSO (in press)

Takayhashi H (2004) Emerging health effects of asbestos in Asia. In: Proceedings of the global asbestos congress, Tokyo, November 19–21, 2004: 2, abstract

Tentes AAK, Trispsiannis G, Markakidis SK et al. (2003) Peritoneal cancer index: a prognostic indicator of survival in advanced ovarian cancer. Eur J Surg Oncol 29:69–73

Vaupel PW (1997) The influence of tumor blood flow and micro-environmental factors on the efficacy of radiation, drugs and localized hyperthermia. Klin Paediatr 209:243–249

Vlasveld LT, Gallee MP, Rodenhuis S et al. (1991) Intraperitoneal chemotherapy for malignant peritoneal mesothelioma. Eur J Cancer 27:732–734

Vogelzang NJ, Rusthoven JJ, Symanowski J et al. (2003) Phase III study of pemetrexed in combination with cisplatin versus cisplatin alone in patients with malignant pleural mesothelioma. J Clin Oncol 21:2636–2644

Wagner JC, Sleggs CA, Marchand P (1960) Diffuse pleural mesothelioma and asbestos exposure in the North Western Cape Province. Br J Ind Med 17:260–271

Whitaker D (2000) The cytology of malignant mesothelioma. Cytopathology 11:139

Witkamp AJ, de Bree E, Kaag MM et al. (2001) Extensive cytoreductive surgery followed by intra-operative hyperthermic intraperitoneal chemotherapy with mitomycin-C in patients with peritoneal carcinomatosis of colorectal origin. Eur J Cancer 37:979–984

Xia C, Xu Z, Yuan X et al. (2002) Induction of apoptosis in mesothelioma cells by antisurvivin oligonucleotides. Mol Cancer Ther 1:687–694

Xu M, Myerson RJ, Straube WL et al. (2002) Radiosensitization of heat resistant human tumour cells by 1 hour at 41.1 degrees C and its effect on DNA repair. Int J Hyperthermia 18:385–403

Yan TD, Haveric N, Carmignani CP et al. (2005a) Abdominal computed tomography scans in the selection of patients with malignant peritoneal mesothelioma for comprehensive treatment with cytoreductive surgery and perioperative intraperitoneal chemotherapy. Cancer 103:839–849

Yan TD, Haveric N, Carmignani CP et al. (2005b) Computed tomographic characterization of malignant peritoneal mesothelioma. Tumori 91:394–400

Younan R, Kusamura S, Baratti D et al. (2005) Bowel complications in 203 cases of peritoneal surface malignancies treated with peritonectomy and closed-technique intraperitoneal hyperthermic perfusion. Ann Surg Oncol 12:910–918

14 Advances in the Management of Gastric Cancer with Peritoneal Dissemination

Yutaka Yonemura, Taiichi Kawamura, Etsurou Bandou, Gorou Tsukiyama, Masayuki Nemoto, Yoshio Endou, Masahiro Miura

14.1 Results of Previous Clinical Studies in Carcinomatosis of Gastric Origin

Prognosis of patients with peritoneal carcinomatosis (PC) from gastrointestinal cancer is poor, with a median overall survival of only 3 months [1, 2], and a 5-year survival rate of less than 1% [3]. Furthermore, no survival advantage was found after gastrectomy and lymph node dissection in this context, and therefore simple gastrectomy without additional lymphadenectomy is the optimal strategy for patients with PC [4]. In addition, there is no standard treatment and no effective anticancer drug for peritoneal dissemination. At present, intravenous 5-fluorouracil (5-FU) has been used alone [5] or in combination with other anticancer drugs FAM [6] and FAMTX [7] for chemotherapy of advanced gastric cancer. However, systemic chemotherapy does not improve the survival of patients with peritoneal dissemination [8, 9], because only a small amount of drug reaches the peritoneal cavity after intravenous administration. The reasons for this are the limited drug distribution due to the existence of the peritoneal–blood barrier and the scanty number of subperitoneal blood vessels [9–11].

In contrast, intraperitoneal chemotherapy offers potential therapeutic advantages over systemic chemotherapy by generating high local concentrations of drugs [12, 13[. Armstrong et al. reported a significant survival benefit after intraperitoneal cisplatin and paclitaxel compared with systemic chemotherapy in patients with optimally debulked stage III ovarian cancer [17].

Hyperthermic intraperitoneal perfusion chemotherapy (HIPEC) has been introduced to improve the treatment of gastric cancer with PC. The combination of hyperthermia and chemotherapy has shown synergism in the case of anticancer drugs such as cisplatinum (CDDP), mitomycin C, adriamycin and etoposide [14–16]. In addition, Los et al. reported that chemohyperthermia resulted in a higher anticancer drug concentration in experimental peritoneal tumors after the combined treatment than after chemotherapy alone [18]. The increased tumor platinum (Pt) concentrations, rising from 1.3 µg Pt/g tumor at 37°C to 5.4 µg Pt/g tumor at 41.5°C for CDDP and from 0.2 µg Pt/g tumor to 0.7 µg Pt/g tumor at 41.5°C for carboplatin (CBDCA), contributed considerably to enhanced numbers of CDDP or CBDCA DNA adducts. As a result of the latter, intraperitoneal chemotherapy combined with regional hyperthermia led to an increase in tumor growth delay after increasing the temperature to 41.5°C for CDDP and CBDCA [17].

In the clinical setting, Fujimoto et al. reported pathological changes in cancer cells harvested from patients with PC from gastric cancer after HIPEC, and gastric cancer cells in the abdominal effusion and/or lavage vanished [19]. However, HIPEC treatment did not kill all the gastric cancer cells, which had penetrated deeply into subperitoneal layers.

To confirm the efficacy of HIPEC, Verwaal et al. performed a randomized, controlled study in patients with PC from colorectal cancer [20]. One-hundred and five patients were assigned to receive either standard treatment consisting of systemic chemotherapy (fluorouracil-leucovorin) with or without palliative surgery or experimental therapy consisting of aggressive cytoreduction with HIPEC, followed by the same systemic chemotherapy regimen. After a median follow-up period of 21.6 months, the median survival was 12.6 months in the standard therapy arm and 22.3 months in the experimental therapy arm. There was a statistically significant difference between the two groups. If the cytoreduction was macroscopically complete, the median survival was also significantly better than if patients had limited or extensive residual disease. Accordingly, cytoreduction followed by HIPEC improves survival in patients with peritoneal carcinomatosis of colorectal origin [20].

Yonemura et al. reported the efficacy of HIPEC in 83 gastric cancer patients with PC [21]. After aggressive resection of the primary tumor, lymph nodes and peritoneal metastases, a warmed saline solution containing 30 mg of mitomycin C, 150 mg of etoposide, and 300 mg of cisplatinum was introduced into the peritoneal cavity via a closed HIPEC circuit and kept for 60 min, maintaining the abdominal temperature at 42°–43°C. Among 43 evaluable patients with residual peritoneal seeding, eight (19%) and nine (21%) exhibited complete response and partial response, respectively. The overall 1- and 5-year survival rates were 43% and 11%, respectively. Patients who underwent complete resection survived significantly longer than those with residual disease, and those with complete response had a significantly better prognosis than those with partial response and nonresponders. One-year survival rates for complete response, partial response, and nonresponders were 88%, 27%, and 22%, respectively. Accordingly, HIPEC is an effective therapy for selected patients with gastric cancer with PC [21]. HIPEC is indicated for peritoneal tumors less than 2–3 mm in diameter, because penetration of HIPEC is limited to a depth of 1–2 mm from the peritoneal surface [18]. The effectiveness of anticancer agents has an inverse relationship with the tumor burden. The best time to perform HIPEC is the period immediately after cytoreductive surgery. Accordingly, surgical resection of large tumors is required for any improvement of survival with the use of HIPEC.

Jeung et al. reported the feasibility of using intraperitoneal chemotherapy to treat gastric cancer with PC after palliative gastrectomy with maximal cytoreduction [22]. Early postoperative intraperitoneal chemotherapy started on the day of operation with 5-FU 500 mg/m2 and cisplatin 40 mg/m2 (days 1–3) over a 4-week interval. The progression-free survival (PFS) of the 49 patients was 7 months, and the overall survival was 12 months. In multivariate analysis, performance status was the only significant defining factor for PFS. The predominant toxicity was neutropenia and nausea/vomiting. Performance status emerged as a major determining factor for prognosis and patient selection for early postoperative intraperitoneal chemotherapy in patients with advanced gastric cancer after maximal cytoreductive surgery [22].

Traditionally, no surgical procedure was available to remove all the peritoneal tumor nodules in cases with PC. However, in 1995, peritonectomy was first described as a new surgical procedure to perform complete cytoreduction in these cases [23]. Despite the high morbidity rates after peritonectomy, it resulted in downstaging of peritoneal dissemination and improved survival [2]. At present, this approach is being performed as a treatment modality for PC from colon cancer, gastric cancer, and pseudomyxoma peritonei [24–26].

14.2 Rationale and Results of Neoadjuvant Intraperitoneal-Systemic Chemotherapy

According to the recent literature, complete removal of PC is an independent prognostic factor for good prognosis [25]. However, the rate of complete cytoreduction in gastric cancer patients with PC is low [26]. In colon cancer, patients with 0 to 5 of the 7 regions of the abdominal cavity involved by tumor at the time of cytoreduction had a significantly better survival than patients with 6 or 7 affected regions. However, patients with involvement of 6 or more regions of the abdominal cavity, or grossly incomplete cytoreduction, still had a grave prognosis [20]. In contrast, complete resection is associated with improved survival and is the most important prognostic indicator in colorectal and gastric carcinomatosis [27].

Neoadjuvant chemotherapy is known to reduce tumor burden and induce downstaging, which could result in the increase of the incidence of complete cytoreduction. We developed a new neoadjuvant intraperitoneal-systemic chemotherapy protocol (NIPS) in order to increase the rate of complete cytoreduction [6]. If neoadjuvant chemotherapy could induce a reduction in the number of the regions involved by peritoneal carcinomatosis, the rate of complete cytoreduction by peritonectomy might increase, resulting in a survival improvement. NIPS could attack PC from both sides, not only from the peritoneal cavity but also from the subperitoneal blood vessels.

14.2.1 Methods and Results of NIPS

A peritoneal port system was introduced into the abdominal cavity under local anesthesia, and the tip placed on the cul-de-sac of Douglas. After the cytological diagnosis of peritoneal dissemination by peritoneal lavage through port system, 30 mg/m2 of Taxotere and 100 mg /m2 of carboplatin (CBDCA) with1,000 ml of saline were introduced through the port. On the same day, 100 mg /m2 of methotrexate (MTX) and 600 mg/m2 of 5-FU were injected via a peripheral vein (Fig. 14.1). This regimen is repeated weekly for two to six courses. Before and after NIPS, 500 ml of saline is injected into the peritoneal cavity through a port, and the recovered fluid is studied for cytology.

Potentially, in vitro chemosensitivity testing is a good predictor of clinical chemosensitivity [28]. From the results of chemosensitivity tests using a collagen gel method [29], carboplatin, Taxotere, and 5-FU showed high cytotoxicity against 165 clinically obtained primary gastric cancers and therefore were selected for NIPS. MTX is used to enhance the cytoxicity of 5-FU.

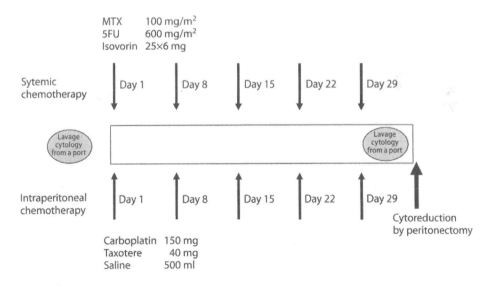

Fig. 14.1 Neoadjuvant intraperitoneal-systemic chemotherapy (NIPS). NIPS weekly chemotherapy is done for more than four cycles. Aims of NIPS are to kill peritoneal free cancer cells (achievement of containment), to increase the incidence of complete cytoreduction, to preserve wider intact peritoneum, and to know the chemosensitivity

The distribution and size of peritoneal metastases were obtained from laparoscopic or surgical charts. Effects of NIPS were evaluated by comparing the size of PC before and after NIPS. In the nonoperable patients, the effects of NIPS were evaluated by barium enema, laparoscopy, or CT scan. The stage of peritoneal dissemination was determined by The Japanese General Rules for Gastric Cancer Study: metastasis to the adjacent peritoneum (P1), a few metastases to distant peritoneal sites (P2), and numerous metastases to the distant peritoneum (P3) [30].

Sixty-nine patients with P3 dissemination from gastric cancer were treated with NIPS. Lavage cytology had been positive in 35 patients before NIPS and changed to be negative in 24 (68%) patients after NIPS. Regarding the number of NIPS cycles, positive cytology before NIPS changed to be negative in 18 (75%) of 24 patients after more than 4 cycles of NIPS. Accordingly, the optimal number of cycles for NIPS is 4. Among 31 patients with ascites, it disappeared in 14 (45%) patients after NIPS. Forty-four patients (64%) showed partial response after NIPS.

After NIPS, 37 patients (including 16 recurrent cases) were operated, and the other 32 patients did not undergo operation because of the progression of disease or refusal of operation. P3 status changed to P2 in two patients.

During NIPS, level 3 or 4 side-effects were found in five patients (16%). Bone marrow suppression and diarrhea were found in three and two patients, respectively. Bone marrow suppression developed after three cycles in two patients and after six cycles in one patient.

14.2.2 Peritonectomy After NIPS and Results

The technique to remove peritoneal dissemination, the so-called peritonectomy procedure, was developed by Sugarbaker and Yonemura [23, 26]. Peritonectomy consists of two separate procedures, parietal and visceral peritonectomy. For the complete removal of the visceral peritoneum bearing cancer, total gastrectomy, subtotal colectomy, and/or resection of small intestine are performed. If the small bowel mesentery is involved, nodules are removed with or without the resection of small bowel wall. The final goal of peritonectomy is the complete removal of all nodules.

Peritoneum covering the diaphragm is removed by electrosurgical dissection between the peritoneum and the diaphragmatic muscle. The whole peritoneum covering the diaphragm is removed [26] (Fig. 14.2).

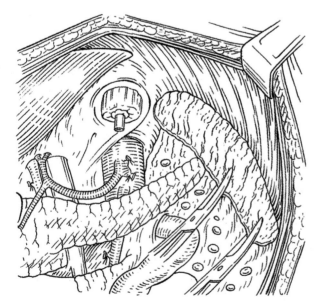

Fig. 14.2 Peritonectomy of left subdiaphragmatic region. Peritoneum covering the left diaphragm is dissected with an electrosurgical technique

Pelvic peritonectomy is carried out by stripping the pelvic peritoneum covering the bladder, and the cul-de-sac is completely removed with the rectum. In females, the uterus is removed with the pelvic peritoneum combined with bilateral salpingo-oophorectomy (Fig. 14.3).

Thirty-one patients underwent peritonectomy, and the resected organs and peritoneum are shown in Table 14.1. Gastrectomy was performed in 21 primary cases. A variety of supplemental procedures were performed to achieve tumor debulking, and the common procedures for visceral peritonectomy were subtotal colectomy (n=24), total hysterectomy in combination with bilateral salpingo-oophorectomy (n=15), resection of small bowel mesentery (n=15), and small bowel resection (n=15). Fulguration of peritoneal nodules was used as an adjunctive surgical technique in 31 patients. Left and right subdiaphragmatic peritonectomy was performed in 16 and 14 patients, respectively. Pelvic peritonectomy was performed in 19 patients. Local peritonectomy is defined as the resection of less than two peritoneal parts shown in Table 14.1. More than three peritoneal parts were resected in general peritonectomy. Complete cytoreduction was achieved in 18 of 37 patients (49%).

Postoperative complications were found in six patients after peritonectomy. Pneumonia developed in two patients, and renal failure occurred in one patient. Surgical complications included two instances of anastomotic leakage. The overall operative mortality rate was 4.5% (1/24), and the cause of death was multiple organ failure with renal failure, hepatic coma, and sepsis.

Median survival time (MST) of all patients was 14.9 months, with a 2-year survival of 19%. MST of patients who received peritonectomy was 19.3 months, and that of patients who

Table 14.1. Surgical procedures in 31 patients treated with peritonectomy

Primary/recurrent	15/31
Gastrectomy	19
Subtotal colectomy	24
Salpingo-oophorectomy	15
Small bowel resection	15
Left diaphragmatic peritonectomy	16
Right diaphragmatic peritonectomy	14
Resection of Douglas's pouch	19
Resection of small bowel mesentery	15
Local peritonectomy/general peritonectomy	13/18

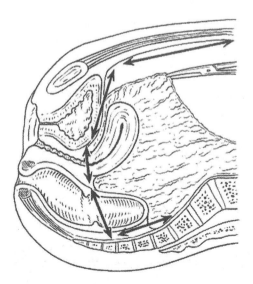
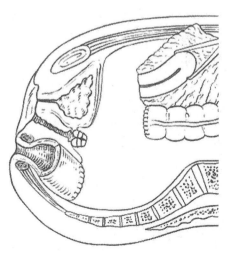

Fig. 14.3 Peritonectomy of pelvic peritoneum

did not receive an operation was 9.6 months (Fig. 14.4). There was a significant survival difference between the two groups (P<0.05). Patients who received a complete resection had a MST of 28.8 months, and MST of patients who had an incomplete cytoreduction was 15.6 months (Fig. 14.5).

14.3 Conclusions and Directions for Future Clinical Research

Independent prognostic indicators of patients with PC from colon cancer are cancer histopathology (invasive or expansive progression), lymph node metastasis, the extent of PC, and the completeness of cytoreduction [31, 32]. Among these prognosticators, completeness of cytoreduction is the most powerful indicator. To achieve a complete cytoreduction, new treatment modalities consisting of peritonectomy and perioperative intraperitoneal chemotherapy are proposed [33].

In the surgical treatment of PC, complete cytoreduction is considered to be the only significant prognostic factor [27]. Culliford et al. reported a 5-year survival of 54% for complete cytoreduction and 15% for incomplete cytoreduction [27]. Furthermore, Glehen et al. reported that the 2-year survival rate was 79% for patients with macroscopic complete resection

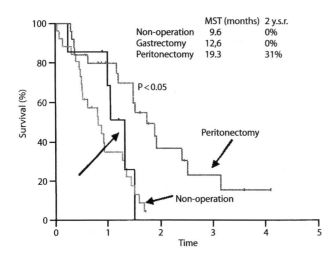

Fig. 14.4 Survival of patients after NIPS. Patients treated with peritonectomy survived significantly better than the patients who underwent gastrectomy alone or no operation

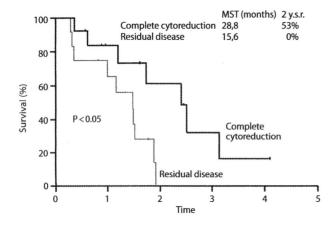

Fig. 14.5 Survival of patients who underwent cytoreductive surgery after NIPS. Patients who received complete cytoreduction survived significantly better than those with residual disease after peritonectomy

and 44.7% for patients without macroscopic incomplete cytoreduction [24]. In PC from gastric cancer, patients receiving a complete cytoreduction had a significantly higher survival than did those with residual disease [33]. However, the biological behaviors of colon and gastric cancer are different: Macroscopic complete cytoreduction in PC from gastric cancer is more difficult to achieve than in colon cancer. In addition, it is very difficult to achieve in P3 dissemination even by peritonectomy, especially when the small bowel mesentery is diffusely involved.

To increase the rate of complete cytoreduction and to preserve the intact peritoneum as much as possible, NIPS was developed. NIPS can downstage large volume peritoneal dissemination of gastric cancer. When NIPS was combined with peritonectomy, a complete cytoreduction was possible in one-quarter of the patients who had been expected to undergo an incomplete cytoreduction [33].

The other aims of NIPS are to eradicate peritoneal free cancer cells before operation and to know the drug sensitivities. Free intraperitoneal cancer cells can be detected in 65% of patients with peritoneal dissemination [3]. The peritoneal free cancer cells are viable and may be trapped on the peritoneal wound created by the surgical procedures. Accordingly, the free cancer cells should be eradicated before peritonectomy.

After NIPS, positive cytology became to be negative in 24 (67%) of 35 patients. NIPS, therefore, may eradicate intraperitoneal free cancer cells prior to peritonectomy.

According to Cunliffe [34], for intra-abdominal metastasis, nutrition can be derived from both the peritoneal surface as well as the blood supply. In NIPS, peritoneal dissemination is attacked from both sides not only through intraperitoneal but also intravenous therapy. Generally, systemic chemotherapy has little effects on PC [35], and intraperitoneal chemotherapy alone showed a response rate of about less than 30% [19, 36]. NIPS showed a fairly good response rate of 65%. Accordingly, the two-route chemotherapy may be the best option for preoperative chemotherapy in PC of gastric origin.

References

1. Sadeghi B, Arvieux C, Glehen O et al. (2000) Peritoneal carcinomatosis from non gynecologic malignancies: results of the EVOCAPE a multicentric prospective study. Cancer 88:358–363
2. Chu DZ, Lang NP, Thompson C et al. (1989) Peritoneal carcinomatosis in nongynecological malignancy. A prospective study of prognostic factors. Cancer 63:364–367
3. Bando E, Yonemura Y, Takeshita Y et al. (1999) Intraoperative lavage for cytological examination in 1,297 patients with gastric carcinoma. Am J Surg 178:256–262
4. Wu CC, Chen JT, Chang MC et al. (1997) Optimal surgical strategy for potentially curable serosa-involved gastric carcinoma with intraperitoneal free cancer cells. J Am Coll Surg 184:611–617
5. Cullinan SA, Moertel CG, Fleming TR et al. (1985) A comparison of three chemotherapeutic regimens in the treatment of advanced pancreatic and gastric carcinoma. Fluorouracil vs. fluorouracil and doxorubicin vs. fluorouracil, doxorubicin, and mitomycin. JAMA 253:2061–2067
6. MacDonald JS, Schein PS, Woolley PV et al. (1980) 5-Fluorouracil, doxorubicin and mitomycin (FAM) combination chemotherapy for advanced gastric cancer. Ann Intern Med 93:533–536
7. Wils JA, Klein HO, Wagener DJ et al. (1991) Sequential high-dose methotrexate and fluorouracil combined with doxorubicin–a step ahead in the treatment of advanced gastric cancer: a trial of the European Organization for Research and Treatment of Cancer Gastrointestinal Tract Cooperative Group. J Clin Oncol 9:827–831
8. Ajani JA, Ota DM, Jessup JM et al. (1991) Resectable gastric carcinoma: an evaluation of preoperative and postoperative chemotherapy. Cancer 68:1501–1506
9. Sugarbaker PH, Yonemura Y (2000) Clinical pathway for the management of resectable gastric cancer with peritoneal seeding: best palliation with a ray of hope for cure. Oncology 58:96–107
10. Sugarbaker PH et al. (1993) Studies of the peritoneal-plasma barrier after systemic mitomycin C administration. Reg Cancer Treat 4:188–194
11. Jacquet P, Sugarbaker PH (1996) Peritoneal-plasma barrier. In: P.H. Sugarbaker (ed) Peritoneal carcinomatosis: principles of management. Kluwer Academic Publisher, Boston, pp 53–63
12. Yonemura Y, Endou Y, Bando E et al. (2004) Effect of intraperitoneal administration of docetaxel on peritoneal dissemination of gastric cancer. Cancer Lett 210:189–196
13. Markman M (1991) Intraperitoneal chemotherapy Semin Oncol 18:248–254
14. Wallner KE, Banda M, Li GC (1987) Hyperthermic enhancement of cell killing by mitomycin C in mytomycin-resistant Chinese hamster ovary cells. Cancer Res 47:1308–1312

15. Herman TS (1983) Temperature dependence of adryamicin, cis-diammindichloroplatinum, bleomycin, and 1,3-bis(2-chloroethyl)-1-nitrosourea cytotoxicity in vitro. Cancer Res 43:517–520
16. Yonemura Y, Fujimura T, Fushida S et al. (1991) Hyperthermo-chemotherapy combined with cytoreductive surgery for the treatment of gastric cancer with peritoneal dissemination. World J Surg 15:530–536
17. Armstrong DK, Bundy B, Wenzel L et al. (2006) Gynecologic Oncology Group. Intraperitoneal cisplatin and paclitaxel in ovarian cancer. N Engl J Med 354:34–43
18. Los G, van Vugt MJ, Pinedo HM et al. (1994) Response of peritoneal solid tumours after intraperitoneal chemohyperthermia treatment with cisplatin or carboplatin. Br J Cancer 69:235–41
19. Fujimoto S, Takahashi M, Kobayashi K et al. (1993) Relation between clinical and histologic outcome of intraperitoneal hyperthermic perfusion for patients with gastric cancer and peritoneal metastasis. Oncology 50:338–343
20. Verwaal VJ, van Ruth S, de Bree E et al. (2003) Randomized trial of cytoreduction and hyperthermic intraperitoneal chemotherapy versus systemic chemotherapy and palliative surgery in patients with peritoneal carcinomatosis of colorectal cancer. J Clin Oncol 15:3737–3743
21. Yonemura Y, Fujimara T, Nishimura G et al. (1996) Effects of intraoperative chemohyperthermia in patients with gastric cancer with peritoneal dissemination. Surgery 119:437–444
22. Jeung HC, Rha SY, Jang WI et al. (2002) Treatment of advanced gastric cancer by palliative gastrectomy, cytoreductive therapy and postoperative intraperitoneal chemotherapy. Br J Surg 89:460–466
23. Sugarbaker PH (1995) Peritonectomy procedures. Ann Surg 21:29–42
24. Glehen O, Mithieux F, Osinsky D et al. (2003) Surgery combined with peritonectomy procedures and intraperitoneal chemohyperthermia in abdominal cancers with peritoneal carcinomatosis: a phase II study. J Clin Oncol 21:799–806
25. Sugarbaker PH (1999) Successful management of microscopic residual disease in large bowel cancer. Cancer Chemother Pharmacol 43:S15–S25
26. Yonemura Y et al. (1999) Peritonectomy as a treatment modality for patients with peritoneal dissemination from gastric cancer. In: Nakashima T, Yamaguchi T (eds) Multimodality therapy for gastric cancer. Springer-Verlag, Tokyo, pp 71–80
27. Culliford AT, Brooks AD, Sharma AS et al. (2001) Surgical debulking and intraperitoneal chemotherapy for established peritoneal metastases from colon and appendix cancer. Ann Surg Oncol 8:787–795
28. Kubota T, Sasano N, Abe O et al. (1995) Potential of the histoculture drug-response assay to contribute to cancer patient survival. Clin Cancer Res 1:1537–1543
29. Tanaka M, Sasaki T (1992) Cell culture (collagen gel matrix) and its application for chemosensitivity test. Gan To Kagaku Ryoho 19:743–748
30. Japanese Research Society for Gastric Cancer (1995) The general rules for gastric cancer study. 1st English edn. Kanehara Shuppan, Tokyo
31. Glehen O; Kwiatkowski F, Sugarbaker PH et al. (2004) Cytoreductive surgery combined with perioperative intraperitoneal chemotherapy for the management of peritoneal carcinomatosis from colorectal cancer. A multi-institutional study of 506 patients. J Clin Oncol 15:3284–3292
32. Sugarbaker PH (1999) Management of peritoneal surface malignancy: the surgeon's role. Langenbecks Arch Surg 384:576–587
33. Yonemura Y, Kawamura T, Bandou E et al. (2005) Treatment of peritoneal dissemination from gastric cancer by peritonectomy and chemohyperthermic peritoneal perfusion. Br J Surg 92:370–375
34. Cunliffe WJ (1991) The rationale for early postoperative intraperitoneal chemotherapy for gastric cancer. In: Sugarbaker P (ed) Management of gastric cancer. Kluwer Academic Publishers, Boston, pp 143–157
35. Ajani JA, Ota DM, Jessup JM et al. (1991) Resectable gastric carcinoma: an evaluation of preoperative and postoperative chemotherapy. Cancer 68:1501–1506
36. Hirose K, Katayama K, Iida A et al. (1999) Efficacy of continuous peritoneal perfusion for the prophylaxis and treatment of peritoneal metastasis of advanced gastric cancer. Oncology 57:106–114

15 Intraperitoneal Chemotherapy in the Management of Ovarian Cancer

Maurie Markman

15.1 Intraperitoneal Chemotherapy: Historical Perspective

The delivery of antineoplastic agents directly into the peritoneal cavity as a management strategy for patients with malignancies principally (or exclusively) confined to this body compartment was initially examined in the earliest days of the modern chemotherapeutic era (Weisberger et al. 1955; Green 1959; Suhrland and Weisberger 1965). The major focus of these efforts was on the control of malignant ascites formation.

Although evidence of biological activity was observed, specifically a reduction in the rate of reaccumulation of ascites, objective tumor regressions were very infrequent. Furthermore, with the drugs employed in these early days local toxicity was common.

In the absence of data even suggesting the possible superiority of intraperitoneal drug delivery compared to systemic administration, this strategy became focused on those settings in which an individual patient's ascites was a major clinical issue. For example, intraperitoneal bleomycin has been employed as a palliative management approach in this setting (Ostrowski and Halsall 1982), but it remains uncertain whether any of the apparent benefit of this approach has anything to do with a direct antineoplastic influence of the cytotoxic agent, as opposed to a sclerosing effect of this drug.

Over the ensuing years the intraperitoneal route has been employed for delivery of radioisotopes, including being examined in phase III randomized trials. However, there was essentially no interest in employing this route for the administration of cytotoxic agents.

15.2 Theoretical Rationale for Intraperitoneal Chemotherapy

In the late 1970s, investigators at the National Cancer Institute (Bethesda, MD) presented a provocative modeling study that suggested that the intraperitoneal delivery of certain antineoplastic agents would result in a rather striking increase in the concentration of the drugs in contact with tumor present in the peritoneal cavity (Dedrick et al. 1978; Dedrick 1985). The investigators further proposed this route of delivery as a possible management strategy for patients with ovarian cancer. A number of clinical and biological factors influenced the development of this model (Table 15.1).

First, it has long been recognized that ovarian cancer remains largely confined to the peritoneal cavity, at least from the perspective of its major clinical manifestations, for most of its natural history (Bergman 1966; Dauplet et al. 1987). Second, as drug uptake from the peritoneal cavity proceeds through the portal circulation before entry into the systemic compartment (Kraft et al. 1968; Lukas et al. 1971), agents known to undergo extensive metabolism during first passage through the liver would

Table 15.1 Rationale for intraperitoneal chemotherapy in ovarian cancer

1. Opportunity to increase concentration of drugs that slowly exit from the peritoneal cavity and are rapidly cleared from the systemic circulation after regional delivery

2. Biological activity of a number of cytotoxic agents has been demonstrated to be enhanced in ovarian cancer by increasing the peak concentration or total exposure over time.

3. Significantly increased contact of the peritoneal cavity to agents that are rapidly and extensively metabolized during first passage through the liver

4. Ovarian cancer remains largely confined to the peritoneal cavity in most patients for the majority of its natural history.

be predicted to have a profound pharmacokinetic advantage for cavity exposure following regional delivery. Finally, the slower an agent is cleared from the peritoneal cavity, and the more rapidly it is cleared from the systemic circulation, the greater will be the pharmacokinetic advantage associated with intraperitoneal drug delivery.

For example, the "Dedrick analysis" specifically "modeled" the intraperitoneal delivery of the cytotoxic drug cytarabine (a standard agent employed in the management of acute leukemia). After intraperitoneal treatment it was hypothesized that tumor present within the peritoneal cavity would be exposed to 1,000-fold higher concentrations of this drug compared to that achieved in the systemic circulation (Dedrick et al. 1978).

Other important theoretical considerations in the selection of antineoplastic agents to be examined for a potential role when delivered by the intraperitoneal route include (Table 15.1) (a) substantial inherent biological activity of the drug against the particular malignancy (e.g., cisplatin in ovarian cancer); (b) evidence for concentration-dependent cytotoxicity in preclinical in vitro or in vivo systems that may be exploited at the clinical level with the drug concentrations possibly attainable after regional delivery; and (c) absence of vesicant or sclerosing properties of the agent when in direct contact with the peritoneal lining.

15.3 Preclinical Evaluation of Intraperitoneal Chemotherapy

Publication of this interesting theoretical analysis led several investigative teams to examine the potential for intraperitoneal chemotherapy in preclinical systems. In addition to confirming the validity of the basic pharmacokinetic analysis, these studies reinforced the risk of local toxicity associated with regional treatment (e.g., doxorubicin) and revealed that the cytotoxic activity of a number of agents with known activity in ovarian cancer could be substantially enhanced at the extremely high concentrations possibly safely achievable within the peritoneal cavity after intraperitoneal delivery, but not after systemic administration (Litterst et al. 1982a, b; Alberts et al. 1985).

Furthermore, a variety of reports revealed perhaps the major limitation associated with intraperitoneal antineoplastic drug therapy: the limited ability of drugs (e.g., cisplatin, doxorubicin, methrotrexate, 5-fluorouracil) to penetrate directly into tumor tissue (Ozols et al. 1979; West et al. 1980; Durand 1981; Nederman and Carlsson 1984; Los et al. 1989, 1991). Thus, although extremely high drug concentrations might bathe the surface of the peritoneal lining, increased tissue levels (compared to what could be attained after systemic drug delivery) were found only a few millimeters from the surface of the tumor.

These data would suggest that although intraperitoneal drug administration may be an effective management strategy for a particular malignancy, its role will be essentially limited to a subset of those patients with very small-volume macroscopic cancer, or microscopic disease only, when the treatment program is initiated.

(It is important to note here that although this conclusion from data generated in preclinical systems appears justified, the actual human situation is more complex. Thus a woman with ovarian cancer who receives cisplatin-based primary chemotherapy may start her treatment program with relatively large-volume disease within the peritoneal cavity, but if a major response develops, the volume of residual disease present in this body compartment may be considerably less at the time of the second or third cycle of the planned treatment program. At this point, after shrinkage of the tumor in response to drug delivered through the vascular compartment, the potential benefits of local therapy may become quite relevant.)

15.4 Objections to the Use of Intraperitoneal Therapy

15.4.1 Theoretical Concerns

In addition to the issue of the limited direct penetration of drug into tumor (or normal tissue), a second theoretical concern with this basic management approach is the potential for an actual reduction in overall therapeutic efficacy of a treatment program due to a lower concentration of an agent reaching the cancer by capillary flow after regional administration, compared to standard systemic delivery. However, if a particular drug is administered by the intraperitoneal route and the active (nonmetabolized) form subsequently reaches the systemic compartment at concentrations equivalent to that attainable with systemic delivery, there should be no compromise associated with drug delivery by capillary flow (Howell et al. 1982; Casper et al. 1983; Lopez et al. 1985; Pretorius et al. 1983; Degregorio et al. 1986; Elferink et al. 1988).

Conversely, if an agent administered regionally produces a degree of local toxicity such that the concentration ultimately reaching the systemic compartment is lower than that achieved with intravenous infusion, the potential impact of this result on the outcome of the therapeutic regimen must be understood (Ozols et al. 1982; Markman et al. 1992b; Francis et al. 1995). A reasonable solution to this theoretical objection to intraperitoneal delivery of such agents would be to treat patients by both the intraperitoneal and systemic routes to take advantage of both high local concentrations and drug delivery by capillary flow.

15.4.2 Practical Concerns

There are a number of practical aspects associated with intraperitoneal drug delivery that also must be considered (Table 15.2). These include (a) unique toxic effects (e.g., abdominal pain, bowel obstruction) that might be observed when an established anticancer agent, which is routinely administered systemically, is now infused regionally (e.g., doxorubicin); (b) development of a safe and cost-effective method for drug delivery (e.g., indwelling catheters attached to subcutaneous devices) (Walker et al. 2006); (c) the risk of intraperitoneal infectious episodes associated with the frequent access to the cavity required (Kaplan et al. 1985); and (d) the need to ensure adequate drug distribution throughout the area being treated.

Table 15.2 Practical concerns associated with intraperitoneal chemotherapy

1. Unique toxic effects (e.g., pain, bowel obstruction) following regional drug delivery
2. Requirement for establishment of a safe, and cost-effective, delivery system
3. Risk of intraperitoneal infectious episodes
4. Added time, effort, inconvenience, and cost associated with regional treatment

A number of reports have examined relevant technical aspects of intraperitoneal drug delivery and the unique toxicities associated with regional treatment (Walker et al. 2006; Makhija et al. 2001). However, it is clear that there needs to be further research effort in this area. For example, important concerns such as the optimal type of catheter to employ for intraperitoneal treatment (e.g., a Tenckhoff-type device used for peritoneal dialysis versus the "much thinner" and flexible indwelling intravenous catheters) and the advisability of inserting catheters at primary surgical cytoreduction when a bowel resection has been performed are matters that will need to be further investigated before definitive recommendations can be made to clinicians considering this management approach in routine practice (Walker et al. 2006).

15.4.3 Adequacy of Drug Distribution

As regards the issue of the adequacy of drug distribution, some have suggested the need to instill radioisotopes or contrast material into the abdominal cavity of each patient after catheter placement to ensure that the drug-containing fluid reaches all areas of the body compartment.

However, as a practical matter, based on experience of a number of centers, it is reasonable to state that if a "standard" treatment volume of 1–2 l can be easily infused into the cavity, there is likely to be an acceptable degree of distribution, such that a formal "distribution study" is not required.

Conversely, if considerable difficulty is encountered in infusing the drug-containing fluid, such that considerable external pressure is required to simply infuse a 1-l bag (e.g., the need to attach a blood pressure cuff to the bag to "speed up the process"), it is highly likely a "distribution study" will be quite abnormal. Thus, under these circumstances, it is reasonable to conclude either that there is a serious problem with the catheter placement or that extensive intra-abdominal adhesions prevent the fluid from adequately entering the cavity.

In general, unless an obvious surgically correctable defect (e.g., kink in the catheter) can be identified, it is appropriate to conclude that such patients may not be able to be treated by the intraperitoneal route, despite being otherwise "good candidates" for this approach (e.g., presence of small-volume residual ovarian cancer following initial surgical cytoreduction). Again, experience would suggest that even if the "catheter is repositioned" or "adhesions are surgically removed," the individual patient's documented response to the presence of this foreign body will simply be repeated, preventing use of this route of drug delivery.

Table 15.3 Pharmacokinetic advantage for intraperitoneal drug delivery associated with selected agents with known activity in ovarian cancer

Agent	Ratio of peritoneal cavity to systemic compartment	
	Peak concentration	AUC
Cisplatin	20	12
Carboplatin		18
Doxorubicin	470	
Paclitaxel	1,000	1,000
Melphalan	93	
Methotrexate	92	

AUC, area under the concentration versus time curve

Additional studies have explored the regional delivery of several combination chemotherapy programs, designed to take advantage of synergistic activity of the drugs suggested in preclinical systems (e.g., cisplatin plus cytarabine, cisplatin plus etoposide).

As predicted by the earlier modeling studies, drugs extensively metabolized in the liver during their first passage through this organ demonstrated the most impressive pharmacokinetic advantage associated with intraperitoneal delivery (e.g., doxorubicin, 5-fluorouracil, paclitaxel) compared to agents that do not undergo such metabolism (e.g., cisplatin, carboplatin) (Markman 1993, 2003).

Furthermore, these studies revealed that certain agents were associated with minimal local toxic effects (e.g., cisplatin, carboplatin), while other agents could lead to considerable abdominal pain (e.g., doxorubicin, mitomycin, paclitaxel) (Markman 1993).

15.5 Phase I Clinical Trials of Intraperitoneal Chemotherapy

Over the past several decades a relatively large number of phase I trials have been conducted that defined both the safety and pharmacokinetic profile of cytotoxic and biological agents when delivered directly into the peritoneal cavity (Table 15.3) (Markman 1993, 2003).

15.6 Phase II Trials of Intraperitoneal Chemotherapy in Ovarian Cancer

Following the conduct of the phase I safety and pharmacokinetic studies, investigators initiated phase II intraperitoneal efficacy trials in ovarian cancer (Markman 1993, 2003). The large majority of these studies focused on the use of this strategy in the "second-line setting," after the completion of primary platinum-based systemic therapy. In most of the studies a surgical end point (i.e., findings at the performance of a third-look laparotomy) was utilized as the measure of efficacy of the treatment program.

Not surprisingly, because of its central role in the management of ovarian cancer, much of the attention in the phase II evaluation of intraperitoneal therapy in this setting was focused on cisplatin, with fewer studies subsequently examining carboplatin or other agents. However, it should be noted that non-cisplatin-based phase II trials in this area have been conducted and reported in the peer-reviewed literature, with evidence of biological activity being observed (Markman 1993; Markman et al. 1990; Markman 1998). Furthermore, a smaller number of phase II primary intraperitoneal chemotherapy strategies, employing both cisplatin and non-cisplatin-based regimens, have also been examined.

[Of interest, despite the fact that accumulating data revealed that cisplatin and carboplatin are equivalent in their cytotoxic effects when delivered systemically in the management of ovarian cancer, very limited preclinical data suggested the superiority of cisplatin for regional treatment (Los et al. 1991), due to higher measured cytotoxic drug concentrations within tumor cells, presumably resulting from greater direct uptake of this platinum agent into tumor from free-surface diffusion. The relevance of this preclinical observation at the clinical level is unknown, since there has yet to be a direct comparison between cisplatin and carboplatin when delivered by the intraperitoneal route. Clearly, such a study needs to be conducted.]

15.6.1 Cisplatin-Based Second-Line Intraperitoneal Chemotherapy of Ovarian Cancer

It is reasonable to summarize the general findings of the cisplatin-based second-line ovarian cancer intraperitoneal trials in the following manner: (a) objective tumor regression, including surgically documented, pathologically confirmed complete responses were observed; (b) patients with very small-volume residual disease (largest residual tumor mass <0.5–1 cm in maximal diameter) were far more likely to demonstrate evidence of an objective response to treatment, compared with individuals with any larger (>1 cm) tumor nodule; (c) patients whose cancers had failed to demonstrate any evidence of biological activity to the prior intravenous platinum-based treatment (e.g., "stable disease" or progression as "best response") rarely showed evidence of an objective response to intraperitoneal cisplatin, even if only very small-volume disease was present at the time of initiation of the second-line treatment program (Markman et al. 1991).

In subsequent reports, several single-institution retrospective analyses described the long-term survival of a subgroup of patients who had received second-line cisplatin-based intraperitoneal chemotherapy (Howell et al. 1987; Markman et al. 1992a; Recio et al. 1998; Barakat et al. 2002). While these data were quite provocative in that a number of patients survived for extended periods of time despite having recurred after primary chemotherapy, in the absence of data from a prospective phase III randomized trial it is completely unknown whether the apparent prolonged survival of these individuals relates to a direct effect of the specific intraperitoneal treatment programs or simply represents the outcome of a group of patients with inherently more favorable clinical and biological characteristics (e.g., very small-volume recurrent, but still highly platinum-sensitive, cancer).

Unfortunately, there has yet to be conducted a randomized phase III trial of second-line chemotherapy of ovarian caner comparing an intraperitoneal cisplatin-based approach to an alternative strategy (e.g., continuation of intravenous platinum-based therapy). Such a trial is clearly urgently needed.

15.7 Phase III Trials of Primary Cisplatin-Based Intraperitoneal Chemotherapy in the Management of Advanced Ovarian Cancer

In contrast to the current situation with second-line therapy of ovarian cancer, the results of three prospective phase III randomized trials of cisplatin-based intraperitoneal chemotherapy employed as primary chemotherapy of advanced ovarian cancer have now unquestionably defined this approach as a "standard of care" in a particular subgroup of patients with this malignancy (Table 15.4). The specific study questions in the individual trials, and their outcomes, are briefly outlined below.

15.7.1 Phase III Trial of Intraperitoneal versus Intravenous Cisplatin, with All Patients Also Receiving Intravenous Cyclophosphamide

The Southwest Oncology Group (SWOG) and the Gynecologic Oncology Group (GOG) compared a primary chemotherapy program for women with "small-volume residual" advanced ovarian cancer, after an attempt at initial surgical cytoreduction, which employed either intraperitoneal or intravenous cisplatin (delivered at a dose of 100 mg/m2 in both study arms) (Alberts et al. 1996).

All patients treated in this trial also received intravenous cyclophosphamide. It should be noted that the size of the maximum residual tumor mass permitted for entry onto this trial was 2 cm.

Patients treated on the intraperitoneal study arm experienced a lower incidence of neutopenia and tinnitus but a somewhat higher incidence of abdominal discomfort (mostly mild or moderate in severity). However, of great relevance, the regional cisplatin-based treatment program was associated with a statistically significant improvement in overall survival, compared to systemic delivery of the agent (median survival 49 months vs. 41 months; $P=0.02$) (Alberts et al. 1996).

15.7.2 Phase III Trial of Intraperitoneal versus Intravenous Cisplatin, with All Patients Also Receiving Intravenous Paclitaxel

While clinicians recognized the importance of the findings of the above-noted study, the large majority of practicing oncologists appeared to conclude that by simply substituting intravenous paclitaxel for intravenous cyclophosphamide, a patient would achieve the same survival benefits, without the technical requirements associated with regional therapy. Thus a second randomized phase III trial was initiated to examine this question.

Table 15.4 Randomized phase III trials of primary cisplatin-based intraperitoneal chemotherapy

	Median progression-free survival		Median overall survival	
	IV "control"	IP regimen	IV "control"	IP regimen
Trial 1 (Alberts et al. 1996)			41 months	49 months ($P=0.02$)
Trial 2 (Markman et al. 2001)	22 months	28 months ($P=0.01$)	52 months	63 months ($P=0.05$)
Trial 3 (Armstrong et al. 2006)	18.3 months	24 months ($P=0.0266$)	50 months	66 months ($P=0.0173$)

Trial 1: IV „control" – IV cisplatin 100 mg/m^2 + IV cyclophosphamide 600 mg/m^2. Q 21 days × 6 cycles.
  IP regimen – IP cisplatin 100 mg/m^2 + IV cyclophosphamide 600 mg/m^2. Q 21 days × 6 cycles
Trial 2: IV "control" – IV cisplatin 75 mg/m^2 + IV paclitaxel 135 mg/m^2 over 24 h. Q 21 days × 6 cycles.
  IP regimen – IV carboplatin (AUC 9) q 28 days × 2 cycles followed by IP cisplatin 100 mg/m^2 + IV paclitaxel 135 mg/m^2 over 24 h. Q 21 days × 6 cycles
Trial 3: IV "control" – IV cisplatin 75 mg/m^2 + IV paclitaxel 135 mg/m^2 over 24 h. Q 21 days × 6 cycles.
  IP regimen – IP cisplatin 100 mg/m^2 + IV paclitaxel 135 mg/m^2 over 24 h + IP paclitaxel 60 mg/m^2 (day 8) q 21 days × 6 cycles

In this study, patients were randomized to receive either the "new standard" systemic regimen for advanced ovarian cancer, cisplatin (75 mg/m2) plus paclitaxel (135 mg/m2 over 24 h) (McGuire et al. 1996), or an "experimental program" containing intraperitoneal cisplatin (100 mg/m2) plus intravenous paclitaxel (Markman et al. 2001). Further, in an effort to initiate the regional treatment program in individual patients with the smallest possible volume of disease, in this trial the investigative intraperitoneal regimen was started after two cycles of moderately high-dose single-agent intravenous carboplatin (AUC 9). It was hoped the systemic therapy would "chemically debulk" any residual macroscopic tumor masses, enhancing the opportunity for a favorable effect of the subsequently delivered intraperitoneal cisplatin (Shapiro et al. 1997).

It should also be noted that in this study the maximum size of the largest residual tumor mass permitted for study entry was 1 cm (compared to 2 cm in the previously discussed trial).

Unfortunately, the initial two cycles of "moderately high-dose" intravenous carboplatin were associated with an unacceptable incidence of severe, and persistent thrombocytopenia, resulting in an inability of many patients to complete the subsequently planned regional treatment program. In fact, 19% of patients randomized to the "experimental" study arm received two or fewer courses of intraperitoneal cisplatin (Markman et al. 2001).

However, despite this unanticipated toxicity, treatment with the regional treatment program was still associated with a statistically significant improvement in both progression-free (median: 28 months vs. 22 months; P=0.01) and overall survival (63 months vs. 52 months; P=0.05). Thus, of great clinical relevance, even though all patients in this study received intravenous paclitaxel, the use of intraperitoneal cisplatin (compared to intravenous cisplatin) was associated with a further improvement in the ultimate outcome of therapy.

Since the publication of this second phase III intraperitoneal study, some have argued that perhaps the two cycles of "moderately high-dose" intravenous carboplatin were at least partially responsible for the favorable impact of the treatment regimen on survival. This is a most unlikely explanation as, in fact, there have been a number of previously reported randomized trials in ovarian cancer that have completely failed to reveal any evidence that increasing the "dose intensity" of systemically delivered platinum, at the concentrations safely achievable with intravenous administration, will improve survival (Jakobsen et al. 1997; Gore et al. 1998; McGuire et al. 1995; Conte et al. 1996; Wrigley et al. 1996).

The severity of the bone marrow suppression observed in this trial led the study's investigators to conclude that, despite the favorable effect on outcome, this specific intraperitoneal regimen should not be further explored in research trials or employed in routine clinical practice.

15.7.3 Phase III Trial of Intravenous Cisplatin/Paclitaxel Versus Intraperitoneal Cisplatin plus Both Intravenous and Intraperitoneal Paclitaxel

Finally, the most recently reported randomized phase III trial, conducted by the GOG, again compared a standard intravenous cisplatin (75 mg/m^2)/paclitaxel (135 mg/m^2 over 24 h) regimen to an experimental program of intraperitoneal cisplatin (100 mg/m2) plus paclitaxel delivered both intravenously (135 mg/m2 over 24 h) and by the intraperitoneal route (60 mg/m2, day 8) (Armstrong et al. 2006). As in the preceding study, "small-volume residual disease" was defined as all tumor masses persisting in the peritoneal cavity after initial surgery being less than 1 cm in maximal diameter.

Although increased toxicity was again noted in the experimental treatment arm (neurotoxicity, myelosuppression, emesis), there was a highly statistically significant improvement in both time to disease progression (median: 24 months vs. 18.3 months; P=0.0266) and overall survival (66 months vs. 50 months; P=0.0173) associated with the regional treatment strategy. Furthermore, a formal quality-of-life analysis was included in this study, and although the short-term quality-of-life was more adversely affected with intraperitoneal treatment (compared to "all-systemic" therapy), at 12-month follow-up there was no difference in this important parameter between the two study groups.

15.8 Conclusions Regarding Primary Cisplatin-Based Chemotherapy in "Small-Volume Residual" Advanced Ovarian Cancer

The results of these three prospective phase III randomized trials led to the unambiguous conclusion that intraperitoneal cisplatin significantly improves survival in small-volume residual advanced ovarian cancer, compared to systemically delivered cisplatin. Furthermore, while there has not as yet been a direct comparison of intraperitoneal cisplatin-based to intravenous carboplatin-based therapy in this setting, it is known that intravenous cisplatin and intravenous carboplatin are equivalent in efficacy in this malignancy (Covens et al. 2002; du Bois et al. 2003; Ozols et al. 2003).

Thus evaluation of existing evidence-based clinical data leads to the rational inference that intraperitoneal cisplatin is a superior treatment option, compared to intravenous carboplatin-based therapy in women with small-volume residual advanced ovarian cancer.

15.9 What Is the "Optimal" Primary Intraperitoneal Chemotherapy Regimen in Small-Volume Residual Advanced Ovarian Cancer?

Despite the overwhelming evidence supporting the use of intraperitoneal chemotherapy as primary treatment of small-volume residual advanced ovarian cancer, many questions remain. For example, it might be asked: (a) if intraperitoneal carboplatin can be substituted for intraperitoneal cisplatin; (b) if it is necessary to administer intraperitoneal cisplatin at a dose of 100 mg/m^2; or (c) if it is required that intraperitoneal paclitaxel be administered, along with intraperitoneal cisplatin, to achieve maximum clinical benefit.

Based on existing data revealing a major survival benefit associated with intraperitoneal cisplatin in this setting, it would be inappropriate to conclude that intraperitoneal carboplatin can simply be substituted for intraperitoneal cisplatin.

Conversely, with both the safety and pharmacokinetic advantage previously demonstrated for intraperitoneal carboplatin (similar to that of cisplatin), it would be reasonable to suggest that if an individual patient is unable to tolerate the systemic toxicity associated with cisplatin after regional delivery (particularly emesis), use of intraperitoneal carboplatin might be an appropriate option (Fujiwara et al. 2005). Limited trial data have shown that it is possible to safely combine intraperitoneal carboplatin, delivered at an AUC of 6, with intravenous paclitaxel (175 mg/m^2 over 3 h).

Understanding that the advantage of regional cisplatin relates to the major pharmacokinetic differences between the intravenous and intraperitoneal routes of administration, and not specifically to the delivered dose, leads to the logical conclusion that lowering the dose of intraperitoneal cisplatin from 100 mg/m^2 to 75 mg/m2 or 80 mg/m^2 would almost certainly not negatively influence the benefits of regional delivery, but might substantially improve patient tolerance to the regimen because of the resulting somewhat lower systemic drug concentrations. Based on this consideration, it would be appropriate to argue that use of this lower dose of intraperitoneal cisplatin, combined with intravenous paclitaxel, would be a most reasonable standard treatment option, outside the setting of a clinical trial.

The question of the importance of intraperitoneal paclitaxel to the success of a primary regional treatment program in the management of ovarian cancer remains unanswered. Although the final phase III trial noted above included paclitaxel delivered regionally (Armstrong et al. 2006), and this program was associated with the greatest improvement in overall survival among the three randomized studies, the previous two trials (which did not include intraperitoneal paclitaxel) also revealed a statistically significant favorable impact on survival (Alberts et al. 1996; Markman et al .2001). Furthermore, it is likely (although not definitively proven) that much of the increased local toxicity observed in this recent study was due to the paclitaxel (Markman et al. 1992b), as this route of administration of the agent has been shown to cause abdominal discomfort.

One potential option in clinical practice would be to administer the initial cycle of intraperitoneal chemotherapy with only the cisplatin delivered by this route, and with the paclitaxel delivered exclusively systemically. If the first cycle is reasonably well tolerated, without the development of significant abdominal discomfort, it may be appropriate to add intraperitoneal paclitaxel to the second and subsequent treatment cycles.

Table 15.5 Additional settings where IP chemotherapy is a rational management strategy

1. Patient with advanced ovarian/primary peritoneal cancer receiving neoadjuvant chemotherapy who achieves an excellent response after 3–4 cycles of platinum-based systemic chemotherapy (documented at an interval surgical cytoreductive procedure)
2. Patient with advanced ovarian cancer found to have a pathologically negative, or microscopically positive (only), second-look laparotomy or laparoscopy
3. Primary chemotherapy for high-risk early stage (e.g., stage IC, stage II) ovarian cancer

15.10 Use of Intraperitoneal Chemotherapy in Ovarian Cancer in Other Clinical Settings

The lack of data from prospective phase III randomized trials does not permit definitive conclusions regarding other settings in which intraperitoneal chemotherapy should be employed in women with ovarian cancer. However, existing information from nonrandomized studies led to the suggestion that regional drug delivery would be a rational strategy in several additional areas of patient management (Table 15.5).

Ultimately, randomized phase II trials will be required to determine whether intraperitoneal therapy improves survival in any of these settings (Barakat et al. 1998). However, until such data are available, it may be quite appropriate in selected patients to consider this management option, being certain the individual has been informed of the current absence of definitive evidence-based data to prove the clinical utility of this management approach.

Of particular appeal in this regard is the use of regional therapy in an ovarian cancer patient who initiates systemic therapy with extensive intra-abdominal disease, and who at the time of a surgical reassessment (e.g., interval cytoreductive procedure; second-look laparotomy) is found to have no, or only microscopic, residual cancer. Unfortunately, in such patients, it is well established that the ultimate risk of relapse of the disease is extremely great.

However, as the malignant cells in this particular patient have now been shown to be exquisitely sensitive to platinum-based treatment, it is realistic to hypothesize that the very high concentrations of platinum in direct contact with residual cancer that are achievable after subsequent intraperitoneal drug delivery in this specific setting may be translated into genuine long-term control of the disease process. Again, in the absence of definitive phase III trial data, it is rational to consider management of such a patient with this novel approach.

15.11 Conclusion

The results of extensive preclinical investigation, phase I and phase II clinical trials, and now definitive phase III randomized studies have clearly demonstrated that intraperitoneal cisplatin-based chemotherapy should be considered the new standard of care in the primary treatment of small-volume residual advanced ovarian cancer. Future research efforts in this arena will hopefully define the optimal intraperitoneal treatment strategy: drugs, dosages, and delivery techniques.

References

Alberts DS, Young L, Mason N, Salmon SE (1985) In vitro evaluation of anticancer drugs against ovarian cancer at concentrations achievable by intraperitoneal administration. Semin Oncol 12 [Suppl 4]:38–42

Alberts DS, Liu PY, Hannigan EV, O'Toole R, Williams SD, Young JA, Franklin EW, Clarke-Pearson DL, Malviya VK DuBeshter B (1996) Intraperitoneal cisplatin plus intravenous cyclophosphamide versus intravenous cisplatin plus intravenous cyclophosphamide for stage III ovarian cancer. N Engl J Med 335:1950–1955

Armstrong DK, Bundy B, Wenzel L, Huang HQ, Baergen R, Shashikant L, Copeland LJ, Walker JL, Burger RA (2006) Phase III randomized trial of intravenous cisplatin and paclitaxel versus an intensive regimen of intravenous paclitaxel, intraperitoneal cisplatin and intraperitoneal paclitaxel in stage III ovarian cancer: a Gynecologic Oncology Group Study. N Engl J Med 354:34–43

Barakat RR, Almadrones L, Venkatraman ES, Aghajanian C, Brown C, Shapiro F, Curtin JP, Sprigs D (1998) A phase II trial of intraperitoneal cisplatin and etoposide as consolidation therapy in patients with Stage II–IV epithelial ovarian cancer following negative surgical assessment. Gynecol Oncol 69:17–22

Barakat RR, Sabbatini P, Bhaskaran D, Revzin M, Smith A, Venkatraman E, Aghajanian C, Hensley M, Soignet S, Brown C, Soslow R, Markman M, Hoskins WJ, Spriggs D (2002) Intraperitoneal chemotherapy for ovarian carcinoma: results of long-term follow-up. J Clin Oncol 20:694–698

Bergman F (1966) Carcinoma of the ovary: a clinicopathological study of 86 autopsied cases with special reference to mode of spread. Acta Obstet Gynecol Scand 45:211–231

Casper ES, Kelsen DP, Alcock NW, Lewis JL Jr (1983) IP cisplatin in patients with malignant ascites: pharmacokinetic evaluation and comparison with the iv route. Cancer Treat Rep 67:235–238

Conte PF, Bruzzone M, Carnino F, Gadducci A, Algeri R, Bellini A, Boccardo F, Brunetti I, Catsafados E, Chiara S, Foglia G, Gallo L, Iskra L, Mammoliti S, Parodi G, Ragni N, Rosso R, Rugiati S, Rubagotti A (1996) High-dose versus low-dose cisplatin in combination with cyclophosphamide and epidoxorubicin in suboptimal ovarian cancer: a randomized study of the Gruppo Oncologico Nord-Ovest. J Clin Oncol 14:351–356

Covens A, Carey M, Bryson P, Verma S, Fung MFK, Johnston M (2002) Systematic review of first-line chemotherapy for newly diagnosed postoperative patients with stage II, III, or IV epithelial ovarian cancer. Gynecol Oncol 85:71–80

Dauplat J, Hacker NF, Nieberg RK, Berek JS, Rose TP, Sagae S (1987) Distant metastases in epithelial ovarian carcinoma. Cancer 60:1561–1566

Dedrick RL (1985) Theoretical and experimental bases of intraperitoneal chemotherapy. Semin Oncol 12:1–6

Dedrick RL, Myers CE, Bungay PM, DeVita VT Jr (1978) Pharmacokinetic rationale for peritoneal drug administration in the treatment of ovarian cancer. Cancer Treat Rep 62:1–9

Degregorio MW, Lum BL, Holleran WM, Wilbur BJ, Sikic BI (1986) Preliminary observations of intraperitoneal carboplatin pharmacokinetics during a phase I study of the Northern California Oncology Group. Cancer Chemother Pharmacol 18:235–238

du Bois A, Luck HJ, Meier W, Adams HP, Mobus V, Costa S, Bauknecht T, Richter B, Warm M, Schroder W, Olbricht S, Nitz U, Jackisch C, Emons G, Wagner U, Kuhn W, Pfisterer J (2003) A randomized clinical trial of cisplatin/paclitaxel versus carboplatin/paclitaxel as first-line treatment of ovarian cancer. J Natl Cancer 95:1320–1329

Durand RE (1981) Flow cytometry studies of intracellular adriamycin in multicell spheroids in vitro. Cancer Res 41:3495–3498

Elferink F, van der Vijgh WJ, Klein I, Bokkel Huinink WW, Dubbelman R, McVie JG (1988) Pharmacokinetics of carboplatin after intraperitoneal administration. Cancer Chemother Pharmacol 21:57–60

Francis P, Rowinsky E, Schneider J, Hakes T, Hoskins W, Markman M (1995) Phase I feasibility and pharmacologic study of weekly intraperitoneal paclitaxel: a Gynecologic Oncology Group Pilot study. J Clin Oncol 13:2961–2967

Fujiwara K, Markman M, Morgan M, Coleman RL (2005) Intraperitoneal carboplatin-based chemotherapy for epithelial ovarian cancer. Gynecol Oncol 97:10–15

Gore M, Mainwaring P, A'Hern R, MacFarlane V, Slevin M, Harper P, Osborne R, Mansi J, Blake P, Wiltshaw E, Shepherd J for the London Gynaecological Oncology Group (1998) Randomized trial of dose-intensity with single-agent carboplatin in patients with epithelial ovarian cancer. J Clin Oncol 16:2426–2434

Green TH (1959) Hemisulfur mustard in the palliation of patients with metastatic ovarian carcinoma. Obstet Gynecol 13:383–393

Howell SB, Pfeifle CL, Wung WE, Olshen RA, Lucas WE, Yon JL, Green M (1982) Intraperitoneal cisplatin with systemic thiosulfate protection. Ann Intern Med 97:845–851

Howell SB, Zimm S, Markman M, Abramson IS, Cleary S, Lucas WE, Weiss RJ (1987) Long-term survival of advanced refractory ovarian carcinoma patients with small-volume disease treated with intraperitoneal chemotherapy. J Clin Oncol 5:1607–1612

Jakobsen A, Bertelsen K, Andersen JE, Havsteen H, Jakobsen P, Moeller KA, Nielsen K, Sandberg E, Stroeyer I (1997) Dose-effect study of carboplatin in ovarian cancer: a Danish Ovarian Cancer Group study. J Clin Oncol 15:193–198

Kaplan RA, Markman M, Lucas WE, Pfeifle C, Howell SB (1985) Infectious peritonitis in patients receiving intraperitoneal chemotherapy. Am J Med 78:49–53

Kraft AR, Tompkins RK, Jesseph JE (1968) Peritoneal electrolyte absorption: Analysis of portal, systemic venous and lymphatic transport. Surgery 64:148–153

Litterst CL, Collins JM, Lowe MC, Arnold ST, Powell DM, Guarino AM (1982a) Local and systemic toxicity resulting from large-volume IP administration of doxorubicin in the rat. Cancer Treat Rep 66:157–161

Litterst CL, Torres IJ, Arnold S, McGunagle D, Furner R, Sikic BI, Guarino AM (1982b) Absorption of antineoplastic drugs following large-volume IP administration of rats. Cancer Treat Rep 66:147–155

Los G, Mutsaers PHA, van der Vijgh WJF, Baldew GS, de Graaf PW, McVie JG (1989) Direct diffusion of cis-diamminedichloroplatinum(II) in intraperitoneal rat tumors after intraperitoneal chemotherapy: a comparison with systemic chemotherapy. Cancer Res 49:3380–3384

Los G, Verdegaal EM, Mutsaers PH, McVie JG (1991) Penetration of carboplatin and cisplatin into rat peritoneal tumor nodules after intraperitoneal chemotherapy. Cancer Chemother Pharmacol 28:159–165

Lukas G, Brindle S, Greengard P (1971) The route of absorption of intraperitoneally administered compounds. J Pharmacol Exp Ther 178:562–566

Makhija S, Leitao M, Sabbatini P, Bellin N, Almadrones L, Leon L, Spriggs DR, Barakat R (2001) Complications associated with intraperitoneal chemotherapy catheters. Gynecol Oncol 81:77–81

Markman M (1993) Intraperitoneal therapy for treatment of malignant disease principally confined to the peritoneal cavity. Crit Rev Oncol Hematol 14:15–28

Markman M (2003) Intraperitoneal antineoplastic drug delivery: rationale and results. Lancet Oncol 4:277–283

Markman M, George M, Hakes T, Reichman B, Hoskins W, Rubin S, Jones W, Almadrones L, Lewis JL Jr (1990) Phase II trial of intraperitoneal mitoxantrone in the management of refractory ovarian cancer. J Clin Oncol 8:146–150

Markman M, Reichman B, Hakes T, Jones W, Lewis JL Jr, Rubin S, Almadrones L, Hoskins W (1991) Responses to second-line cisplatin-based intraperitoneal therapy in ovarian cancer: influence of a prior response to intravenous cisplatin. J Clin Oncol 9:1801–1805

Markman M, Reichman B, Hakes T, Lewis JL Jr, Jones W, Rubin S, Barakat R, Curtin J, Almadrones L, Hoskins W (1992a) Impact on survival of surgically defined favorable responses to salvage intraperitoneal chemotherapy in small-volume residual ovarian cancer. J Clin Oncol 10:1479–1484

Markman M, Rowinsky E, Hakes T, Reichman B, Jones W, Lewis JL Jr, Rubin S, Curtin J, Barakat R, Phillips M, Hurowitz L, Almadrones L, Hoskins W (1992b) Phase I trial of intraperitoneal taxol: a Gynecologic Oncology Group Study. J Clin Oncol 10:1485–1491

Markman M, Brady MF, Spirtos NM, Hanjani P, Rubin SC (1998) Phase II trial of intraperitoneal paclitaxel in carcinoma of the ovary, tube, and peritoneum: a Gynecologic Oncology Group study. J Clin Oncol 16:2620–2624

Markman M, Bundy BN, Alberts DS, Fowler JM, Clark-Pearson DL, Carson LF, Wadler S, Sickel J (2001) Phase III trial of standard-dose intravenous cisplatin plus paclitaxel versus moderately high-dose carboplatin followed by intravenous paclitaxel and intraperitoneal cisplatin in small-volume stage III ovarian carcinoma: an intergroup study of the Gynecologic Oncology Group, Southwestern Oncology Group, and Eastern Cooperative Oncology Group. J Clin Oncol 19:1001–1007

McGuire WP, Hoskins WJ, Brady MF, Homesley HD, Creasman WT, Berman ML, Ball H, Berek JS, Woodward J (1995) Assessment of dose-intensive therapy in suboptimally debulked ovarian cancer: a Gynecologic Oncology Group study. J Clin Oncol 13:1589–1599

McGuire WP, Hoskins WJ, Brady MF, Kucera PR, Partridge EE, Look KY, Clarke-Pearson DL, Davidson M (1996) Cyclophosphamide and cisplatin compared with paclitaxel and cisplatin in patients with stage III and stage IV ovarian cancer. N Engl J Med 334:1–6

Nederman T Carlsson J (1984) Penetration and binding of vinblastine and 5-fluorouracil in cellular spheroids. Cancer Chemother Pharmacol 13:131–135

Ostrowski MJ (1986) An assessment of the long-term results of controlling the reaccumulation of malignant effusions using intracavitary bleomycin. Cancer 57:721–727

Ozols RF, Locker GY, Doroshow JH, Grotzinger KR, Myers CE, Young RC (1979) Pharmacokinetics of adriamycin and tissue penetration in murine ovarian cancer. Cancer Res 39:3209–3214

Ozols RF, Young RC, Speyer JL, Sugarbaker PH, Greene R, Jenkins J, Myers CE (1982) Phase I and pharmacological studies of adriamycin administered intraperitoneally to patients with ovarian cancer. Cancer Res 42:4265–4269

Ozols RF, Bundy BN, Greer BE, Fowler JM, Clarke-Pearson D, Burger RA, Mannel RS, DeGeest K, Hartenbach EM, Baergen R (2003) Phase III trial of carboplatin and paclitaxel compared with cisplatin and paclitaxel in patients with optimally resected stage III ovarian cancer: a Gynecologic Oncology Group Study. J Clin Oncol 21:3194–3200

Pretorius RG, Hacker NF, Berek JS, Ford LC, Hoeschele JD, Butler TA, Lagasse LD (1983) Pharmacokinetics of IP cisplatin in refractory ovarian carcinoma. Cancer Treat Rep 67:1085–1092

Recio FO, Piver MS, Hempling RE, Driscoll DL (1998) Five-year survival after second-line cisplatin-based intraperitoneal chemotherapy for advanced ovarian cancer. Gynecol Oncol 68:267–273

Shapiro F, Schneider J, Markman M, Reichman BS, Venkatraman E, Barakat R, Almadrones L, Spriggs D (1997) High-intensity intravenous cyclophosphamide and cisplatin, interim surgical debulking, and intraperitoneal cisplatin in advanced ovarian carcinoma: a pilot trial with ten-year follow-up. Gynecol Oncol 67:39–45

Suhrland LG Weisberger AS (1965) Intracavitary 5-fluorouracil in malignant effusions. Arch Intern Med 116:431–433

Walker JL, Armstrong D, Huang HQ, Fowler J, Webster K, Burger R, Clarke-Pearson D (2006) Intraperitoneal catheter outcomes in a phase III trial of intravenous versus intraperitoneal chemotherapy in optimal stage III ovarian and primary peritoneal cancer: a gynecologic oncology group study. Gynecol Oncol 100:27–32

Weisberger AS, Levine B, Storaasli JP (1955) Use of nitrogen mustard in treatment of serious effusions of neoplastic origin. JAMA 159: 1704–1707

West GW, Weichselbau R, Little JB (1980) Limited penetration of methotrexate into human osteosarcoma spheroids as a proposed model for solid tumor resistance to adjuvant chemotherapy. Cancer Res 40:3665–3668

Wrigley E, Weaver A, Jayson G, Ranson M, Renninson J, Prendiville J, Dobson M, Collins CD, Swindell R, Buckley CH, Radford JA, Crowther D (1996) A randomised trial investigating the dose intensity of primary chemotherapy in patients with ovarian carcinoma: a comparison of chemotherapy given every four weeks with the same chemotherapy given at three week intervals. Ann Oncol 7:705–711

Printing: Krips bv, Meppel
Binding: Stürtz, Würzburg